Springer Series on
Health Care and Society

PATIENT EDUCATION:
An Inquiry into the State of the Art

Wendy D. Squyres, Ph.D., Editor
with contributors

Springer Publishing Company

New York

Springer Publishing Company, Inc.
200 Park Avenue South
New York, New York   10003

80 81   82   83   84 / 10   9   8   7   6   5   4   3   2   1

Library of Congress Cataloging in Publication Data

Main entry under title:

Patient education

   (Springer series on health care and society; 4) Includes bibliographical ref-
   erences and index.   1. Patient education. I. Squyres, Wendy D.
II. Series. [DNLM: 1. Patients—Education. W1
SP685S v. 4 / W85 P2977]
R727.4.P37   610'.7   79-27556
ISBN 0-8261-3120-4
ISBN 0-8261-3121-2 pbk.

Printed in the United States of America

This book is dedicated to the memory of Lawrence M. Allport. His greatest talent was also his calling—he lived to serve others.

Contents

Foreword

Those of us who are engaged in providing continuing education for health science professionals spend a good deal of time seeking to assist health care providers to keep abreast of the most recent developments in clinical practice and related scientific discovery. Indeed, continuing education is often referred to as the vehicle by which good medical science becomes good clinical care.

Occasionally, there is an opportunity to observe and in some modest way to facilitate the identification and dissemination of ideas that are relevant to an emerging body of knowledge and a particular field of study and will effect good clinical care. The series of symposia out of which this volume grew provided such an opportunity.

The programs brought together a wide range of health practitioners, persons particularly concerned with health policy and possessed of the patience to inquire into the teaching and learning process as it happens in, effects, and is effected by the health care milieu. It is my belief that the inquiry was a fruitful one. It was conducted by thoughtful people who brought to the exploration a lively curiosity and critical ability that enriched the dialogue and strengthened the points of both agreement and conflict. There was an intellectual vitality in the symposia that is also present herein. I commend Dr. Wendy D. Squyres and her colleagues for their good work and highly recommend it to your use.

Lucy Ann Geiselman, Ph.D.
Dean, Continuing Education in
Health Sciences
University of California
San Francisco, 1979

Preface

Over the past three years practitioners, policy makers, teachers, and students have met together in a series of annual, national symposia devoted to the examination of current issues in patient education. Physicians, nurses, health educators, pharmacists, health planners, dieticians, social workers, physical therapists, respiratory therapists, administrators, dentists, librarians, media specialists, as well as patients (people who are having or have had experience with disease) have exchanged information on the planning, implementation, and evaluation of patient education programs in a variety of health care settings, such as inpatient, outpatient, private office, community clinic, health maintenance organizations (HMOs), voluntary health, and governmental agency settings.

The reciprocal effects of such a national interchange became more apparent each year. That is, as patients grew willing and able to build or rebuild skills in disease management, health maintenance, and the effective use of the health care system, providers were experiencing the need to reexamine the patient-provider relationship and roles, quality of care issues, health employee training, as well as innovative explorations into what constitutes a health care team. Representatives from organizations such as hospitals, clinics, HMOs, and community health agencies talked not only about intra-agency changes but also about interagency collaboration.

The surge of interest in patient education in the last decade, accompanied by uneven administrative support or limited resource allocations, has left many patient educators feeling isolated and forced to reinvent the wheel every time a program is needed or called for. In response, almost as a grass-roots act, during or as a result of the symposia, practitioners, academicians, students, and patients began forming regional networks to exchange information and materials, cooperate on program efforts, and provide peer support.

Over seventy-five people acted as symposia faculty. They high-lighted national policy relevant to patient education, showcased model programs, described staff training needs, identified organizational and societal forces and barriers to effective efforts, laid out theoretical models, and described empirical results of research related to the practice of patient education. This book is intended to capture the experiences of those symposia faculty and of the more than 1,100 participants who came together from all over the United States (including Alaska and Hawaii), Puerto Rico and Canada, and to serve as a resource to practitioners, policy makers, researchers, teachers and students of patient education. It will be a resource to the extent that it reflects the current state of the art, cites and directs people to the literature, reports recent research efforts, and raises questions for future research.

Each chapter introduces a theoretical rationale for the issue under consideration, a review of the literature, one or more case studies to show how the conceptual thesis is useful in the practice of patient education, and finally, references for further investigation and study. The Appendix provides a resource guide for patient education materials, and there is also an annotated bibliography of works central to the major themes of the book.

It should be noted that the authors have been selected from a large and competent pool of nationally prominent individuals in the field. Several prospective authors were so committed to their practices and patients that they were unable to give time to writing. Therefore this book does not necessarily reflect the collective views of the entire faculty, the symposia planners, or all of the symposia participants. It is heavily influenced by the interests of the authors who were willing to accept the challenge of this book under numerous constraints; nevertheless, every effort has been made to direct people to the literature in areas not dealt with in great detail.

Wendy D. Squyres, Ph.D.
Baltimore, Maryland
April 1979

Acknowledgments

Preparation of this book was supported in part by National Institutes of Health, U.S. Department of Health, Education, and Welfare grants HL22934 and HL07180 on which Dr. Squyres was a postdoctoral fellow, Dr. Green is director, Mr. D'Altroy and Ms. Hebert are predoctoral fellows, and Dr. Mullen was a postdoctoral fellow, all working at the Johns Hopkins University, School of Hygiene and Public Health, Division of Health Education, from August 1978 through July 1979.

For their contribution to chapter 4, the editor expresses her gratitude to Susan Hammerstad, R.N., B.S.N., Inservice Instructor at Stanford University Hospital, as well as Joan Mersch, R.N., M.S., Clinical Nursing Coodinator of the Coronary Care Unit at Stanford and her staff, and Joanne Denham, R.N., B.S.N., for their preparation, use, and written documentation of the sample protocol.

The author of chapter 8 gratefully acknowledges Dr. Lawrence W. Green, Dr. Mayhew Derryberry, and Ms. Karyl Shanks for their helpful comments on a draft of this manuscript.

Chapter 11 appears in this book with the permission of the American Journal of Nursing Company; it appeared in the March 1978 issue of *Nursing Outlook*.

The basic principles for the Taking Charge Program, and the Daily Behavior Record were reprinted with permission from the Bull Publishing Company. The Smoking Diary was reprinted with permission from Prentice-Hall, Inc. The Stress Log was reprinted by permission of Virginia A. Price, Stanford University.

The Appendix was prepared with the assistance of Mary Hess-Mussell, Linda McAffee-Bilsborough, and Leslie L. Wheeler of the Human Services Center staff, the California State University, Chico.

The editor gratefully acknowledges the pivotal role of the symposia's chief sponsor, the University of California at San Francisco's

xiv   *Acknowledgments*

Office of Continuing Education in the Health Sciences, for sharing the
vision for such an annual event, and for being willing to take the risk
before such meetings came into vogue. Their vision came from a
deep commitment to the consumers of health care services as well
as to the advancement of quality in people's lives. Many thanks are
extended to the other sponsors of the National Symposia on Patient
Education: the University of California at San Francisco's School
of Medicine, School of Dentistry, School of Nursing, School of Pharmacy, and Hospitals and Clinics; the American Nurses Association,
Division of Practice and Community Health Nursing; The American
Hospital Association; the American Nurses Association-Congress for
Nursing Practice; the Society for Public Health Education; the Bureau of Health Education; the National Center for Health Education, Inc.; and the American Dental Association.

                                                              —W. S.

Contributors

MARIAN ULRICH ADCOCK holds a B.S. in nursing and in psychology from Macalester College, St. Paul, Minnesota, and a master's degree in public health (health education) from the University of Minnesota, Minneapolis. Ms. Adcock is the President of Adcock and Associates, a health education consulting firm in St. Paul, Minnesota. She also has held, or currently holds, academic appointments at Yale University, University of Michigan, University of Missouri, and the University of Minnesota. A major goal of Ms. Adcock throughout her career has been to integrate health education into patient care.

ELIZABETH BERNHEIMER started her professional career as an oboist, receiving her bachelor's degree from the New England Conservatory of Music. She later became a health professional, receiving an M.P.H. from the University of Hawaii with a major in health education and a minor in medical care. She has designed, implemented, and evaluated a system-wide approach to patient education in a large hospital in San Francisco; written extensively on patient education; and received the Ann Wilson Haynes Award in 1977 for her work in this field. Currently, she is Assistant Professor in the Department of Family and Community Medicine at the University of Nevada, serving as director of the Preceptorship Program.

LAWREN H. D'ALTROY has been employed by the Johns Hopkins Oncology Center Cancer Control Program as Patient Educator and is currently a consultant to the center. In these capacities he has developed and evaluated education protocols for staff and patient education materials on chemotherapeutic medications for outpatients, for aplastic inpatients, and for parents of children with cancer. His doctoral work in health education at the Johns Hopkins University School of Hygiene and Public Health, Division of Health Education, emphasizes application of the behavioral sciences to health education problems and evaluation in the social sciences (including experimental design and biostatistics). Before going to Johns Hopkins, he was Coordinator of Special Projects in the Health Education Department of United Hospitals of St. Paul, Minnesota, where he coordinated the development and administration of a patient drug self-administration program and developed both an educational curriculum in patient teaching skills for hospital care givers, and rehabilitation and education programs for chronic obstructive lung disease patients.

JEANNE FLYNTZ DEJOSEPH is currently the Assistant Director of Nurses/Perinatal at Stanford University Hospital, Stanford, California. She received her undergraduate degree at Boston College School of Nursing and earned her M.S., C.N.M., and Ph.D., at the University of Utah. She has practiced obstetric and gynecologic nursing for fifteen years and has taught obstetrics for six years. She also organizes and participates in many academic and community programs in women's health.

DOROTHY JOAN DEL BUENO currently holds a joint position with the University of Pennsylvania and the Hospital of the University of Pennsylvania, Philadelphia. Previously she was Associate Director of Nursing, Director of Staff Development at Columbia Presbyterian Medical Center. She has served as a consultant on evaluation, human resource development, and competency-based education for many hospitals, colleges, universities, industry and government agencies. A prolific author, she also presents numerous workshops and conferences for individuals in the health care services. Dr. del Bueno is the chairperson of the American Nurses Association Council on Continuing Education and was a board member of the American Society for Hospital Education and Training.

CAROL N. D'ONOFRIO has her doctorate in public health and is Associate Professor of Public Health at the University of California at Berkeley. Her interests are concentrated on the development of health programs responsive to the needs of disadvantaged consumer groups and those at high risk for disease, and on the corresponding implications for the educational aspects of health policy, program planning, service delivery, and evaluation. She has published articles on these subjects and has served as a consultant to numerous health agencies. Her current work is focused on the prevention and early detection of cancer, and on strengthening educational programs within health maintenance organizations.

JARED I. FINE holds doctor of dental surgery and master's in public health degrees. He is currently Lecturer in the Division of General Dentistry, School of Dentistry, University of California at San Francisco; Assistant Chief at the Dental Health Bureau, Alameda County Health Care Services Agency; and Site Administrator for the National Preventive Dentistry Demonstration Program in Hayward, California. His research work is in the areas of the relationship of attitudes, values, and personality traits to preventive health behavior; the relative efficacy of population-specific preventive interventions; and the cost effectiveness of school-based dental health programs.

THOMAS G. FLORA, ED.D., is presently the Director of the Human Services Center at California State University, Chico, California. His academic background includes graduate preparations in health education and education curriculum design. He has worked as a consultant to rural hospitals in the development of both individual patient education programs and the development of institution-wide instructional systems. His present activities include the establishment of a regional support network for patient education in rural northeastern California.

LAWRENCE W. GREEN received his master's and doctoral degrees in public health from the University of California at Berkeley, then served on the faculty there for two years as Coordinator of Doctoral Training in Health Education, and two years in Bangladesh on their family planning project with the Ford Foundation. In 1970, he migrated to Baltimore where he established the graduate programs in health education and the continuing education program of the Johns Hopkins University School of Hygiene and Public Health. He is now Professor in the Departments of Health Services Administration, Population Dynamics, Behavioral Sciences, and Oncology; head of the Health Education Division; and Director of Health Education Studies for the Center for Health Services Research and Development of the Johns Hopkins Medical Institutions. The recipient of three international awards for his research in health education, he has also served as consultant to the World Health Organization, the National Center for Health Services Research, the National Academy of Sciences, the National Institutes of Health, and numerous other health agencies and foundations. He is the author of articles and books on health behavior, the former editor of *Health Education Monographs*, and currently on the editorial boards of four other journals. This year he received the Distinguished Career Award of the Public Health Education Section of the American Public Health Association and has accepted the surgeon general's request for him to take a leave of absence from Johns Hopkins to direct the Office of Health Information and Health Promotion of the U.S. Department of Health, Education, and Welfare in Washington.

BARBARA HEBERT is a doctoral student in the Division of Health Education, the Johns Hopkins University School of Hygiene and Public Health, Baltimore, Maryland. She received a Master of Public Health degree in health education from the University of Michigan School of Public Health in 1973. For the next two years she was employed as a health educator for Teamsters Local 688 in St. Louis, Missouri. She then joined the Veterans Administration as Patient Health Education Coordinator for five VA hospitals in the District of Columbia-Maryland area.

ROBERT HECHT studied Communication Arts at Seton Hall University in New Jersey, earning a B.A. degree in 1963. Realizing that he would never become a good jazz musician, he went on to do newspaper reporting and to produce various radio programs in the New Jersey area. He continued his communications studies as a field communications crewman at Fort Dix, New Jersey. He later did public relations writing for the Chase Manhattan Bank, taught English at Newark Academy, moved to northern California to work as a free-lance photographer, and subsequently became a media specialist at Stanford University. He is presently Coordinator of the Division of Instructional Media at Stanford University Medical School. He has written and produced numerous media programs in health science and is the author of several articles.

LOWELL STERN LEVIN is Associate Professor, Department of Epidemiology and Public Health, Yale University School of Medicine. He received his M.A. from Stanford University, his Ed.D. in education administration from Harvard University, and his M.P.H. in Health Education from Yale University. He is a member of the Advisory Panel on Health Education for the J.E. Fogarty International Center, a member of the consultant panel to the National Center for Health Education, and an educational planning consultant for the Joint Center for Studies of Health Programs, Institute of Social Medicine, University of Copenhagen, Denmark. He is an internationally known speaker and author on self-care and consumer participation in health services.

PATRICIA DOLAN MULLEN was graduated from the University of California at Berkeley with degrees in public health education (M.P.H. and Dr.P.H.), librarianship (M.L.S.), and English literature (A.B.). She spent two years in Ethiopia with the Peace Corps, which stimulated her interest in health education, with an emphasis on community development and social change. She has held faculty positions at the University of California at Berkeley and the University of Washington. Most recently she was Associate Director and Evaluation Specialist for the Department of Health Education, Group Health Cooperative of Puget Sound. Currently, she works for the Office of Health Information and Health Promotion of the U.S. Department of Health, Education, and Welfare in Washington. Her professional concerns include civil rights, health care for the disadvantaged, development of alternatives to the fee-for-service medical care delivery system, qualitative research approaches, the social psychology of chronic illness, health care provider behavior, and health education programs in health maintenance organizations.

DOROTHY S. ODA holds R.N., M.S., and D.N.S. degrees. She is Assistant Professor in the Department of Mental Health and Community Nursing, School of Nursing, University of California at San Francisco; Program Director of the Multilevel School Nurse Preparation Program; a consultant to the Robert Wood Johnson Foundation for school health programs; and a board member of the Nursing Dynamics Corporation. Her research work is in school health, school nursing and dental referral outcome, and specialized nursing role development.

LINDA ORMISTON received her Ph.D. in psychology from Stanford University under Professor Albert Bandura. She has taught behavioral self-management programs and trained others to teach them. Her extensive work with weight management programs includes being Assistant Director of the Diet and Weight Control Classes, Stanford Heart Disease Prevention Program, Stanford University School of Medicine, from 1976 to 1978. Also interested in parenting, she has served as a consultant to the Committee on Children's Television, San Francisco. Currently she is working as a private consultant, teaching at West Valley College, Saratoga, California, and conducting a clinical internship at the West Valley Community Mental Health Center in Los Gatos, California.

SHERYL BURT RUZEK holds a B.A. from San Francisco State University and received an M.A. and Ph.D. in sociology from the University of California at Davis. She is currently Community Coordinator, Program for Women in Health Sciences, University of California, San Francisco. She is also Research Associate and Member of the Advisory Board, Center for the Study of Women, Institute for Scientific Analysis, San Francisco. She co-chairs the national Sociologists for Women in Society committee on health. She is the author of *The Women's Health Movement: Feminist Alternatives to Medical Control, Women and Health Careers: A Guide for Career Exploration*, "Women and Health: A Bibliography with Selected Annotation," and articles on medical self-help and client-professional relations. Currently she is writing a book on volunteerism in health and beginning a cross-national study of health services to families with infants.

KEITH W. SEHNERT received his B.A. at the University of South Dakota and M.D. at the Case Western Reserve University in Cleveland, Ohio. He is President of Health Activation Systems, Inc.; a consultant for Health Promotion Programs at InterStudy; and Clinical Professor of Public Health at the University of Minnesota. A pioneer in the concepts of self-care and self-health, he developed the nation's first medical self-care class in 1970. While Director of the Center for Continuing Health Education at Georgetown University, he expanded the concept into the Course for Activated Patients (CAP), which has now been taught in nearly every state in the United States and in foreign countries. He is author of the best selling book *How To Be Your Own Doctor . . . Sometimes.*

WENDY D. SQUYRES, editor of this volume, received her Ph.D. in health sciences and education psychology from the University of Utah College of Health. She received a postdoctoral fellowship from the Johns Hopkins University School of Hygiene and Public Health, Division of Health Education, where she participated in the design of behavioral self-management interventions to reduce adolescent hypertension. She was previously the Education and Development Manager, Stanford University Medical Center, and the Training Consultant and Coordinator, University of California at San Francisco, Hospitals and Clinics. She also conceived of and directs the National Symposia on Patient Education and is currently the Regional Director of Health Education, Northern California Kaiser-Permanente Medical Centers.

1

Introduction

Wendy D. Squyres

The words *patient education* are often used interchangeably with the words *health education, patient teaching, patient counseling, patient information,* and *patient communication,* and occasionally with such terms as *self-care, compliance education, self-management,* and *behavior modification.* The position taken in this book is that the list of words just presented are not synonymous. Instead the authors of this book use *patient education* specifically to refer to planned combinations of learning activities designed to assist people who are having or have had experience with illness or disease in making changes in their behavior conducive to health (Green, Kreuter, Partridge, & Deeds, 1979). These learning activities are not limited to patient-provider interactions in hospitals but include educational efforts in ambulatory settings, private offices, free-standing clinics, voluntary health agencies, health maintenance organizations, and community settings. In spite of the vast number of settings in which patient education programs are offered, and in spite of considerations that can be given to a common process of health education planning, it should be kept in mind that many factors influence the unique and specialized quality that programs should reflect. These factors include:

1. *The nature of the health problems.* Programs geared to chronic, asymptomatic disease management, for example, will be quite different in their approach from programs geared to preparing people for surgery.
2. *The specific characteristics and needs of the target population.* University students, for example, often require different considerations than geriatric residents of an extended care facility.

3. *The health behaviors requiring change.* Health education approaches needed for adding new behaviors are different from those needed to change old ones.
4. *The administrative dilemmas.* For example, health education programs offered after long waiting periods in clinic reception areas will be received much differently than programs scheduled promptly with little or no waiting time.

There is an increasing demand on health care delivery institutions to provide health promotion and health maintenance programs for well populations in the communities they serve. Yet, regardless of the benefit such programs have, they do not alleviate the need for specialized efforts geared to people and their families who are consumers of health services and who are experiencing illness or disease. It is a fundamental premise here that special considerations need to be given to the powerful influence that illness has on the lives of individuals and their families, and that the new or changed behaviors and skills required for disease management and a return to health require sensitive and complex interventions. These interventions are both educational and therapeutic. The health educator in this setting, then, not only needs the ability to apply the behavioral sciences to health self-management but needs to understand the many roles of health providers in medical organizations, the unique climate of medical care, and the complexity of recovery and rehabilitation in this society.

It is the purpose of this book to present a conceptualization of the state of the art of patient education and to highlight selected issues for study. A review of the literature from the last decade teaches us that the successful patient education programs are the ones that have both a philosophical and a programmatic context. The philosophical position that this book embraces reflects one that is often described as a "patient-centered" position. Simonds spoke for all of us when he outlined the following foundation values (Lesparre, 1970):

1. Patients shall be respected and cared for as human beings.
2. Patients shall be recognized as having unique sociopsychological, cultural, and familial backgrounds relevant to their conditions.
3. Patients shall have the opportunity to obtain the information and the guidance they need and shall have the support to help them use the information once it is obtained.

4. Patients shall be provided an active and participatory role in their own care to the extent they choose and are able.
5. Patients shall be stimulated and guided through effective educational means to acquire new knowledge, attitudes, and actions that will promote their ability to care for themselves more adequately and to maintain their health at an optimum level.
6. Patients shall be cared for through services designed and organized to promote and support learnings and behaviors that are appropriate to their care and to the maintenance of their care.

There are numerous program development protocols available for the health practitioner who is interested in a comprehensive, well thought-out patient education program. One of them, which is paraphrased here in part, comes from a three-year study conducted by the Community Health Education Project of the American Public Health Association (Martin, 1977):

1. Providers, administrators, and funding sources, as well as consumers, must be involved in developing and implementing the program in order to ensure that it receives adequate support including budget, equipment, supplies, space, time, and the cooperation of all personnel.
   a. Staff agreement and support for an activity are essential if it is to be undertaken successfully.
   b. Because provider resistance to the program may be strong, special efforts should be made to identify elements of the health education program that will be useful in promoting, not disrupting, each staff member's work.
   c. The documentation of program success is an important tool for gaining and maintaining this support.
2. One person with knowledge of educational approaches should be given the responsibility for the overall planning and development of the health education program.
   a. This position should be located within a component of the administrative hierarchy, which will ensure coordination of all programs and a delegation of power sufficient to implement them.
3. The resources of the organization's professional personnel are utilized most fully and effectively if the educational ac-

tivities are an integral part of the total of health services provided, and take place in a systematic, coordinated, and centrally guided way.

   a. This requires clear allocation of health education functions and responsibilities to the entire staff, and the development of clear goal statements for all educational activities.
   b. Resources, including money, should be designated specifically for the health education program.

4. A team approach should be utilized and all personnel should be involved in the development and implementation of health education activities.

   a. The physician must be included, often before other staff can be involved successfully.
   b. Inservice training should be provided to teach the principles and methods of health education. This training should include not only the use of educational materials but also the development of communication skills, acknowledgment of the patients' right to make their own decisions, and an understanding of the complex factors that affect health behavior.
   c. Because physicians and nurses are more apt to be accustomed to working with patients on a one-to-one basis, they are likely to require additional training in group process skills.

5. The planning and development of the program should involve both consumers and providers and follow the basic steps of program planning—assessment of educational needs, definition of goals, selection of appropriate methods, effective implementation, and evaluation.

   a. A broad range of staff including all levels of personnel should be included from the very beginning, when initial plans are developed.

6. The planning and implementation of a comprehensive health education program may take from two to five years.

   a. Although some positive results may come quickly, everyone, including funding sources, must recognize that significant effects, such as lasting behavioral changes, are achieved very slowly.

7. Sound health behavior is encouraged most effectively when providers and consumers are actively involved in the educational process.

a. Educational objectives must be made clear and must be communicated to and accepted by all involved—staff, patients and their families, and funding sources.

b. Health education must be a process of interaction rather than merely a flow of predetermined information from provider to consumer.

8. It is essential that health messages be repeated consistently throughout the patient care process.

a. Changes in individual behavior are complex and often require long periods of time. Because the provision of information alone seldom results in behavior changes, the message must be repeated and reinforced utilizing a variety of educational approaches, not just one isolated activity.

9. The goal of the program may or may not be behavioral change.

a. The individual should receive all the information and support necessary to make an informed decision. It is still his prerogative, however, to make a decision that ultimately may adversely affect his health status.

10. Because it is difficult to change individual behavior, emphasis should be placed on providing an environment that supports such change and minimizes the barriers the individual encounters.

a. Providers should first focus on those activities that they, themselves, can take part in which will encourage the desired behavior change, e.g., attractive facilities, convenient hours, continuity of care, and nonsmoking by staff.

11. Since organizations differ from one another in a variety of aspects, each should develop its own clearly defined approach to health education rather than utilize an inappropriate model.

12. While some aspects of an organization's educational program may be general, others may have to be tailored specifically to the needs of particular patients, etc., hypertensives, diabetics, and individuals with minimal reading skills.

a. Approaches must have personal relevance for the individual and be closely related to his own goals and experiences.

b. Emphasis must be placed not just on content but on the

method of presentation in order to generate enthusiasm and interest.

    c. Techniques that utilize small groups and individual counseling should be emphasized.

    d. Coercion is not an acceptable method.

13. While most of an organization's health education is likely to be addressed to patients, efforts should also extend into the community as a potential pool of future patients, and also to help residents protect themselves against avoidable illness that could transform them into new or returning patients.

14. Evaluation of all health education activities is a necessary element for ensuring that present approaches and methods are effective, and for generating ideas to render them more effective.

    a. The primary aim of health education is to assure sound health-related habits on the part of the consumer. The final measure of educational effectiveness, therefore, is to be found in consumer behavior, although measures of knowledge, attitudes, and motivations will be useful for certain purposes. Evaluation activities should include techniques that document behavior change.

15. In order to monitor an organization's educational program, assure its optimal effectiveness, and identify weaknesses, it is necessary to introduce systematic recording procedures, periodic reviews, and regular discussions of health education at staff meetings.

    a. Emphasis must be placed not on reporting that activities have or have not been engaged in but on their effectiveness in promoting behavior change.

    b. Flexibility in a program is essential to ensure that activities can be modified or eliminated when their ineffectiveness is documented.

This book is the product of national meetings designed to survey the field, to discuss issues relevant to the study and practice of the field, and to discover what's working and what isn't working in patient education; hence, it is not built around a single, central thesis. Nevertheless as symposia faculty began submitting papers, one unsolicited theme emerged; a theme that often appears in rhetoric but seldom in practice: the concept of active patient participation. There are undoubtedly numerous reasons why assuring active patient participation is more difficult than merely enjoining colleagues to provide activities during national meetings. Some will cite the "system" as the villain, or the ambiguity (sometimes sheer negativism) of administrators, or the actual ambivalence of consumers of health products and services toward assuming responsibility, or the attitudes of providers. A few will cite the more subtle, but probably more powerful, influence—the blind faith in simplistic definitions of education. Over the past quarter of a century the health and medical profession has succumbed to the temptation to deify education, to assume that it automatically improves the quality of lives, yields roused and motivated individuals, and most commonly, leaves people with the desire to go home and do exactly what the professional feels is best. The result of all this has been the assumption that medically recommended complex behavior changes can be accomplished through simple educational interventions such as dispensing pamphlets or showing films. Furthermore some health and medical care providers would have been tempted to hope that mastery of diagnostic and therapeutic clinical skills would automatically carry the ability to alter patient behaviors. Effective patient education requires more than the best clinical skills, more than rapport, and more than articulate information sharing.

So far there is agreement on what the purpose of patient education is: that specific aspects of personal health behavior have an important influence on morbidity and mortality, and that recuperation from illness, and specifically prevention of subsequent recurrence of illness, depends on the patient taking charge and changing certain risk behaviors. The problem occurs when well-meaning health and medical practitioners decide that simply reporting the "what" to patients automatically describes the "how." When patients are able to repeat back the instructions they were given regarding what they need to do to get well or stay well, practitioners rave about the success of their patient education efforts. Unfortunately the patient may be worlds away from actually making the changes. Knowing what to do doesn't ensure that people will actually take the necessary steps.

Patient education resembles the complexity of an electrical circuitry board. Once one point is activated, the next stage is triggered. The end product, whether it is a light bulb flashing or a bell ringing, won't take place if any of the stations along the board are not activated in sequence. Human behavior circuitry is so much more complex. Although knowledge may be a requisite for skill acquisition, knowledge on its own will not necessarily lead to behavior change.

The entire process is further complicated by the fact that there are usually numerous ways to minimize health risks. Algorithms, or decision trees, are helpful if there are very few choices available. Usually, however, a healthy, enriched life is a maze of hundreds of small country roads leading to the same general destination. It isn't difficult to get agreement on the fact that the patient needs to take responsibility for choosing the road; what is difficult, however, is the way the health professional can be most helpful. Does the patient need a vehicle, or a map, or some provisions for the journey? How are the decisions made? Sometimes the patients need guided practice under supervision so that, once they are told they are doing the procedure correctly, they can go home and repeat it with confidence. In other cases there is an aspect of the environment at home that keeps the patients from practicing the new or altered behavior (e.g., a physical barrier such as stairs, an emotional barrier such as critical parents, or a cultural belief such as dietary taboos). In most cases a forty-five-minute classroom presentation on anatomy and physiology fails to take into consideration these additional reasons why the behavior circuit board is not completed.

On the one hand, then, the knowledge of the disease process and medical therapeutics alone falls short of providing the full support patients need for making health behavior change. On the other hand the most empathetic, genuinely caring perspective of patients and their families doesn't necessarily lead to an understanding of human behavior either. An understanding of human behavior on its own—without an understanding of health, illness, and health care systems and organizations, too—also comes short of the desired balance of skills required to build the bridge between health learning and health performance. It is easy to see at the outset that preparing a single professionally trained architect for the construction of such a bridge would be inappropriate at this time. Instead of one species of architects we need to train numerous subspecies of architects to join together, including the one who will actually march across the bridge (the patient), to participate in a team approach to accomplish the task. It will be necessary for each member to bring to the team his or her special area of expertise, but in addition each needs to know that the blueprints for the bridge bear a great resemblance to the electric circuit board. Electrical contacts at just one point of the board will not turn on the light. Simplistic or single educational interventions will not lead to long-term, or necessarily even short-term, changes.

This book emphasizes the role of the patient in the patient-provider relationship. It also emphasizes the skills that the members of the health care team need in order to be effective patient educators. It makes the case for calling attention to the health behavior dimensions and the setting and population dimensions of health behavior change (see chapter 2). It also makes the case for changes required of both the health care delivery system and the training of health care providers. Numerous examples are given to highlight these issues and to demonstrate their utility and application to the practice of patient education. Instead of succumbing to the temptations of placing false hopes in simplistic views of education, this book not only articulates the "what" required for active patient participation but also identifies, in part, the "how."

References

Green, L. W., Kreuter, M., Partridge, K. B., & Deeds, S. G. *Health education planning: A diagnostic approach.* Palo Alto: Mayfield, 1979, p. 7.

Lesparre, M. The patient as a health student. *Hospitals,* March 16, 1970, pp. 75–80.

Martin, E. D. *A guide to health education in ambulatory care settings* (U.S. Department of Health, Education, and Welfare, Health Services Administration, Bureau of Community Health Services, February 7, 1977), pp. 87–91.

2

What Do Recent Evaluations of
Patient Education Tell Us?*

*Lawrence W. Green, Wendy D. Squyres,
Lawren H. D'Altroy, Barbara Hebert*

To learn what recent evaluations of patient education are revealing to practitioners, administrators, and policy makers, a review of the published literature from 1974 to present was conducted.[1] The review is in three parts; the first part asks how the authors of these studies defined *success* for their programs, and whether a state-of-the-art profile can be drawn from the successes and failures identified in this review. The second part restates the questions for future evaluations of patient education. The third re-

*Preparation of this chapter was supported by National Institutes of Health research training grant HL07180 on which Green is director, Squyres is a post-doctoral fellow, D'Altroy and Hebert are predoctoral fellows, Division of Health Education, Department of Health Services Administration, School of Hygiene and Public Health, the Johns Hopkins University, 615 N. Wolfe Street, Baltimore, Maryland 21205. The chapter was presented as a paper at the Second Annual National Symposium on Patient Education, University of California Medical Center, San Francisco, October 22, 1978.

[1]Based on empirical studies retrieved by MEDLINE & MEDLAR search for 1974–1978, using A(1) "patient education"; (2) "evaluation"; B(3) hospitals; (4) nursing homes; and (5) long-term care facilities as key terms, on August 28, 1978. Of the 134 citations retrieved, one-third were usable for this review. Of the remaining, one-third were not of patient education, one-fifth were not completed empirical evaluations; and nine were unavailable in regional library holdings. MEDLINE & MEDLARS were utilized because of their generally accepted use by clinicians in hospital, clinic, and private office settings. The observations of this review, therefore, are limited by the absence of the patient education literature from data sources such as *Psychological Abstracts, ERIC,* and *Social Science Citations Index.*

views selected studies in greater depth to illustrate some of the methods and principles drawn from the first two parts.

Evaluation is defined as the comparison of an object of interest against a standard of acceptability (Green, 1974). The review includes those published reports designed to appraise the acceptability of a patient education program as the object of interest. Only those studies evaluating programs using impact on patients or patient outcomes as standards of acceptability were selected.

A Profile of Published Patient Education Evaluations, 1974-1978

Definitions of "Success"

In contrast to earlier reviews of the patient education literature (Gillum & Barsky, 1974; Green and Figa-Talamanca, 1974; Young, 1968), most reported outcomes have transcended the knowledge-only category and now include attitudinal, behavioral, biomedical, and cost-effectiveness measures. The following amplifications of each standard of acceptability summarize reported criteria of success in recent patient education evaluations.

KNOWLEDGE GAIN. Five (23%) of the twenty-two studies reviewed defined success solely on the criterion of patient increase in knowledge (Black & Mitchell, 1977; Caron & Roth, 1977; Hassell & Medved, 1975; Teuscher & Heidecker, 1976; Rahe, Scalzi, & Shine, 1975). Knowledge change was determined by pre- and postscores on written questionnaires (fig. 2-1).

Nine (41%) of the twenty-two studies reviewed defined success as the combination of knowledge gained with behavior change (Kay & Hammond, 1978; Sly, 1975; Lawson, Traylor, & Gram, 1976), with attitude change (Alkhateeb, Lukeroth, & Riggs, 1975; Laugharne & Steiner, 1977), with more effective utilization of hospital facilities (Laugharne & Steiner, 1977), with performance of a certain category of health provider as a source of health knowledge (Solfin, Young, & Clayton, 1977), with biomedical improvements (Jones, Turner, & Slowie, 1976), and with the comparative performance of certain media (Alkhateeb et al., 1975; Bracken, Bracken, & Landry, 1977; Vignos, Parker, & Thompson, 1976).

Figure 2-1.
Patient knowledge as a criterion of
success in twenty-two evaluations
of patient education between 1974
and 1978.

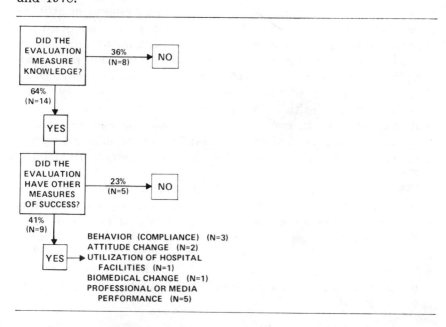

ATTITUDE CHANGE.   One-fourth of the studies reviewed defined
success in terms of change in patient attitudes. The affective categories include reduction of anxiety (Roter, 1977; Wallace & Wallace,
1977), reduction of anger (Roter, 1977), appreciation of care given
(Wallace & Wallace, 1977), motivation (Alkhateeb et al., 1975), satisfaction with services received (Lazes, 1977), the degree to which
the educational program was seen as interesting and beneficial to the
patient (Alkhateeb et al., 1975), the degree to which the patient liked
the educational program (Salzer, 1975), and the degree to which the
patient felt that the educational content was unique (Salzer, 1975).

Attitude change was always combined with at least one other
outcome category. In two studies the educational outcome actually
increased anxiety (Roter, 1977; Wallace & Wallace, 1977) and anger
(Roter, 1977). In one study there was an accompanying positive behavior change (Roter, 1977). In the other the postmyocardial patients whose anxiety increased with education expressed gladness

nevertheless that they received the educational intervention (Wallac & Wallace, 1977). Another program with postmyocardial patients did not change the high anxiety of patients, but after behavioral changes the patients had low anxiety six months postdischarge (Pozen, Stechmiller, Harris, Smith, Fried, & Voigt, 1977).

One caution, which will be discussed further in the observations on the state of the art, is that six of the seven measures of attitude change were provider centered (e.g., patient satisfaction with the educational program). Only one measured attitudes toward the prescribed behavior that might be directly motivational. An implicit assumption is that positive attitudes toward the educational effort or toward the provider of the medical care setting necessarily would lead to improved health behaviors (fig. 2-2). Roter's study showed that patients could be made *less* satisfied with their encounter with the physician as a result of an educational intervention in the waiting room yet decrease their subsequent broken appointments (Roter, 1977).

Most of the studies reporting favorable attitudes toward the program did not go on to study behavioral change. We are left to wonder whether attitude changes are necessary or important steps in the behavioral change of patients; and if so, whether the object of the attitudes should be the providers, the institution, the prescribed behavior, or the health problem; and if it is the provider or the institution, whether negative attitudes might not be just as useful as positive attitudes.

BEHAVIORAL CHANGE. Ten percent of the studies (fig. 2-2) defined success solely in terms of behavioral change (Bryant, Stender, Frist, & Somers, 1976; Jesudasan, George, Chacko, Taylor, Kurian, & Job, 1976). Over one-third used a combination of behavioral change and biomedical change (Green, Werlin, Schauffler, & Avery, 1977; Johnston, Cantwell, & Fletcher, 1976; Witschi, Singer, Wo-Lee, & Stare, 1978), attitudinal change (Roter, 1977; Salzer, 1975), or increased knowledge (Kay & Hammond, 1978; Sly, 1975) as the standards of acceptability.

Behaviors that were described in the studies included care of joints of the body, getting more rest, using medications (Kay & Hammond, 1978); dietary management (Johnston et al., 1976; Lazes, 1977; Salzer, 1975; Witschi et al., 1978); increased question asking (Roter, 1977); heart patients returning to work and stopping smoking (Johnston et al., 1976; Pozen et al., 1977); diabetic patients taking urine tests, exercise, applying appropriate first aid, and going for periodic eye examinations (Salzer, 1975); management of the environment by asthma patients (Sly, 1975); and appropriate utilization of health care facilities (Green et al., 1977; Kay & Hammond, 1978; Lazes, 1977; Roter, 1977). Most of the behavioral changes were measured by self-report questionnaires rather than through observation or other forms of record keeping.

Figure 2-2.
The implied assumption of causal relationships in
most evaluations measuring patient satisfaction.

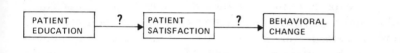

COST EFFECTIVENESS AND USE OF HEALTH SERVICES. Less than 10 percent of the studies explicitly identified cost effectiveness as a criterion of success (Green et al., 1977; Laugharne & Steiner, 1977). One used a shared service approach to diabetes education. Three hospitals pooled their resources to develop a cooperative diabetes education center (Laugharne & Steiner, 1977). Even though the outcome measures were stated in terms other than cost effectiveness, the three studies reporting improved utilization of health care facilities, and the one study reporting improved health work force utilization, were considering implicitly the cost/benefit ratio of the methodologies under question (Laugharne & Steiner, 1977; Lazes, 1977; Pozen et al., 1977; Solfin et al., 1977).

Improved utilization patterns included outpatient rather than inpatient services (Laugharne & Steiner, 1977), increased number of appointments kept (Lazes, 1977), clinic rather than emergency room use by venereal disease patients (Bryant et al., 1976), and self-care rather than emergency room utilization by asthmatic patients (Green et al., 1977). In the health work force utilization category, one study suggested that an individualized medication education program delivered by a pharmacist was more effective than traditionally delivered patient education programs (Solfin et al., 1977). The other study suggested that the group-teaching approach utilizing audiovisual materials for patients with diabetes reduced the dietitian's time to less than half of what was formerly needed (Hassell & Medved, 1975).

In summary, empirical reports of patient education programs

published in the medical and health journals carry hopes that informed patients who have positive attitudes about the quality of their care and the educational programs conducted in their behalf go on to change their behaviors. Adherence to medical regimens usually receives primary attention, with some attention given to changes in life-styles or personal health behaviors. Few, less than one-fifth, used biomedical improvements as their standards of acceptability.

Some Observations on the State of the Art

What can be expected from a standard medical search procedure? From 134 computer-generated references on patient education and evaluation, 22 percent were *not* evaluation studies designed to determine whether the program "worked." Most could not even be described as case studies in any formal sense. Instead, they described the most salient features of their program, extolled the values of patient education, and rallied hospitals and other health care delivery settings to incorporate patient teaching into their delivery of care. Such exhortations add little to our understanding of what works, and they undermine the credibility of patient education to the extent that they remain so prevalent in the literature.

Such articles calling for more inpatient education are probably only marginally useful in stimulating the development of programs when compared to similar articles five or ten years ago. It is generally agreed that the message has been heard. A comparison of the results of two American Hospital Association surveys shows a substantial rise (15 to 46.4%) in hospitals with patient education services from 1972 to 1975 (American Hospital Association, 1977a, 1977b). A number of books, proceedings, special journal issues, and papers devoted to the subject of design and organization of patient education services has been published in the last few years (Redman, 1976, 1978; Simmons, 1975; Slepcevitch, 1974).

Another 31 percent were not reports of patient education efforts but of staff education programs designed to prepare health professionals to carry out patient education strategies, or medical or nursing procedures. Few of the articles mentioned or developed the idea of health care team cooperation in the implementation of inpatient education programs. Attitudes about team work range from that expressed in an article for librarians suggesting ways that their training and position could be used to complement and enhance the team approach to education (Harris, 1978), to that expressed in an article for pharmacists, which concludes that they should provide ambulatory clinical services as independent practitioners equal to other clinicians (Gardner & Trinca, 1978).

Only two articles dealt with the nonhospital institutionalized population. One concluded that there is growing interest on the part of long-term care staff in patient and family education and that programs in these areas are worth developing (Rosenberg & Judkins, 1976).

Most of the articles actually reporting hospital patient education programs failed to describe the educational and behavioral change techniques employed. Instead, the writers described how educational services had been organized at their facilities.

Of the 134 MEDLINE & MEDLARS references retrieved on patient education and evaluation, less than one-third actually were of patient education programs that included an evaluation component. One generalization that could be drawn is that an automated search for evaluation as an integral part of patient education programs will yield one-third nonpatient programs and one-fifth nonempirical evaluations. Much of what is being written and indexed under these headings is still off the target of patient education and evaluation.

An analysis of the studies reveals some common pitfalls in patient education diagnosis, planning, implementation, evaluation, and analysis. The following problems have been discussed previously in the literature in one form or another (Deeds, 1976; Green, 1974, 1977; Green & Figa-Talamanca, 1974; Green, Levine, & Deeds, 1975; Green et al., 1977; Werlin & Schauffler, 1978). Nevertheless the literature reviewed from the last four years reveals that many patient education programs and studies continue to succumb to these traps:

OVERSIMPLIFYING THE BEHAVIORAL TASKS. Most clinicians and evaluators acknowledge that health education is a process necessarily linked to health behavior, but little attention was given in the studies reviewed to differentiating the behavioral and nonbehavioral determinants of a health problem, or to giving priority to health behaviors based on a critical assessment of their relative importance and potential changeability. There was a tendency to oversimplify the multiple influence of attitudes, beliefs, values, perceptions, social supports, physical barriers, financial barriers, and the behaviors of health providers on the patient's health behavior. These several omissions and simplifications result in concentration of equal resources on important as well as trivial behaviors, on simple as well as complex behaviors, and on prevalent as well as rare attitudes or beliefs. The indiscriminate allocation of scarce educational resources results in a poor return in outcomes relative to apparent investment of effort.

ATHEORETICAL ASSUMPTION ABOUT CAUSE. In several of the studies reviewed, methods or programs were tried and tested, and assumptions were made about *why* outcomes did or did not happen. These assumptions usually were not tested, seldom were related to formal theory, and often were not even made explicit so that they could be questioned. The hypothesized cause-effect relationship between patient education interventions and health outcomes needs to be made explicit in a systematic approach to patient education planning (Green, Kreuter, Partridge, & Deeds, 1979; Green et al., 1975). Interventions need to be preceded by behavioral and educational diagnoses. It is this diagnostic approach that sets the stage for appropriate analysis of outcomes of patient education programs. Those programs in this review that utilized a combination of approaches, and that measured a number of immediate, intermediate, and long-range outcomes, reflected this preferred, systematic approach to planning and evaluation.

EVALUATING A TECHNIQUE OR METHOD BY COMPARISON WITH ITS ABSENCE. Health education theory and research have warned that no single educational input should be expected to have significant, lasting impact on health behavior unless it is supported by other educational inputs. Some of the evaluations sought to evaluate a method of education by comparing a group of patients who received that method with control patients who received no planned health education. It is suggested that evaluations be designed to test multiple methods in a comprehensive program by using factorial designs with various combinations of two or more methods so that their independent and interactive effects can be analyzed.

PREOCCUPATION WITH A FAVORITE METHOD OR MEDIUM. Success with a method of patient education in one setting for one population of patients does not guarantee success with all patients in all settings. Health education theory and research suggest that the best combination of educational methods, media, and messages for some patients is not necessarily the best combination for others. The recent studies reviewed showed some sensitivity to this principle in planning, but it was often ignored in drawing conclusions and generalizations from successful or unsuccessful results. Analysis of patient education evaluations should attempt to show major differences

in the effectiveness of methods with different groups of patients identified by characteristics such as age, sex, socioeconomic level, and
other demographic measures.

How The Question Should Be Posed

The profile of recent evaluation efforts in patient education demonstrates the pitfalls in oversimplifying or ignoring the influences on
health and behavior. Reliance on any single educational method usually leads to negligible effects, or to short-term improvements not
sustained over time. Such findings lead to frustration and to skepticism on the part of clinicians that health education has anything
to offer in the management and control of health problems. Many
patient education efforts have been based both on inadequate assessments of the behavioral problems to which they are addressed and
on insufficient attention to the need for a variety of educational interventions in influencing and sustaining behavior change.

One conclusion that is safely drawn from the literature on health
behavior and behavior change is that there are no universal determinants of success. There is no formula for behavior change that is
universally applicable for all populations, settings, health problems,
or health behaviors. There are, however, certain elements that must
be taken into account in designing any educational program. This
presentation focuses on two dimensions of these elements: (1) the
health-behavioral dimension and (2) the setting-population dimension. Greater attention to these dimensions should improve the quality of educational diagnosis and prevent most of the pitfalls described
earlier.

Health-behavioral Dimension

Health problems generally require some behavioral response on the
part of the people experiencing them. The behavioral response can be
as simple as taking aspirin for a headache or as complex as reorder-
ing diet, exercise, work, and social habits while undergoing dialysis
for kidney malfunction. The appropriateness of behavioral responses
is, in any case, a function of the health problem. Types of behavioral
responses vary with types of health problems. Chronic diseases require different, more numerous, and more complex behavioral responses than do acute or self-limiting diseases. Asymptomatic health
problems such as hypertension produce especially troublesome be-

havioral demands in contrast to symptomatic health problems, because the individual usually feels no distress or receives no relief from the treatment procedure. In the case of hypertension, the treatment regimen may actually make the individual feel worse.

Not only do different types of health problems produce requirements for different behavioral responses, but a given health problem may require multiple behavioral responses. Three classifications of behavioral patterns have been formulated to describe this relationship. These classifications may be as useful in identifying the multiple behavioral demands of a given health problem as they are in distinguishing between the demands resulting from different types of health problems.

A sociologic dimension of behavioral patterns has been classified into: (1) health behavior, (2) illness behavior, (3) sick-role behavior, and (4) the at-risk role (Baric, 1969; Kasl, 1974; Kasl & Cobb, 1966). Health behavior is described as "any activity undertaken by a person who believes himself to be healthy, for the purpose of preventing disease or detecting disease in an asymptomatic stage" (Kasl & Cobb, 1966), while illness behavior is viewed as "any activity undertaken by a person who feels ill, for the purpose of defining the state of his health and of discovering a suitable remedy" (Kasl & Cobb, 1966). Sick-role behavior is characterized as "the activity undertaken by those who consider themselves ill, for the purpose of getting well" (Kasl, 1974). The at-risk role describes a person who feels well but knows that one or more risk factors are present (Baric, 1969). The boundaries between these behavioral patterns often are blurred. All of the patterns may not be evident for a specific health problem, nor will they be evident for all individuals with the same health problem or health goal. Role classifications, however, have provided a conceptual framework for many studies of health behavior; analysis of role patterns may suggest fruitful program interventions.

A second classification, grounded theory, uses a form of comparative analysis to identify characteristic patterns of patient responses to the problems illness poses (Mullen & Reynolds, 1978). The focus of attention is the personal calculus of the process of decision making by which people adjust to the demands of health problems. The grounded theory perspective has been applied most frequently to chronic diseases and other health problems requiring long-term life-style changes (Strauss & Glaser, 1975; Mullen, 1977). Results of these studies indicate that using this approach enables practitioners to understand and predict behavioral responses to the set of conditions imposed by various health problems.

A third classification, more behavioristic in origin, sorts behavioral demands along five dimensions: (1) frequency—the regularity with which a behavior occurs, (2) persistence—the duration over which the behavior change is sustained, (3) promptness—the reduction of delay in adopting a behavior, (4) quality—the appropriateness of choice in health actions, and (5) range—the variety or complexity of a set of health behaviors (Green, 1978, 1979). This classification makes no assumptions about the sociology or psychology of behavioral change, but it is particularly useful in assessing the behavioral goals of a patient education program insofar as it allows for finer distinctions among behaviors than the other two classifications. Measuring behavioral changes on these dimensions would lend greater specificity and comparability to evaluations of patient education.

Discussion of the health-behavioral dimension has focused on the relationship between health problems and behavior: namely, that health problems generally require behavioral responses. Behavioral responses vary with the type of health problem: acute versus chronic or symptomatic versus asymptomatic. Behavioral responses themselves can be classified by expected social roles, by the degree of behavior change required, or by the dimensions of behavior change. Both the health and the behavioral problems, however, are defined partially by the setting and population in which they are found.

Setting/Population Dimensions

For purposes of this discussion, settings can be classified as inpatient or outpatient. Subsumed under the inpatient setting are a variety of institutions: general medical and surgical or psychiatric hospitals, community and teaching hospitals, long-term care facilities, and nursing homes. Outpatient settings include free-standing clinics and health centers; ambulatory care, specialty clinic or outpatient services of hospitals; hospital maintenance organizations (HMOs); and some types of group or private practices.

Certain characteristics of the setting will influence the range and amount of educational activities.

1. *Institutional characteristics.* Size, physical structure, location, affiliations with educational institutions such as medical and nursing schools, complexity of the organizational structure, and membership in a multifacility system
2. *Management characteristics.* Degree of administrative con-

trol, patterns of interdepartmental communication and collaboration, tolerance for change or innovation, presence or absence of incentives for educational activities

3. *Health services characteristics.* Primary versus tertiary, ambulatory versus inpatient, specialized versus comprehensive, or combinations thereof

4. *Client characteristics.* Specific patient groups (e.g., veterans or children); residential proximity and referral patterns within a geographic service area; membership in a specific occupational group (e.g., union workers or students); socioeconomic, demographic, and literacy distributions

5. *Resource characteristics.* Level of existing support for educational activities (personnel, space, equipment, funds), potential for future allocation, access to educational resources of other agencies.[2]

Population or community characteristics must also be taken into consideration in planning educational programs. In addition to the client characteristics mentioned earlier, the important community characteristics include: (1) demographic composition (age, race, and sex distributions, socioeconomic structure, and educational level; (2) existence of social support systems (family, friends); (3) psychosocial and cultural variables including prevalent knowledge, attitudes, beliefs, values, and skills; and (4) epidemiologic profile of mortality, morbidity, and disability.

Taking both the health-behavioral dimension and the setting-population dimension into consideration, the question of "what works" thus becomes a question of which educational interventions are effective in a given getting for a particular population in influencing specific behavioral responses to specific health problems. Clearly, the planning of patient education along these several dimensions will be more complex than simply "improving compliance" or "teaching patients."

Recent Evaluations of Exemplary Programs

In this section, six studies are presented in detail in two groups. The programs selected have been drawn from the recent literature in medical and health care journals. They show some heartening results for

[2]This classification was prepared for the American Public Health Association's Committee on Revision of the Patient Education Planning Model, 1978.

patient education, and they demonstrate some of the more promising approaches to program design and evaluation discussed in the previous sections.

Self-care Discharge Education

A number of studies have attempted to measure changes effected by hospital education in specific, labor-intensive, self-care techniques for chronic problems that require frequent or extended hospitalization. Four programs are reviewed here in some depth to demonstrate the potential impact of patient education on utilization of health services. The target populations included renal patients requiring dialysis, hemophiliacs, and children with neurogenic bladder disease requiring frequent catheter changes. The behavior demands of the diseases are similar in that they require much skilled handling of paraphernalia such as needles, intravenous tubing, catheters, and blood products. These procedures normally would be carried out by trained hospital personnel. The patients and their families were taught to perform the procedures to give them more responsibility for their own care, to reduce the cost of care, and to reduce the time both staff and patients had to commit to care.

In one program the staff of the Nashville (Tennessee) VA Hospital taught home dialysis to patients in a six-week in-hospital course (Latos, Spannuth, & Stone, 1977). Patients in this program roomed together, in part to provide each other with support. Teaching methods included lectures by members of the medical team to small groups of patients, individual counseling, and regular follow-up after discharge. A booklet on home dialysis was provided. Finally, a technician modified the electrical and plumbing systems in each patient's residence to support the dialysis unit. A dialysis assistant (usually the patient's spouse) had to be present and taught during the last three weeks of training.

Between 1969 and 1977, 182 patients were given this course. The five-year survival rate for home dialysis was 91 percent; for renal transplant, 59 percent; and for center dialysis, 51 percent. Mortality for the first two years was 6 percent for the home dialysis group versus 26 percent for the center dialysis group. The members of each group were not randomly assigned, which subtracts from the significance of the results. The authors did attempt to address the question of group differences by noting that patients in all groups were substantially (although not completely) alike in terms of other complications. Indeed, the renal transplant patients were selected from among the healthier members of the population, and 70 percent had been on home dialysis prior to the transplant.

The authors note: "In our experience, the main factor preventing patients from entering home dialysis has not been the underlying medical condition but whether they have someone at home who is able to assist with the dialysis procedure." The authors cite a 50 percent completion rate for their training course compared with 28 percent nationally. With approximately 22,000 people on hemodialysis in the United States in 1976, they considered their program to have potential for wide application. This program illustrates the value of addressing the several predisposing, enabling, and reinforcing factors related to patient behavior.

Another article reported on a program at the VA hospital in Tampa, Florida, in which patients learned to do their own dialysis at the hospital. A total of 220 nursing hours was used to teach each pair of patients. Included in the course were sessions designed to reduce anxiety and to teach nondominant hand use (for insertion of needles), body chemistry, medications, and how the machine worked. Patients (and partners when available) had to pass a series of six exams. The author noted that twice as many patients were now being cared for by the same number of nurses.

In an Ohio hospital pilot program, a 14-year-old hemophiliac and his family were taught in the hospital to self-administer medications and blood products by a team consisting of a medical intern, a nurse, and a pharmacist (Fudge & Vlasses, 1977). The patient's past history was used as the control. Comparing the year before the teaching program to the year after, hospital days were reduced from 103 to 24, school attendance rose 15 percent, and cost savings were $20,230. Twenty-three patients were on the program as of August 1977, with the pharmacist's instruction services reimbursed at $40 per patient by Blue Cross and Medicaid.

In another program, children with neurogenic bladder dysfunction were taught self-catheterization, based on Lapides' work showing that frequency of catheter changing is more important than sterile technique in reducing incidence of infection (Altshuler, Meyer, & Butz, 1977). Learning time ranged from three to seven days in the hospital. Parents spent from twenty-four to forty-eight hours free of charge in the hospital to observe and learn. Teaching and learning steps included observation, modeling, catheterization of a doll, and finally self-catheterization. Anatomic illustrations and a review instruction sheet were also used. Hospital staff provided follow-up in the patients' homes and schools, with the family doctors, and with public health nurses. Patients periodically returned to the hospital. From 1973 to 1976 a total of fifty-five patients (twenty-two males and twenty-three females) participated in the program. Success rates are displayed in table 2-1. One-third of the children were infection-free; one-third were on suppressive antibiotics; and one-third were treated for culture-demonstrated infections. No control group was reported.

Table 2-1.
Self-catheterization Program Outcomes
(Altshuler, Meyer & Butz, 1977)

OUTCOME	NO. PATIENTS (22 boys, 33 girls)
Success: child dry more than 80% of the time	37
Partial success: child dry less than 80% of the time	6
Total failure: child dry less than 80% of the time or family found program unacceptable	11
Death: (Hydrocephalic child with obstructed shunt)	1
TOTAL	55

Copyright 1977, American Journal of Nursing Company. Reproduced with permission from the American Journal of Nursing, January, Vol. 77, No. 1.

Besides teaching patients labor-intensive technical skills normally performed by hospital personnel, what do these four programs have in common? First, the newly acquired behaviors were expected to become permanent. Teaching was thorough, in all cases lasting from days to weeks, and done in the hospital by members of a medical team, with attention to the patients' psychological needs, knowledge of the disease process, and mastery of technical skills. Family members were included to provide for long-term support and reinforcement in all three cases in which the behavior was to be performed at home; in the fourth, the nurse remained the reinforcing person for patients who performed self-dialysis in the center.

In terms of the dimensions of behavior and setting, the health problems are chronic and symptomatic: The types of behavioral demands are prescriptive, and the key dimension is persistence. The elements of program design included an intensive, in-hospital education program involving multiple staff, a variety of education techniques and interventions, postdischarge follow-up, and reinforcement from a support person, usually a family member.

What was lacking in these reports? None of them had a control population, and only one analyzed the data statistically. Encouraging as the results are, the deficiencies in design and analysis threaten the credibility of the results and limit the contributions to patient education practice that better designed studies might have achieved.

Evaluation of Education for Cardiac Patients

Education for cardiac patients has provided several exemplary programs. One program in the Baltimore City Hospital examined a nurse rehabilitator's impact on patients with myocardial infarction (MI) (Pozen et al., 1977). The 102 patients with MI were divided into high-risk and low-risk groups. These patients were then randomly assigned to control or study groups that were subsequently found to be similar in demographic characteristics. The study group received an educational program from a nurse rehabilitator. All patients received the care routinely provided by coronary care unit (CCU) physicians and nurses. The program consisted of the following:

1. Daily 20–30 minute individual sessions to reduce anxiety and to explain procedures and events in the CCU.
2. Individual and group meetings for 45–60 minutes on alternate days, in which the nurse rehabilitator helped the patients to improve their knowledge of MI and its treatment, cope with anxiety, and plan for return to work. This phase started after patients had left the intensive care unit and entered a postcoronary care unit. The informal group therapy sessions included discussion of diet, medications, risk factors, prescribed activity, and prevention symptoms.
3. Written supplemental materials provided each patient.
4. Weekly contact with patients by telephone or in person after discharge. The nurse rehabilitator reinforced information, responded to new problems, and acted as liaison between patient and physician.
5. Two informal family sessions with the nurse rehabilitator

during the patient's hospital stay. The family was also present at the discharge planning conference with the patient, the nurse rehabilitator, and two physicians.

Results showed a significant increase in knowledge (about causes of MI and medications) by the time of discharge among study patients versus controls ($p < .01$). Postdischarge smoking was reduced significantly ($p < .05$); in fact 70 percent of the program patients quit. Also the return-to-work rate was significantly higher among high-risk program participants ($p < .05$), ranging from 75 percent in the low-risk group to 81 percent in the high-risk group (see table 2-2).

Table 2-2.
Rates of Post-MI Return to Work by
High-risk and Low-risk Patients in the
Baltimore Study (Pozen, Stechmiller,
Harris, Smith, Fried, & Voight, 1977)

HIGH RISK		LOW RISK	
STUDY	CONTROL	STUDY	CONTROL
81%	61%	75%	67%

There was a strong correlation between increased knowledge and return to work; yet the study group forgot most of its newly gained knowledge by one month postdischarge. The authors suggest that early knowledge and the nurse rehabilitator liaison led patients to a decision to take health and life matters into their own hands. This attitude of responsibility outlasted specific knowledge gains. Finally the authors note that there was no difference between study and control groups in anxiety, which was high at admission, high at discharge, and low at six months postdischarge.

Altogether the evaluation was well designed, with random assignment of patients to control and study groups, cross-tabulation of data (e.g., return to work), and use of statistical tests to analyze the significance of the data.

A patient education program in a St. Paul, Minnesota, hospital was designed to effect behavior change in one aspect of the cardiac patient's regimen: medication taking (D'Altroy et al., 1978; Beardsley, 1977). Patients on a post-CCU and a medical-surgical unit were recruited into a drug self-administration program. A matched set of patients from other units were recruited as a control group. Tests showed no difference between the two groups. Although the program was not limited to cardiac patients, 60 percent fell into this category.

While the control group received normal instruction about post-discharge medication taking, the study group received an education program as follows: (1) The physician told the patients they were being put on the program, which was further explained verbally and in writing by a nurse. (2) The pharmacist took their drug histories and taught the patients about their medications during an average of three 25-minute sessions. Written handouts on each drug, and medication organization schedules were supplied and their use explained. (3) In a series of three steps, patients moved from the usual dependence on hospital staff for medication taking to full responsibility for self-administration of drugs left at the bedside. In the first stage, every time a medication was to be taken, the nurse brought all a patient's medications and asked the patient which he or she was to take and what its purpose was, correcting incorrect choices and reinforcing correct choice. In the second stage, patients, using their own medication schedules, called for their own drugs. Again the nurse brought all of them and asked which was to be taken and what its purpose was, correcting wrong choices and reinforcing correct ones. This gradual reinforcement took place twenty-four hours a day, so that most patients eventually knew the names of their drugs, their timing, side effects, contraindications, good storage practices, and so forth, quite well. In the final stage, the patients took their own medications, which were left at the bedside. They had been given the opportunity to achieve some control over their care in the hospital, to learn medication information gradually with immediate feedback, and to perfect their medication-taking behavior under professional guidance in the hospital instead of at home.

Admission and predischarge tests showed a significant increase during hospitalization in study patients' knowledge about their drugs compared with the control group, but there was a considerable loss of knowledge on the part of study patients by one month postdischarge. A thirty-day postdischarge home visit showed significantly greater compliance with the medication regimens in the study group compared to the control group (as shown in table 2-3). Although increased knowledge accounts for part of the difference in compliance (Spearman correlation, $r = .54$), participation in the program process itself accounts for most of the change in knowledge and in compliance.

A later study of the same population showed a significant reduction in rehospitalization days over the next seven months for patients rated compliant at the thirty-day postdischarge interview versus those rated noncompliant (D'Altroy, Beardsley, & Werlin, 1978).

Table 2-3.
A Comparison of Compliance between Self-administration Program Patients and Control Group Patients in the St. Paul Study (Beardsley, 1977; D'Altroy, Blissenbach, Lutz, Beardsley, Cain, & Mandt, 1978)

	Patients	%	Patients	%
Compliant(0-2 days error in pill count 29 days post discharge)	24	71	9	30
Partially compliant (3-4 days error)	10	29	14	47
Noncompliant(5 or more days error)	0	0	7	23
TOTALS	34	100	30	100

significant differences between groups: x^2 = 30.3, df = 1, p = .02

Reprinted, with permission, from *Hospitals, Journal of the American Hospital Association,* vol. 52, no. 21, November 1, 1978, p. 136.

The Baltimore and St. Paul studies show some interesting commonalities and differences. They both dealt with post-MI populations (60% cardiac in the St. Paul study) and tried to effect postdischarge behavior change. Although one program used a single nurse rehabilitator as the teacher and the other used a team approach of physician, pharmacist, and multiple nurses, both had in common a reliance on a series of educational interventions occurring during the hospital stay, using written material to supplement individual teaching. Both measured an increase in knowledge about disease processes and treatment from admission to discharge, with a drop in knowledge from discharge to the follow-up test. Despite the drop in knowledge at the follow-up, both showed a significant correlation between knowledge gain during hospitalization and subsequent behavior change. Both used experimental designs and statistically analyzed the health education program's effect on postdischarge behavioral changes beneficial to the patients. Both used doctoral students (Pozen, Beardsley) to help make the studies more rigorous, in contrast to most of the other studies reported in the recent health care and medical literature on patient education. The use of interested research specialists in departments of health education and behavioral sciences at local universities, as consultants in program design and evaluation, is suggested to improve the quality of program efforts and the usefulness of findings to the field.

Recent evaluations of patient education in ambulatory settings support the findings from the in-patient studies reviewed in the preceding pages. Taken together, the series of randomized control studies in hypertension (Brucker, 1977; Siyne, 1976), asthma (Green et al., 1978; Harris, Goodfriend, & Weingarten, 1978; Maiman, Green, & Gibson, 1979), and obesity (Kirscht, Becker, Haefner, & Maiman, 1978; Maiman, 1977) point to the central importance of selected health belief model variables and the marginal importance of locus of control variables as predisposing factors; to the need for frequent and intense contacts initially to clarify the regimen and train the patient in its adoption as enabling factors; and to periodic follow-up visits and involvement of a family member or significant other person in support of the patient as reinforcing factors. These three sets of factors appear to be the crucial elements in long-term ambulatory management of chronic conditions, especially when the prescribed regimen is painful, bothersome, or complex.

Summary and Conclusions

The superficial review of 134 published evaluations and the more detailed examination of a few exemplary studies reveal some strengths and weaknesses in the state of the art of patient education. The strengths are a rapidly growing empirical literature, increasing rigor being applied in evaluations, increasing sophistication of educational methods being employed and tested, and some useful findings emerging to strengthen the scientific base of practice in patient education. The continuing weaknesses are oversimplification of behavior and the causes of behavior that must be influenced through patient education, a persistent failure to make explicit the theoretical or assumptive connection between educational interventions and behavioral or health outcomes, and severely limited analyses leaving many questions untouched that would have been answerable with further analyses of the data available or a simple modification of the experimental design.

When we contrast these evaluations published in the medical and health care journals with evaluations of smoking cessation and obesity control methods published in the psychology journals, we see the foregoing strengths and weaknesses somewhat balanced. Weaknesses of the patient education evaluations reviewed in this chapter are to a large extent the strengths of the psychological studies. The evaluations by psychologists suffer, on the other hand, from inadequate generalizability. What they gain in theoretical sophistication and internal validity of their more rigorous designs, they lose in external validity because their very methodologies make their results as much a function of the research interventions as of the educational interventions. Most of the patient education evaluations have been conducted under less artificial circumstances.

This reassuring balance in the experimental literature is further supported by a growing body of theoretical, descriptive, and correlational research in medical sociology, health education, and health psychology. Together these various sources of data and theory provide a scientific base for the planning of patient education that should enable practitioners to approach their task with greater confidence and with more testable hypotheses than were justified in earlier years. Our conclusion from this review is that recent evaluations of patient education are telling us that we have turned the corner from mostly art, ideology, and intuition to a road that allows us to develop the next generation of programs and evaluations with a greater sense of continuity with scientific evidence and educational theory.

References and Bibliography

Alkhateeb, W., Lukeroth, C. J., & Riggs, M. A comparison of three educational techniques used in a venereal disease clinic. *Public Health Reports,* March-April 1975, *90;* 150–64.

Altshuler, A., Meyer, J., & Butz, M. K. Even children can learn to do clean self-catheterization. *American Journal of Nursing,* January 1977, *77;* 97–101.

American Hospital Association. *Hospital inpatient education: Survey findings and analyses, 1975.* Atlanta: U.S. Public Health Service Center for Disease Control, Bureau of Health Education, 1977.

American Hospital Association. Research Capsule No. 7. *Hospitals,* December 1, 1977, *46,* 102.

American Public Health Association, Public Health Education Section, Committee on Educational Tasks in Chronic Illness. *A model for planning patient education.* Rockville, Md.: Health Resources Administration, 1972.

Baric, L. Recognition of the "at-risk" role: A means to influence health behavior. *International Journal of Health Education,* 1969, *12,* 24–34.

Beardsley, R. *Evaluation of a patient drug self-administration program.* Unpublished doctoral dissertation, University of Minnesota College of Pharmacy, 1977.

Black, L. F., & Mitchell, M. M. Evaluation of a patient education program for chronic obstructive pulmonary disease. *Mayo Clinic Proceedings,* February 1977, *52,* 106–11.

Bracken, M. B., Bracken, M., & Landry, A. B. Patient education by videotape after myocardial infarction: An empirical evaluation. *Archives of Physical Medicine Rehabilitation,* May 1977, *58,* 213–219.

Brucker, P. C. Assuring patient compliance by health care contracts: Final summary report (Grant No. HL17230). Bethesda National Heart, Lung and Blood Institute, April 15, 1977.

Bryant, N. H., Stender, W., Frist, W., & Somers, A. R. VD hotline: An evaluation. *Public Health Reports,* May-June 1976, *91,* 231–235.

Caron, H. S., & Roth, H. P. An evaluation of a program for teaching clinic patients the rationale of their peptic ulcer regimen. *Health Education Monographs,* Spring 1977, *5,* 25–49.

D'Altroy, L. H., Beardsley, R. S., & Werlin, S. H. *Compliance with drug regimens, rehospitalization, and patient education: Some correlations.* Unpublished manuscript, 1978.

D'Altroy, L. H., Blissenbach, H., Lutz, D., Beardsley, R., Cain, H., Mandt, R., & Quarn, J. Drug self-administration can affect compliance. *Hospitals,* November 1, 1978, *52,* pp. 31–36.

Deeds, S. G. *Overview of evaluation.* Paper presented at the *National Conference on Hospital-Based Patient Education,* Atlanta, August 9–10, 1976. Published by Bureau of Health Education, Atlanta, Georgia 30333.

Flowers, R. V. *Effects of social support on adherence to therapeutic regimens.* Unpublished doctoral dissertation, the University of Michigan, 1978.

Fudge, R. P., & Vlasses, P. H. Third-party reimbursement for pharmacist instruction about anti-hemophilic factor. *American Journal of Hospital Pharmacy.* August 1977, *34,* 831–834.

Gardner, M. E., & Trinca, C. E. The pharmacy clinic: A new approach to ambulatory care. *American Journal of Hospital Pharmacy,* April 1978, *35,* 429–431.

Gillum, R. F., & Barsky, A. J. Diagnosis and management of patient non-compliance. *Journal of American Medical Association,* June 17, 1974, *228,* 1,563–1,567.

Gillum, R. F., Solomon, H. S., Kranz, P., Boepple, P. & Creighton, M. Improving hypertension detection and referral in an ambulatory setting. *Archives of Internal Medicine,* May 1978, *138,* 700–703.

Green, L. W. Toward cost-benefit evaluations of health education: Some concepts, methods and examples. *Health Education Monographs,* 1974, *2* (Suppl. 1), 34–64.

Green, L. W. Evaluation and measurement: Some dilemmas for health education. *American Journal of Public Health,* February 1977, *67,* 155–161.

Green, L. W. Determining the impact and effectiveness of health education as it relates to federal policy. *Health Education Monographs,* 1978, *6* (Suppl.), 28–66.

Green, L. W. Educational strategies to improve compliance with therapeutic and preventive regimens: The recent evidence. In R. B. Haynes, D. Sacket, & W. Taylor (Eds.), *Compliance in health care.* Baltimore: Johns Hopkins University Press, 1979.

Green, L. W., & Figa-Talamanca, I. Suggested designs for evaluation of patient education programs. *Health Education Monographs,* Spring 1974, *2,* 54–71.

Green, L. W., Kreuter, M., Partridge, K. B., & Deeds, S. G. *Health education planning: A diagnostic approach.* Palo Alto: Mayfield, 1979.

Green, L. W., Levine, D. M., & Deeds, S. G. Clinical trials of health education for hypertensive outpatients: Design and baseline data. *Preventive Medicine,* December 1975, *4,* 417–425.

Green, L. W., Werlin, S. H., Schauffler, H. H., & Avery, C. H. Research and demonstration issues in self-care: Measuring the decline of medicocentrism. In *Consumer self-care in health* (DHEW Pub. No. [HRA] 77-3181). Washington, D.C.: National Center for Health Services Research, August 1977.

Harris, C. L. Hospital-based patient education programs and the role of the hospital librarian. *Bulletin of the Medical Librarian Association,* April 1978, *66,* 210–217.

Harris, C., Goodfriend, S., & Weingarten, V. *Reduction of emergency and walk-in visits by asthmatic children in a controlled study of group education.* Manuscript submitted for publication, 1978.

Hassell, J., & Medved, E. Group/audiovisual instruction for patients with diabetes: Learning achievements and time economics. *Journal of the American Dietetic Association,* May 1975, *66,* 465–470.

Jesudasan, K., George, B., Chacko, C. J., Taylor, P. M., Kurian, P. V., & Job, C. K. An evaluation of the self-administration of DDS in Gudiyatham Taluk. *Lepr India,* October 1976, *48,* 668–676.

Johnston, B. L., Cantwell, J. D., & Fletcher, G. F. Eight steps to inpatient cardiac rehabilitation: The team effort—methodology and preliminary results. *Heart and Lung*, January-February, 1976, *5*, 97–111.

Jones, R. J., Turner, D. F., & Slowie, L. A. The educational diagnosis in nutrition counseling for serum cholesterol reduction. In J. Tillotston, (Ed.), *Proceedings of the Nutrition-Behavioral Research Conference.* Bethesda, Md.: National Institutes of Health, 1976.

Kasl, S. V. The health belief model and behavior related to chronic illness. *Health Education Monographs*, 1974, *2*, 433–454.

Kasl, S. V., & Cobb, S. Health behavior, illness behavior and sick-role behavior. *Archives of Environmental Health*, February 1966, *12*, 246–266; April 1966, *12*, 531–541.

Kay, R. L., & Hammond, A. H. Understanding rheumatoid arthritis: Evaluation of a patient education program. *Journal of the American Medical Association*, June 1978, *239*, 2,466–2,467.

Kirscht, J. P., Becker, M. H., Haefner, D. P., & Maiman, L. A. Effects of threatening communication and mothers' health beliefs on weight change in obese children. *Journal of Behavioral Medicine*, June 1978, *1*, 147–157.

Latos, D. L., Spannuth, C. L., & Stone, W. J. Home dialysis program of the Nashville VA Hospital. *Southern Medical Journal*, December 1977, *70*, 1,431–1,435; 1,439.

Laugharne, E., & Steiner, G. Tri-Hospital Diabetes Education Centre: A cost effective, cooperative venture. *Canadian Nurse*, September 1977, *73*, 113–119.

Lawson, V. K., Traylor, M. N., & Gram, M. R. An audio-tutorial aid for dietary instruction in renal dialysis. *Journal of the American Dietetic Association*, October 1976, *69*, 390–396.

Lazes, P. M. Health education project guides outpatients to active self-care. *Hospitals*, February 1977, *51*, 81–86.

Maiman, L. A. *The health belief model and prediction of dietary compliance: A field experiment employing a fear-arousal intervention.* Unpublished doctoral dissertation, the Johns Hopkins University, 1977.

Maiman, L. A., Green, L. W., & Gibson, G. Randomized trials of health education for asthmatic patients. *Journal of American Medical Association*, 1979, *241*, 1919–1922.

Mullen, P. D. *Cutting back after a heart attack: An overview.* Paper presented at the conference on the Future of Community Health Education, Farmington, Maine, December 4–8, 1977.

Mullen, P. D., & Reynolds, R. The potential of grounded theory for health education research: Linking theory and practice. *Health Education Monographs*, Fall 1978, *6*, 280–294.

Pozen, M. W., Stechmiller, J. A., Harris, W., Smith, S., Fried, D.D., & Voigt, G. C. A nurse rehabilitator's impact on patients with myocardial infarction. *Medical Care*, October 1977, *15*, 830–837.

Radius, S. M., Becker, M. H., Rosenstock, I. M., Drachman, R. H., Schuberth, K. C., & Teets, K. C. Factors influencing mothers' compliance with a medication regimen for asthmatic children. *Journal of Asthma Research,* April 1978, *15,* 133–147.

Rahe, R. H., Scalzi, C., & Shine, K. A teaching evaluation questionnaire for postmyocardial infarction patients. *Heart and Lung,* September-October 1975, *4,* 759–766.

Redman, B. *The process of patient teaching in nursing.* St. Louis: Mosby, 1976.

Redman, B. Patient teaching. *Nursing Digest,* Spring 1978, *6* (Whole Issue).

Rosenberg, S., & Judkins, B. A. Federal programs make education an integral part of patient care. *Hospitals,* May 1, 1976, *50,* 62–65.

Roter, D. L. Patient participation in the patient-provider interaction: The effects of patient question asking on the quality of interaction, satisfaction and compliance. *Health Education Monographs,* Winter 1977, *5,* 281–315.

Salzer, J. E. Classes to improve diabetic self-care. *American Journal of Nursing,* August 1975. *75,* 1,324–1,326.

Simmons, J. J. (Ed.). Making health education work. *American Journal of Public Health,* October 1975, *65* (Suppl.).

Slepcevitch, E. (Ed.). *Rx: Education for the patient: Who, what, where, why . . . and at what cost?* (Conference proceedings). Southern Illinois University at Carbondale, June 25–26, 1974.

Sly, R. M. Evaluation of a sound-slide program for patient education. *Annuals of Allergy,* February 1975. *34,* 94–97.

Solfin, D., Young, W. W., & Clayton, B. D. Development and evaluation of an individualized patient education program about digoxin. *American Journal of Hospital Pharmacy,* April 1977, *34,* 367–371.

Stecke, S. B., & Swain, M. Contracting with patients to improve compliance. *Hospitals,* December 11, 1977, *51,* 81–84.

Strauss, A. L., & Glaser, B. G. *Chronic illness and the quality of life.* St. Louis: Mosby, 1975.

Syine, L. *Hypertension education program in a low income community* (NHLBI Grant No. R25 HL16959, Final Rep.). Berkeley: University of California, School of Public Health, July 31, 1976.

Teuscher, A., & Heidecker, B. Evaluation of an instruction programme on diabetes diet by means of a teaching machine. *Medical Education,* November 1976, *10,* 508–511.

Vignos, P. J., Parker, W. T., & Thompson, H. M. Evaluation of a clinic education program for patients with rheumatoid arthritis. *Journal of Rheumatology,* June 1976, *3,* 155–165.

Wallace, N., & Wallace, D. C. Group education after myocardial infarction: Is it effective? *Medical Journal of Australia,* August 1977, *2,* 245–247.

Werlin, S. H., & Schauffler, H. H. Structuring policy development for consumer health education. *American Journal of Public Health,* June 1978, *68,* 596–597.

Witschi, J. D., Singer, M., Wo-Lee, M., & Stare, F. J. Family cooperation and effectiveness in a cholesterol-lowering diet. *Journal of the American Dietetics Association,* April 1978, *72,* 384–389.

Young, M. A. C. Reviews of research and studies on health education (1961–66): Patient education. *Health Education Monographs,* 1968, *1*(26), 1–64.

3

The Rationale and Application of a Needs Assessment in Patient Education

Marian Ulrich Adcock

The purpose of this chapter is to present a rationale for including a needs assessment in patient education and a case study of how United Hospitals of St. Paul, Minnesota, has incorporated assessment into patient education services.

Rationale

A major goal of patient education is to encourage and enable patients to become as self-sufficient as possible in managing their health affairs (Adcock, Ettenheim, & D'Altroy, 1979). It is hoped that the patient will acquire "those ideas and skills that will help him to cope with his immediate medical problems and even, perhaps, to maintain his health and avoid disease" (Levin, 1978b). An equally important goal of health education, for patients as well as healthy people, is to find "effective ways to help [people] protect [themselves] against preventable disease and the abuses of medical services provided by institutions" (Levin, 1978a) and individuals such as medical doctors, nurses, and dentists. One of the challenges facing both health care workers and patients is to determine how they can work together to realize these goals.

For years researchers have been attempting to explain and predict compliance with health and medical care recommendations. Efforts have been made to develop models for "predicting such seemingly diverse activities as preventive health actions, medical care utilization, delay in seeking care, and compliance with medical regimens (Becker, 1974). The health belief model has been used to predict these types of activities with varying degrees of success (Becker, 1974). Another theory, the locus of control, has also shown some promise in predicting and explaining specific health-related behaviors (Wallston & Wallston, 1978). Common to these theories and others is the belief that people exhibit varied degrees of motivation to protect and enhance their health. This motivation is influenced by peoples' perception of their susceptibility to a disease, its seriousness, and the belief that their illness patterns (if they are currently ill) can be altered if they follow medical advice.

Professional health care workers often assume the role of determining the patients' motivation for enhancing their own health and for planning patient education programs that capitalize on specific patients' motivations. Rarely are the patients allowed to decide what their own educational goals are, what the education will consist of, or how their education will be accomplished. In most cases it is the health care workers who assess patients' needs and decide the goals and how they should be met.

Until recently little attention has been paid to self-care education, that area of health education concerned primarily with encouraging patients to protect themselves against iatrogenic disease. Researchers have been posing questions, but little pragmatic work has been done to find methods that would enable patients to adequately protect themselves, especially while they are hospitalized. Current literature contains few, if any, examples that describe assessment tools patients could use in determining how to protect themselves against potential and real mistakes made by health care workers caring for them.

In most cases, a needs assessment in patient education helps health care workers and patients determine the patients' needs in relation to their immediate medical problems. The needs assessment enables the health care workers to judge the patients' learning readiness and set priorities on their needs. Through the assessment the health care workers learn about the context in which these needs will be handled and determine how to encourage patients to follow the medical advice they will be receiving.

A Case Study

United Hospitals has used since 1969 a highly integrated multidisciplinary approach to meet the educational needs of patients. Each of its formalized education programs has the following characteristics:

1. Each encourages patients to become as self-sufficient as possible in managing their health affairs.
2. Each is multidisciplinary in nature.
3. Team planning and teaching are used.
4. The teachers are the professional health workers already caring for the patients' other health needs.
5. Standard methods are used for:
   a. Initiating education for patients and families
   b. Determining the kind of education patients and families need
   c. Setting reasonable behavioral objectives to be attained through education
   d. Delivering the planned educational activities
   e. Evaluating the effectiveness of the education
   f. Making available to patients and families further guidance in self-care after discharge from the hospital, if needed. (Ulrich, 1972)

The following discussion covers the needs assessment component of these characteristics.

Determining Individual Patient Education Needs

In our system patients' learning needs are assessed in several different ways. The attending physician begins the assessment by identifying and incorporating her or his perspective of the patient's health education needs into routine medical care orders, writing the education order in the same manner as an order for any other form of treatment or care (fig. 3-1).

Figure 3-1.
Sample education order.

UNITED HOSPITALS, INC.
CHART COPY
PHYSICIAN'S ORDER FORM
DIABETES EDUCATION

The Inpatient Diabetes Education Program Includes the Following:

      Definition of Disease
      Hypoglycemia; Hyperglycemia; Acidosis
      Urine Testing
      Complications and Good Health Practices
      Exercise
      Diet
      Insulin Administration (when insulin is prescribed)
      Oral Hypoglycemic Agents (when prescribed)

The following services are available at an additional fee:

☐ Assess Patient's Level of Energy Expenditure

☐ Maintain Physical Tolerance While Hospitalized.

      ☐ Maintain Level Expended at Home.   ☐ Decrease Energy Level.

                                                 ☐ Increase Energy Level.

☐ Outpatient Education - Continuation of Program (if not completed during hospital stay).

Treatment Goals:

                                                      PHYSICIAN'S
ANTICIPATED LENGTH OF STAY:_____ DATE:_____ SIGNATURE:_____

CARDIAC EDUCATION

Diagnosis Category: ☐ Angina   ☐ Myocardial Infarct   ☐ Congestive Heart Failure

The Inpatient Cardiac Education Program Includes the Following:

      Symptom Recognition and Prevention
      Medications
      Diet
      Need to Quit Smoking
      Principles of Physical Activity

☐ Participate in the PHYSICAL RECONDITIONING PROGRAM (available at an additional fee)
      (if so, indicate activity level on reconditioning order sheet).

Treatment Goals:

                                                        PHYSICIAN'S
ANTICIPATED LENGTH OF STAY:_____ DATE:_____ SIGNATURE:_____

Developed by the Diabetes Education Planning Group, United Hospitals, Inc., May 1978. Reprinted by permission.

Next, the nurse assigned to care for the patient interviews the patient on the first or second day of the hospital stay, using a standardized format as a guide. This is done to assess:

1. What the patient needs to know about the illness and its treatment (and especially what the patient needs to know upon returning home)
2. What the patient's normal daily routine is, so that necessary changes can be determined
3. Whether the patient intends to follow medical management suggestions or is totally denying the illness and the effectiveness of medical management
4. Whether the patient believes that the illness pattern can be altered if instructions are carried out. (Adcock et al., 1979)

The format the nurse uses when interviewing a patient with a chronic illness contains several important sections:

1. *General information.* This section contains questions about the length of time the patient has had the disease, who else the patient knows who has the disease, and so on.
2. *Physiological control and knowledge about physiological control.* In this section are posed questions to elicit discussion of current problems being experienced in symptom control and of how well the patient thinks she or he is carrying out the prescribed regimen and managing problems related to following the regimen.
3. *Psychological and social adjustment.* In this section the issues discussed relate to how well the patient is coping with the social isolation that may be experienced as a result of the condition and adjusting to changes in the course of the disease, and how comfortable the patient is with her or his attempts to normalize life-style relationships with others and style of life. (Strauss & Glaser, 1975)

Other care givers, such as pharmacists and dietitians, also visit the patient early in the hospital stay to discuss his or her current perception of the illness and the recommended management of it. These exchanges help the health care workers and the patient get to know one another and to begin determining what types of educational help and assistance the patient wants and needs. The pharmacist and dietitian use questions designed to encourage discussion both of how well the patient understands the prescribed regimen and of the patient's ability to carry it out, including handling medical crises.

Once these conversations have taken place, the health workers (nurse, pharmacist, dietitian, occupational therapist, social worker, and others) hold a patient education planning (PEP) conference to pool their information and impressions of the patient and to formulate educational goals for the patient during the remainder of the hospital stay. Goals (listed in order of priority), teaching methods, and time schedules are agreed on and recorded in the patient's chart to guide the care givers when they begin their education work with the patient.

An Analysis

Although each patient's assessment within the education programs encourages interaction between the care givers and the patient and provides valuable information for decision making, the assessment does not address issues of motivation, decision-making rights of the patient, and protection of the patient from iatrogenic disease.

For six months during 1978, as part of an evaluation study, we used another type of interview guide in the protocol of the Patient Drug Self-Administration Program (D'Altroy, 1978). The guide was designed to elicit information from patients concerning locus of control tendencies. This information was then used retrospectively to determine the education approach (participative or authoritative) that would best motivate the patient. Interestingly, we found that persons who showed internal rather than external locus of control tendencies did better with a participative approach.

We anticipated using a similar guide as a routine part of the patient assessment in each of our programs. The information obtained would then be used to help determine educational methods to use with each patient. Unfortunately, the care givers found the locus of control interview time consuming and the data difficult to interpret and understand. In addition, some patients objected to its use and several physicians adamantly opposed its inclusion in the protocol. Consequently, the guide is no longer used in our programs. However, its use during those six months did raise a number of interesting and challenging questions about the different motivational aspects of patients as they assume (or don't assume) active roles in their own health care. The use of locus of control theory in a patient care setting remains a challenging arena where, it may be hoped, more research will be done.

We have also found it difficult to include patients actively in the decision making about what they will be taught and what the priorities are. Although patients are consulted on most issues in the assessment stages of our programs, the care givers, in most cases are opposed to having patients decide their own educational plans. Patients are excluded (in most instances) from the PEP conference where the decisions are made. Care givers say they believe a major goal of patient education is to encourage and enable patients to become as self-sufficient as possible in managing their health affairs; yet they cannot seem to allow, in day-to-day work, the true reduction of patient dependency by giving patients access to information (like their medical charts) and allowing them to make decisions about their care and health education. For these reasons patients remain in a dependent position whenever important decisions are made. They are allowed independence only when it fits into the care givers' educational plans for them.

Only the Patient Drug Self-Administration Program has addressed, to a significant degree, the other important purpose of patient education, namely, finding effective ways to help people protect themselves against preventable disease and the abuses of medical services provided by institutions. The program has been successful in providing enough pertinent information to patients about their medications to give them a basis from which to ask knowledgeable questions about their medicine regimens. Through these questions, errors in the regimen are detected and corrected. The program also puts patients in charge of administering their own medications while hospitalized. This practice prepares patients for managing their medicine regimens at home.

A study of this program revealed a two-and-a-half-fold increase of compliance (30 days postdischarge from the hospital) among program patients versus a matched control group receiving standard instruction about discharge medications ($p = .02$). Program participants who were compliant at the 30-day postdischarge pill count also spent fewer days rehospitalized per 1,000 days discharged than did noncompliant patients ($p < .01$). The relationship between program participation and rehospitalization rates was positive although not significant ($p = .20$) (D'Altroy, Beardsley, & Werlin, 1978).

Conclusion

We have found that, although the rationale for including a needs assessment in patient education is convincing, it has been difficult to use the assessment to actually encourage and enable patients to become self-sufficient in managing their health affairs. More often, the assessment is used by care givers to elicit information from patients so that they have some basis from which to make decisions for the patients about their health education needs. Perhaps some day patients will routinely use the information gathered in the assessments to make their own decisions. They may even, some day, have the opportunity to assess their care givers so that they have better knowledge base for protecting themselves against iatrogenic disease.

References

Adcock, M. U., Ettenheim, T. M., & D'Altroy, L. H. The integration of health education into patient care. In P. M. Lazes (Ed.), *The handbook of health education.* Germantown, Md.: Aspen Systems, 1979.

Becker, M. H. The health belief model and personal health behavior. *Health Education Monographs,* Winter 1974, p. 326.

D'Altroy, L. H. Patient drug self-administration improves regimen compliance. *Hospitals,* November 1, 1978, *52,* 21.

D'Altroy, L. H., Beardsley, R. S., & Werlin, S. H. *Compliance with drug regimens, rehospitalization, and patient education: some correlations.* Unpublished manuscript, 1978.

Levin, L. S. Patient education and self-care: How do they differ? *Nursing Outlook,* March 1978, pp. 170–175. (a)

Levin, L. S. Self care: An emerging component to the health care system. *Hospital and Health Services Administration,* Winter 1978, p. 17. (b)

Strauss, A. L., & Glaser, B. G. *Chronic illness and the quality of life.* St. Louis: Mosby, 1975.

Ulrich, M. R. The hospital as a center for health education. *Health Education Monographs,* Spring 1978, pp. 107–117.

Ulrich, M. R. Patient care includes teaching. *Hospitals,* April 16, 1972, *46,* pp. 59–65.

Wallston, B. S., & Wallston, K. A. Locus of control and health: A review of the literature. *Health Education Monographs,* Spring 1978, pp. 107–117.

4

Writing and Evaluating Educational Protocols

Jeanne Flyntz DeJoseph[*]

Although health is often perceived as a static sense of well-being, it is perhaps better defined as a fluid adjustment to circumstances (Hockey, 1978). The practice of health education, of which patient education is a part, is based on principles that include consideration of the learner, the teacher, and the system. Three of these principles have particular relevance to the writing of protocols for patient education. The first of these is that all learning is motivated (Steuart, 1969). A second principle is that involvement of the teacher as well as the learner is a critical factor in the outcome of health education (Jenny, 1978). The third is that planned behavior change requires a systematic approach (Redman, 1972). The purpose of this chapter is to provide a rationale and offer a suggested procedure for the writing and evaluating of patient education protocols using these principles as building blocks.

Definitions

The term *patient education* incorporates several definitions. In the strict sense it encompasses teaching a patient about the disease

*The author expresses her gratitude to Susan Hammerstad, R.N., B.S.N., Inservice Instructor at Stanford University Hospital, for her help in the preparation of this chapter. Thanks also go to Joan Mersch, R.N., M.S., Clinical Nursing Coordinator of the Coronary Care Unit at Stanford and her staff, and to Joanne Denham, R.N., B.S.N., for their highly commendable preparation, use, and written documentation of the sample protocol, which is reprinted by permission of Stanford University Medical Center, Nursing Service.

process and offering information about coping with the immediate crisis response to a diagnosis (Norris, 1979). In a larger sense it includes sharing information with the patient and the family about a particular disease, working with them to plan strategies for change, and integration of new behaviors into their life-style. In its broadest sense patient education embraces both the assessment of a patient's health within the context of the environmental and social milieu and the joint planning by significant others, the patient, and the health educator to achieve optimal health status and observable behavior change.

For the purposes of this discussion the *patient* is defined as a person who brings to the health education setting a knowledge base of personal needs and feelings and a system of beliefs and values. The *health educator* is defined as a person who comes to the setting with the above as well as with professional expertise and knowledge of the principles and process of learning and teaching and of disease processes and their effect on the patient and the family. The system is defined as those forces that impact the preparation of patient education protocols, such as, for example, budgetary considerations (including computer time for analysis of data) and administrative support.

Two assumptions underlie this discussion of the writing and evaluating of patient education protocols:

1. Patient education depends on reciprocal communication between the learner and the teacher.
2. A structured and systematic approach to patient education leads to increased knowledge as well as to behavior change.

Bridges and Barriers to Patient Education

Patient education is a dynamic process that facilitates the patient's adaptation to an altered state of being. Jenny (1978) has described a strategy for patient education that requires certain skills of the educator including "knowledge, self-concept, role acceptance, initiative, interpersonal skills and teaching abilities" (p. 342). Other bridges to effective patient education include the use of audio, visual, and written aids (Winslow, 1976). Another vital part of the planning of patient education protocols is the inclusion of a provision for evaluation (Green & Figa-Talamanca, 1974). Evaluation of a patient education protocol includes the systematic review of data on patient behavior change as well as the investigation of how well the program has met its stated objectives. Finally, as these bridges are of course two-way, the patient must be motivated to engage to capacity in the process in order to arrive at a meaningful commitment to change. These elements are some of the bridges to effective patient education that are optimally possessed by the learners, the teachers, and the system.

Barriers that interfere with patient education also exist in the system (Redman, 1972; Pohl, 1975; Streeter, 1953; Winslow, 1976). Among them are lack of administrative support or poor communication among the members of the health care team. A barrier inherent in the system is that the amount of teaching needed can rarely be done in the amount of time recommended by the Professional Standards Review Organization (PSRO) for length of patient stay in an acute care facility. The teacher may have insufficient knowledge or preparation to teach, or inadequate time to prepare a protocol. The personal beliefs and values of the teacher influence that person's ability to teach; for example, to the extent that a particular teacher views information sharing as a loss of personal power or status, teaching is less effective. Some barriers are related to the learner, such as a simple unwillingness to request information; on a more complex level the motivational model from which a patient operates has an impact on the ability to engage in the process of education. The health belief model postulates that one major motivational factor in the acceptance of preventive health behaviors is the need to decrease the perceived threat of disease (Becker, 1978). A motivational model that takes milieu as well as personal values and issues into account is the personal choice behavior model (Horn, 1976). In addition to motivation, other barriers include a patient's "educational background, intellectual abilities, and attitudes towards acceptance of responsibility" (Redman, 1972, p. 19). Any of these factors can cause a patient to set up barriers during the process of health education.

When writing a patient education protocol it is important to maximize the bridges to effective patient education. This necessitates careful planning for evaluation, the development of a structured plan (Redman, 1972), and attention to detail in both the assessment of the patient and family and the presentation of the protocol. A health educator who wishes to construct a successful patient education protocol will also attempt, whenever possible, to recognize the barriers in particular settings and situations and to minimize their impact on a particular protocol.

The Nurse as a Health Educator

Although many disciplines participate in the patient education process, nurses are particularly well placed to be a primary resource. Because nurses are so involved in direct patient care and are such a consistent presence to patients, a trust relationship with reciprocal communication may already exist and facilitate the process of patient education. Nurses are also trained in patient assessment and so may act as front-line troubleshooters in the identification of a patient's need for education. In addition nurses should function as referral agents to other members of the health care team to respond to specific patient needs. The American Nurses' Association (1975) has developed a statement about the professional nurse and health education that reaffirms the responsibility and accountability of each nurse to include health education as an integral part of nursing practice.

Preparation of the Protocol

Quality assurance and cost effectiveness are twin barometers of excellence in patient care. Increased emphasis on accountability and legal responsibility for the practice of professional nursing has forced greater attention to be paid to the details of charting and the development of written nursing care plans. The same rationale applies to the delineation of systematic, written, standardized plans for patient education. Steps in the preparation of a patient education protocol include assessment of the patient population, planning and writing of the protocol itself, pilot testing and revision, and use of the revised protocol for patient education. Evaluation is a vital part of the process, as is a provision for periodic review of the protocol for fine tuning while it is in use.

Assessment of the Patient Population

The assessment of patient population is a search for commonalities. The health educator must first review the literature to determine what has been reported about the characteristics, behaviors, needs, or expectations of patients with a particular disease. Utilizing this data base as a start, the health educator can then begin to gather information available in a particular setting, such as the special needs of a group of patients within a cardiac surveillance unit. This step requires keen observation skills. The health educator should survey patients, families, members of the health care team, and other educators in the institution.

Planning and Writing the Protocol

A systematic look at several questions will help the health educator to plan the program. This requires a solid grounding in theory. What are the patient outcomes, stated in behavioral terms? What is the content to be taught? What are the learning experiences that will best meet the goals of this particular group of patients? What audio, visual, and written aids will best serve to emphasize and reinforce the content? What kind of flexibility is provided for different learning styles of patients and different teaching styles of health educators, and, finally, what resources are available? When these data have been obtained, the health educator can make an educational diagnosis and begin writing the protocol. These questions can form a model for the protocol, which might include: Content area, examples of content, teaching and learning activities, patient outcomes, evaluation methods, and resources.

Testing and Revising the Pilot

A very valuable although underutilized tool is the pilot study. Educators, researchers, and health care professionals often develop elegant protocols that are solidly grounded in both empirical data and careful assessment. For a variety of reasons, however, a particular protocol simply may not succeed. A pilot test of the specific protocol on a segment of the patient population can help identify the strengths and weaknesses of that protocol, thereby avoiding potential squandering of resources and pride. In addition the pilot study may also provide baseline data, so necessary to the identification of behavior change. Once the pilot test is complete the health educator can revise the protocol accordingly and implement it.

Evaluation

Planning for evaluation is an integral part of the preparation of an educational protocol. The evaluation process is two-fold. The first aspect is internal, consisting of measuring the patient outcomes. Some observational methods used include checklists, rating scales, and anecdotal notes. Oral or written questioning of the patient and family may also be done (Redman, 1972). In this phase of the evaluation it is important to document actual patient behavior changes, rather than the subjective conclusions of the health educator. For example, "Patient lists the medications she/he is taking" is a description of an observable behavior. To say, "Patient understands medication" is to leave open to question what behaviors are operative or changed. If the objectives are clearly written and stated in behavioral terms, the evaluation flows from them.

The evaluation of the protocol itself is the second, external component of the evaluation process. In this phase the health educator considers the response of a group of patients to a particular protocol. Care must be taken to avoid the inappropriate use of numbers to substantiate the success of a protocol; for example, the number of times a protocol is used does not necessarily imply the amount of learning that has occurred. One indicator of the success of a protocol could be patient responses as measured by a questionnaire given to the patient on a posthospitalization visit to the clinic. The responses can be evaluated against the written educational protocol included in the patient's chart, thereby quantifying in some measure the efficacy of the protocol. The limitation of an inpatient program is that, whereas cognitive and psychomotor behaviors may be identified by the time of a patient's discharge, attitude change is more difficult to measure. The patient may leave the hospital to return to an environment in which new behaviors, skills, and attitudes are not supported or reinforced. Clearly, a followup questionnaire cannot be considered a perfect indicator of the success of an inpatient teaching protocol.

The key to program evaluation is the formulation of realistic program objectives grounded in theory and practice. The health educator can relate both internal and external outcomes to the objectives and so begin to measure and evaluate the success of the protocol.

A Sample Protocol

The following protocol,* which has been in use for two years in a large teaching hospital in northern California, is presented as one example of utilization of the techniques stated in this chapter. It includes:

*Used with permission of Stanford University Medical Center, Nursing Service.

1. A *glossary*, which contains terms of interest to cardiac patients and is discussed during the teaching session
2. The *guidelines* for the nurses who will use the materials
3. The *introduction*, given by the nurse to the patient of the cardiac teaching program

Glossary

1. *Angina:* Chest pain indicating temporary lack of blood to heart muscle
2. *Arteries:* Vessels carrying oxygen-rich blood to tissues
3. *Arteriosclerosis:* Disease in which abnormal amounts of calcium, cholesterol, and other blood elements are deposited on the inner wall of an artery
4. *Cardiac enzymes:* Normally found in the heart muscle and released into the bloodstream when an injury such as myocardial infarction occurs
5. *Cholesterol:* Substance manufactured by body and also present in foods we eat such as egg yolks, organ meats, shellfish, dairy products; when more is taken in than needed by the body, the excess may be deposited in the arteries
6. *Collateral circulation:* As arteries gradually narrow or become obstructed, other small branches of arteries enlarge and form new branches, continuing to bring blood to the heart; often this is enough to provide sufficient oxygen to the heart
7. *Congestive heart failure:* Condition that occurs when heart's ability to pump blood effectively is impaired, causing blood to back up throughout the system
8. *Coronary arteries:* Vessels on surface of heart supplying oxygen-rich blood to heart muscle
9. *Coronary occlusion, coronary thrombosis, myocardial infarction, heart attack:* All terms refer to the same thing—death of the heart muscle due to blockage of blood flow through one or more of the coronary arteries
10. *Electrocardiogram (ECG or EKG):* Recording of the electrical activity of the heart
11. *Ischemia:* Insufficient blood supply to maintain normal function of muscle
12. *Nitroglycerin (NTG):* Medication used to relieve attacks of angina by dilating arteries

13. *Pericardium:* A thin-walled sac surrounding the heart and in which the heart can move
14. *Pulmonary:* Refers to lungs
15. *Sodium:* Causes retention of fluid in body and is commonly found in table salt
16. *Veins:* Vessels bringing oxygen-depleted blood back to the heart

Guidelines

This program has been assembled for the nurse to use in teaching patients recovering from myocardial infarctions. The following are guidelines for using the material:

A. Each section is divided into goals and objectives so that one section may be covered at a time, according to the patient's willingness and learning needs.
B. The material is assembled in this manner in order to cover all aspects of the myocardial infarction; however, flexibility may be used in deciding in which order to introduce each topic, according to the individual needs.
C. Explanation of format
   1. Goal: This is the overall teaching emphasis.
   2. Objectives: These represent specific information to be given in order to accomplish the goal. Remember the patient must also see the need for information in order for the teaching and learning to be effective.
   3. References for nurse preparation: These include sources of information that will aid the nurse prior to beginning the teaching session.
   4. Content: This is the body of knowledge covered under each objective.
   5. Teaching aids: Interesting facts to get the patient's attention or emphasize specific, important points; also includes pamphlets or audiovisual aids that should be given to the patient.
   6. Guide/feedback questions: Questions to ask the patient to solicit information and/or stimulate interest, as giving feedback on the learning process. The nurse may substitute own questions.

Introduction

The nurse should give to the patient the following introduction to the cardiac teaching program:

The cardiac teaching program involves instruction by nurses to patients with coronary artery disease, specifically those with myocardial infarctions and angina.

Upon transferring from the coronary care unit to the cardiac surveillance unit, you will be introduced to your cardiac teaching nurse, who will be involved with you during the remainder of your stay in the hospital. Your nurse will design a teacher program suited specifically to your individual teaching needs and will work closely with you, your family, and other members of the health team.

Upon discharge from the hospital, you will have gained a better understanding of how your heart works and the disease process that has affected it. You will be better able to identify signs and symptoms of your particular health problem and those that necessitate notifying your doctor. Also, prior to leaving the hospital, you will be given instruction on diet, medications, and physical activity, and you will be able to apply this new learning to your own life. Finally, we hope to convey to you an awareness and an understanding of the normal emotional responses to illness.

Through this program, we think you will be able to gain a better understanding of your illness, its medical management, and its assets and liabilities within your personal life.

(See Sample Protocol on pages 54-101.)

Sample Protocol: Cardiac Teaching Program

GOAL I: The patient will be able to understand the anatomical and physiological process involved in cardiovascular health and disease.

OBJECTIVE A: To give general knowledge of the anatomy of the heart.

References for Nurse Preparation	Content	Teaching Aids	Guide Questions to Ask Patients
The CIBA Collection, Vol. 5 —Heart. N.Y., 1968. Pp. 3, 16, 17.	The heart is a four-chambered organ that is located between the lungs, underneath the sternum, mostly to the left side of the body.	Heart is about the size of a closed fist; weighs about 11 ounces.	Ask the patient if he knows how the heart works or what it does.
A Handbook of Heart Disease, Blood Pressure and Strokes. C. A. D'Alonzo, M.D. Gulf Publishing Co., Houston, Texas, 1961. Pp. 24, 45–55.	Most of the heart consists of muscle known as the myocardium.	Heart attack is also called a myocardial infarction, or M.I. for short. Infarction is death of a part of the heart muscle due to lack of oxygenated blood.	
Heart Disease—Diagnosis and Treatment. Stanford University Hospital Booklet, 1978. Pp. 2, 10.	Interior of the heart is divided down the middle by a thick wall called the *septum*.	Right side: Right atrium, right ventricle. Left side: Left atrium, left ventricle.	
The Living Heart. M. DeBakey, M.D., & A. Gotto, M.D. McKay Publishing, 1977. Chap. 4: The Heart and how it works, pp. 31–54.	These two halves of the heart each consist of two compartments, the atria or the upper half, and the ventricles or lower half. The heart is enclosed in a loose-fitting sac called the pericardium.	Use model heart for illustration. Pericarditis is an inflammation of the pericardial sac around the heart; can occur as a complication of the heart attack. Treatment is bed rest, con-	

GOAL I; OBJECTIVE B: To have a general knowledge of the main function of the heart.

References for Nurse Preparation	Content	Teaching Aids	Guide Questions to Ask Patients
	The main function of the heart is to pump oxygenated blood to all parts of the body.	The heart pumps about 5 quarts of blood every minute or 75 gallons of blood every hour.	Stress, muscular exercise, digestion, and illness make the heart work harder.
	The R atrium receives blood, which is bluish in color, from the body, and it is squeezed into the R ventricle.	Show picture of "Your Heart and How It Works." (American Heart Association Pamphlet EM–62 PHE.)	What can the patient do to help the heart rest? What does blood pressure mean?
	The blood returns to the L atrium and is propelled into the L ventricle, which pumps it out through the main artery, the aorta, to all parts of the body.	In between each atria and ventricle lie valves which permit the flow of blood in one direction only. The entire process of blood filling and emptying the heart lasts less than a second.	Systole is the top number and diastole is the bottom number. Examples: $\frac{90}{50}$; $\frac{130}{70}$.
	The heart beat is an electrical impulse that comes from the pacemaker of the heart, located in the R atrium. This causes the heart muscles to contract and "pump" the blood.	The heart beats about 100,000 times a day, or about 65–75 beats per minute. Systole is the contraction phase of the heart.	

55

Sample Protocol: Cardiac Teaching Program

GOAL I; OBJECTIVE B (continued): To have a general knowledge of the main function of the heart.

References for Nurse Preparation	Content	Teaching Aids	Guide Questions to Ask Patients
	Circulation Cycle Blood empties into the R atrium from inferior and superior vena cavas. Sinoarterial node sends electrical impulse, causing muscles to contract in wavelike motion from top to bottom. Pressure forces tricuspid valve open; blood flows into R ventricle; the electrical impulse fired by SA node reaches the atrioventricular node. The impulse is sent along through bundle of His down two branches of the septum causing the R ventricle to contract.	Diastole is the relaxation phase while blood fills atria and ventricles. These two components make up your blood pressure.	

References for Nurse Preparation	Content	Teaching Aids	Guide Questions to Ask Patients
	Tricuspid valve shuts; blood is forced out through pulmonary valve into pulmonary artery. It is oxygenated when it comes in contact with alveoli in lungs. Drains into empty L atrium. L atrium similarly energized by electrical impulse, as was right side. Pressure forces the mitral valve to open and blood fills L ventricle. Mitral valve closes; blood passes through aortic valve into aorta and to rest of the body.		

Sample Protocol: Cardiac Teaching Program

GOAL I; OBJECTIVE C: To be introduced to the coronary circulation and its function, and the healing process after a myocardial infarction.

References for Nurse Preparation	Content	Teaching Aids	Guide Questions to Ask Patients
Heart Attack: New Hope, New Knowledge. M. Prinzmetal, M.D. Simon & Schuster, N.Y., 1958. Chap. 2, pp. 17–19.	Within the heart, there are specialized arteries to supply the heart with oxygenated blood. These are called the coronary arteries. There are two main coronary arteries: (1) the right coronary artery and (2) the left coronary artery. If these small coronary arteries become clogged with fatty substances as in atherosclerosis, an inadequate amount of blood and oxygen is available to the heart muscle. Both right and left coronary arteries have two main branches. The	Coronary arteries require about 20% of the total blood flow. Named coronary because they encircle the heart like a crown. In an adult a coronary artery measures about 4 to 5 inches long. The passageway of the artery is about ⅛ inch in diameter. Give pamphlets from American Heart Association, "After a Coronary," and "The Heart and Blood Vessels."	

References for Nurse Preparation	Content	Teaching Aids	Guide Questions to Ask Patients
	branches of the left coronary artery are (1) anterior descending, supplies branches to L and R ventricles; (2) circumflex artery, supplies branches to L atrium and L ventricle. The branches of the right coronary artery are (1) posterior descending artery, supplies branches to both L and R ventricles; (2) marginal artery, supplies branches to R atrium and R ventricle. Each atrium receives blood from only one source. Two branches supply each ventricle. If this obstruction becomes complete, so that no oxygenated blood can pass through the coronary ar-		

59

Sample Protocol: Cardiac Teaching Program

GOAL I; OBJECTIVE C (*continued*): To be introduced to the coronary circulation and its function, and the healing process after a myocardial infarction.

References for Nurse Preparation	Content	Teaching Aids	Guide Questions to Ask Patients
	tery, the heart muscle dies. This is called a myocardial infarction. Healing process after a heart attack takes about 6–8 weeks. During that time, scar tissue forms over the affected area. *Collateral Circulation* This is the development of small arteries above and below the obstruction to again supply blood flow to previously damaged areas of the heart.	Similar to root structure in a tree; if you cut off a main root, many smaller roots develop to continue nourishing the tree.	

Topic covered more extensively in Disease Process (Goal I; Objective D), and Signs and Symptoms (Goal II).

GOAL I; OBJECTIVE D: Describe the disease processes of coronary artery disease. To give general knowledge of the process of coronary artery disease.

References for Nurse Preparation	Content	Teaching Aids	Guide Questions to Ask Patients
Heart Disease, Blood Pressure and Strokes. A. D'Alonzo, M.D. Gulf Publishing Co., 1961. Pp. 45, 61–72.	Arteriosclerosis occurs as a result of the fatty substances (like cholesterol) building up within the arterial wall in any of its layers. Commonly referred to as "hardening of the arteries." Atherosclerosis is a form of arteriosclerosis in which the deposition of fat (plaque) is rather limited to the lining of the blood vessel wall. Final result of plaque formation is a narrowing of the lumen or center of the blood vessel, which reduces the volume of blood flowing through it. Pain then results when the lumen becomes so obstructed that an ade-	Use diagrams from: 1. *Heart Disease—Diagnosis and Treatment.* Pp. 8 & 12 (Give patient a copy). 2. *The CIBA Collection, Vol. 4—Heart.* 1968. Pp. 213–217. 3. *The Living Heart.* M. DeBakey, M.D., & A. Gotto, M.D. 1977: McKay Publishing Co. P. iii—fig. 65, "Types of Atherosclerotic Lesions." 4. Show American Heart Association A/V tape, "Your Heart Attack and Your Future." 30 minutes.	Before teaching sessions, ask patient if he knows the causes of heart disease or heart attacks.

Sample Protocol: Cardiac Teaching Program

GOAL I; OBJECTIVE D (continued): Describe the disease processes of coronary artery disease. To give general knowledge of the process of coronary artery disease.

References for Nurse Preparation	Content	Teaching Aids	Guide Questions to Ask Patients
	quate amount of oxygen is not available. This is commonly called *angina pectoris*. Atherosclerosis is a form of arteriosclerosis in which the deposition of fat is limited to the lining or the intimal layer. Occurs most often in medium-to-large vessels. The formation of plaque, which occurs initially as focal deposit of lipids within the intimal layer, is the most serious of atherosclerosis involvement. Arteriosclerosis denotes disease affecting one or more of the vessel layers.		

References for Nurse Preparation	Content	Teaching Aids	Guide Questions to Ask Patients
	Steps in the evolution of the atherosclerotic lesions are (1) damage to the endothelial lining, (2) focal assimilation of intimal lipids (3) proliferation of the smooth muscle cells of arterial wall, (4) cell death and injury, (5) formation of necrotic lipid-rich core. Precise interrelationships and causes of these effects are not known.		

Sample Protocol: Cardiac Teaching Program

GOAL I; OBJECTIVE E: To become familiar with risk factors and learn methods of reducing or eliminating them.

References for Nurse Preparation	Content	Teaching Aids	Feedback Questions

The Living Heart. M. DeBakey, M.D., & A. Gotto, M.D. 1977: McKay Publishing Co. "Reduce Your Risk of Heart Attack." American Heart Association pamphlet.	Risk factors are those habits and/or conditions in our lives that seem to be found commonly in persons who have had heart attacks. While there is no scientific evidence that these risk factors produce disease, reducing or eliminating them would seem to be a step toward better health.
	
	For discussion, these risk factors have been classified as follows:
	1. Controllable risk factors:
	  a. Diet
	  b. Overweight
	  c. Inactivity
	  d. Smoking
	  e. Stress
		Common Risk Factors
		1. High blood pressure
		2. High levels of cholesterol or other fatty substances in the blood
		3. Overweight
		4. Diabetes
		5. Lack of exercise
		6. Cigarette smoking
		7. A family history of heart attacks in middle age
		8. Stress
		
		Obesity is a risk factor that tends to aggravate other risk factors, such as high blood pressure and high triglycerides.
			How many risk factors can the patient identify?
			How does the person feel about a change of lifestyle in order to reduce the risk of a second heart attack?

64

References for Nurse Preparation	Content	Teaching Aids	Feedback Questions

	2. Some degree of control:
	  a. High blood pressure (hypertension)
	  b. diabetes mellitus
	3. Incontrollable:
	  a. heredity
	High blood pressure: This is the pressure put on the walls of the arteries as the blood pumps through them. Untreated, it may damage the heart, lungs, kidneys, and brain. Primary risk factors include the following.
	1. Hypertension
	Elevation of systolic blood pressure of 140 mm and a diastolic pressure of 90 mm or over.
	2. Hyperlipidemia
	Excessive levels of cholesterol and triglycerides.
		Reducing high blood pressure may be as simple as eliminating salt from the diet. Sometimes it is necessary to
		1. Take medication
		2. Reduce weight
		3. Eliminate cigarette smoking
		4. Modify stressful living habits
		One should always have regular medical check-ups.
			Does the person know her/his average blood pressure reading?

Sample Protocol: Cardiac Teaching Program

GOAL I; OBJECTIVE E (continued): To become familiar with risk factors and learn methods of reducing or eliminating them.

References for Nurse Preparation	Content	Teaching Aids	Feedback Questions
	Serum cholesterol can be lowered 10–15% by making relatively simple modifications in diet.		
	It is desirable to wait at least three weeks after an M.I. before checking the triglycerides or cholesterol. Testing when the patient is acutely ill often gives an inaccurate level.		
	In America, normal cholesterol level is between 150–250 mgs.%.		
	In countries where the serum cholesterol is less than 150 mg.%, atherosclerosis is practically nonexistent.		
	3. Cigarette smoking		

References for Nurse Preparation	Content	Teaching Aids	Feedback Questions
	Smoking makes the heart beat faster, raises the blood pressure and narrows blood vessels of the skin.	Increases work of the heart; constricts blood vessels, which are not getting enough oxygenated blood in the first place.	Do you smoke? How much? Do you want to stop smoking?
	Smoking increases the carbon monoxide content of the blood and displaces oxygen from hemoglobin, thereby reducing oxygen supply to tissues and cells.		
	Tobacco contains nicotine, tar, and other substances that may produce cancer.	Methods for decreasing: 1. Stop smoking 2. Use set of progressive filters 3. Gradually reduce the number of cigarettes—inhale fewer times or put out before it is at the end 4. Choose a brand with low tar and nicotine content 5. Program of behavior modification	

Sample Protocol: Cardiac Teaching Program

GOAL I; OBJECTIVE E *(continued)*: To become familiar with risk factors and learn methods of reducing or eliminating them.

References for Nurse Preparation	Content	Teaching Aids	Feedback Questions
		Show A/V teaching slide on smoking—"Quit for Life." Give booklet, "What everyone should know about smoking."	
	4. Diabetes mellitus With diabetes, the body does not produce enough insulin—an enzyme, made in the pancreas, which converts sugar and starch into energy. This is also associated with: 1. Rise in fatty substances in the blood 2. Development of atherosclerosis 3. Increased incidence of heart attack. If there exists a family history of diabetes, a	As in any illness, a heart attack can upset a diabetic's usual lifestyle and also his usual blood sugar. It may be necessary to treat with insulin initially, but most people are back on their regular treatment of diabetes when they go home from the hospital. With a diabetic patient, nurse may want to emphasize that they should continue checking the urine for a few weeks	Is the patient a new diabetic? If so, you may want to consult the *Diabetic Teaching Manual* for more detail. How long has the person been a diabetic? What did she/he do to control diabetes? Diet? Weight control? Exercise? Oral medication? Insulin? Does she/he need counseling concerning any aspect of diabetes? Do they test their urine?

References for Nurse Preparation	Content	Teaching Aids	Feedback Questions
			How often? With what results?
	person should have the blood sugar level checked during regular medical checkups.	after returning home, if their diabetes has been unstable.	
	Secondary risk factors include the following: 1. *Diabetes mellitus* Abnormal elevation of blood sugar, hyperglycemia. Pancreas produces insulin and glucagon, two hormones which regulate the level of sugar in the blood. Glucagon causes an elevation of blood glucose through glycogen breakdown by the liver. Insulin causes a decrease in blood sugar by stimulating the uptake of glucose into cells and tissues.		

Sample Protocol: Cardiac Teaching Program

GOAL I; OBJECTIVE E (continued): To become familiar with risk factors and learn methods of reducing or eliminating them.

References for Nurse Preparation	Content	Teaching Aids	Feedback Questions
Use "The Way to a Man's Heart" and "Recipes for Fat Controlled, Low Cholesterol Meals," American Heart Association pamphlets.	*2. Overweight* Being overweight is a risk factor that tends to aggravate other risk factors, such as high blood pressure, high triglycerides, and diabetes. *3. Lack of Exercise* Some scientific studies have shown that men who lead sedentary lives may run a higher risk of heart attack than those who get regular exercise, and there is some evidence	Life expectancy statistics have shown higher mortality from cardiovascular disease in overweight individuals. Lose weight by: 1. Following a balanced diet with fewer calories 2. Learn what works for you and follow that for holding desired weight You should always increase your activity gradually. For patients who are recuperating from a heart attack, or those with angina pectoris, controlled physical activity can be	Ask patients what they would like to weigh. Have they lost weight in the hospital? What kind of hobbies or spare time activities did they do prior to hospitalization? Do they get regular exercise? What form of exercise? What form of exercise sounds most appealing to them?

References for Nurse Preparation	Content	Teaching Aids	Feedback Questions
	to support the claim that the better the physical shape, the more rapidly you may recover from illness.	an important part of the rehabilitation program. Safest exercise is walking; with doctor's approval, may progress to various other forms of activity.	
	Exercise can take almost any form, including 1. Walking 2. Swimming 3. Cycling 4. Tennis 5. Calisthenics	Exercise can also help control obesity, blood pressure, and levels of cholesterol.	
	Should be done 3–5 times weekly for 15–30 minutes.		
	Anyone over 40 should have an exercise ECG or treadmill test before undertaking a program of physical exercise.		
	As patient recovers from an M.I., she/he will be increasing activity gradually.		
	Bedrest-chair-bathroom-walking in room-hall-home.		

Sample Protocol: Cardiac Teaching Program

GOAL I; OBJECTIVE E *(continued)*: To become familiar with risk factors and learn methods of reducing or eliminating them.

References for Nurse Preparation	Content	Teaching Aids	Feedback Questions
	Doctor may do a 24-hour Holter or treadmill to determine exercise tolerance. If patient can walk, he/she should gradually increase the length of walk.		
	More on exercise in later discussion on physical activity guidelines.		
	4. Heredity If you had close relatives who died between ages 40–60 from complications of atherosclerosis, this could mean that a tendency to disease runs in your family. If so, you may develop heart disease too if you add these risk factors	Heredity is one of the uncontrollable risk factors. You may or may not inherit the disease. Way of life has great influence.	Has anyone in your family had heart disease?

References for Nurse Preparation	Content	Teaching Aids	Feedback Questions
	1. Uncontrolled hypertension 2. Being overweight 3. Smoking 4. Diet rich in animal fats and cholesterol 5. Lack of exercise Or, you can turn your family history to good advantage by recognizing the warning early and taking steps to reduce the risks that are within your control. Mother apparently carries dominant gene. When both parents have heart disease, the tendency for the offspring to have disease is particularly strong.		

Sample Protocol: Cardiac Teaching Program

GOAL I; OBJECTIVE F: The patient will be given information describing the difference between angina and a myocardial infarction, and will learn more about the healing process and implications for activity.

References for Nurse Preparation	Content	Teaching Aids	Guide Questions to Ask Patients
Handbook of Heart Disease, Blood Pressure and Strokes. A. D'Alonzo, M.D. 1961: Gulf Publishing Co. Chap. 10, pp. 91–96.	*Angina pectoris* "Angina" means tightness or constriction. "Pectoris" indicates location in the chest under the pectoral muscles. Pain usually starts as a tightness in the chest, usually goes down left arm, sometimes right; may also radiate to back, fingers, or jaw. The pain is usually relieved by resting, and is caused by a temporary lack of supply of oxygenated blood to the heart muscles. This lack of oxygenated blood is called ischemia.	Angina is a common condition, characterized by definite pattern of heart pain. It can be brought on by exercise, emotion, or excitement. Angina is the result of inadequate oxygen supply to heart muscle. If this lack of oxygenated blood persists, acutal heart muscle damage can occur; this is a heart attack or myocardial infarction. Give patient a copy of "If You Have Angina," American Heart Association pamphlet.	Question patient as to whether he/she had any chest discomfort or pain in the few days or weeks before his/her heart attack.

References for Nurse Preparation	Content	Teaching Aids	Guide Questions to Ask Patients
	Treatment of angina is as follows. 1. Rest helps to cut down on workload of heart. 2. Relax; avoid excitement, emotion, or exercise. 3. Nitroglycerin: A small pill used under tongue where it is rapidly absorbed; works by widening coronary blood vessels, enabling heart to get more blood through the clogged arteries.	Nitroglycerine should be taken when pain first occurs. May take 10–20 nitroglycerin pills per day with no harmful effects. This dosage is rarely necessary. After taking nitroglycerin, wait 5 min. before taking another. May take up to 3 tablets, waiting 5 min. between each. If pain persists or has a different pattern, notify doctor at once.	Ask patient if she/he has ever experienced angina, if so: 1. What pattern does the pain follow? 2. What seems to bring on an attack? 3. What does she/he do for it?
Handbook of Heart Disease, Blood Pressure, and Strokes. A. D'Alonzo, M.D. 1961: Gulf Publishing Co. Chap. 7, Coronary Artery Disease, pp. 51–64.	*Myocardial infarction* Prolonged pain caused by inadequate supply of oxygenated blood to heart muscle. Heart muscle affected dies; scar tissues form over the area within approx. 6–8 weeks. Symptoms include (1) un-	CIBA—pages 63–64 (pictures of various infarcts). Show patient a picture of her/his heart attack. Show audiovisual aid, "Signals for Action," after teaching session. Produced by the American Heart Association, Dallas, Texas.	Ask patient how her/his heart attack felt.

Sample Protocol: Cardiac Teaching Program

GOAL I; OBJECTIVE F (*continued*): The patient will be given information describing the difference between angina and a myocardial infarction, and will learn more about the healing process and implications for activity.

References for Nurse Preparation	Content	Teaching Aids	Guide Questions to Ask Patients
	comfortable pressure or vise-like pain in center of chest; radiates to shoulder, arms, jaw, or back; (2) sudden sweating; (3) shortness of breath; (4) nausea, vomiting; and (5) weakness, fatigue.		
	To treat myocardial infarction, rest; call doctor immediately or ambulance paramedic. *Get to the hospital the quickest way you can.*		

GOAL II: The patient will be able to identify signs and symptoms of his particular health problem.

OBJECTIVE A: Have the patient with a myocardial infarction state at least three signs and symptoms of congestive heart failure and know when to alert the physician.

References for Nurse Preparation	Content	Teaching Aids	Question for the Patients
Handbook of Heart Disease, Blood Pressure, and Strokes. A. D'Alonzo, M.D. 1961: Gulf Publishing Co. Pp. 76–80.	Heart Failure ("Pump Failure") defined: The heart muscle is weakened to the extent that it is unable to meet the demands of the body organs for blood.	"Facts about Congestive Heart Failure," American Heart Assoc. pamphlet.	After teaching, ask the patient what he/she considers warning signs of congestive heart failure to be and when he/she would notify physician.
	Cause: For MI patient, part of the heart may become enlarged and unable to contract and effectively pump the necessary volume of blood.		Emphasize importance of daily weighings so patient will be more alert for weight changes.
	Effect: Accumulation of excess blood and fluid in the lungs.		
	Symptoms: Difficult breathing, shortness of breath, weight gain, protrusion of abdomen, swelling or puffiness of ankles and		

Sample Protocol: Cardiac Teaching Program

GOAL II; The patient will be able to identify signs and symptoms of his particular health problem.

OBJECTIVE A *(continued)*: Have the patient with a myocardial infarction state at least three signs and symptoms of congestive heart failure and know when to alert the physician.

References for Nurse Preparation	Content	Teaching Aids	Question for the Patients
	legs, and coughing and wheezing (poor oxygenation). Treatment: Will vary with each person and the stage of heart failure at that point, but will include some of the following. 1. Rest, sleep. 2. Restrict sodium in diet (causes retention, restricts fluids). 3. Oxygen. 4. Medicine that restores pumping capacity of heart and encourages the kidneys to excrete the excess fluid.		

References for Nurse Preparation	Content	Teaching Aids	Question for the Patients
	Notify doctor at first signs of failure, which are sudden weight gain (2–3 lbs/day) and shortness of breath. The earlier treatment is started the better—delays could result in enlarged heart.		What are the negative effects of overweight in the body?
	Reduce caloric intake. 1. Being overweight increases risks to diabetes and high blood pressure and decreases life expectancy. 2. Look at eating habits or patterns to see times of increased caloric intake.	Emphasize foods lower in calories and high in fiber for snacks (i.e., carrots, celery, radish, cucumber, zucchini). Avoid foods high in calories. Limit portion sizes. With doctor's permission, increase exercise.	
	Diet guidelines. 1. Limit eggs to 3 per week, including those in cooking. 2. Use cooking methods that help remove fat: Baking, broiling, roasting, stewing.	For this part of teaching, emphasize what patient should remember for her/his diet.	

79

Sample Protocol: Cardiac Teaching Program

GOAL II: The patient will be able to identify signs and symptoms of his particular health problem.

OBJECTIVE A *(continued)*: Have the patient with a myocardial infarction state at least three signs and symptoms of congestive heart failure and know when to alert the physician.

References for Nurse Preparation	Content	Teaching Aids	Question for the Patients
	3. Use polyunsaturated fats.		
	4. Use fish, poultry, veal for most meals; choose lean cuts of beef, lamb, pork. Trim visible fat before cooking.		

Note: Throughout the patient's hospitalization, the attitude should be to encourage some changes in dietary management and some modification in eating habits and patterns.

GOAL III: To educate patient and family in applicable meal planning guidelines; to promote a nutritionally balanced meal low in saturated fat and cholesterol; to achieve normal weight and/or weight maintenance, as recommended by patient's physician and counseled by a dietician. (The format for this goal includes an introduction and a note to the nurse. This format differs slightly because the primary teaching focus shifts from the nurse to the dietician; however, the teaching/reinforcement remains a collaborative effort and so the instructions to the nurse follow in the unusual format.)

THE DIETITIAN'S ROLE

1. Review the medical record.
2. Interview the patient and/or family.
3. Consult with health-care personnel involved in patient's care.
4. Begin teaching with visual aids and printed pamphlets that emphasize good nutritional planning of meals.
5. Outline suitable individualized sample meal plan, involving patient and family.
6. Give patient booklets, recipes, and any helpful information.
7. Evaluate knowledge comprehension. Review guidelines if necessary.

Note: The dietitian is to be informed by the nursing clerk when diet education is ordered. Diet counseling can be initiated by the physician's orders or on dietitian's recommendation.

The dietitian's approach is to individualize teaching the patient and family the appropriate guidelines for planning meals, marketing, and cooking, by considering the needs of the patient.

The nurse's role, as a member of the team, is to reinforce the dietitian's teaching and to refer questions to the dietitian.

References for Nurse Preparation	Content	Teaching Aids	Question for the Patients
	Emphasize foods lower in calories and high in fiber for snacks (i.e, carrots,	1. Reducing caloric intake a. Being overweight increases risk to dia-	What are the negative effects of overweight in the body?

Sample Protocol: Cardiac Teaching Program

GOAL III (*continued*): To educate patient and family in applicable meal planning guidelines; to promote a nutritionally balanced meal low in saturated fat and cholesterol; to achieve normal weight and/or weight maintenance, as recommended by patient's physician and counseled by a dietician. (The format for this goal includes an introduction and a note to the nurse. This format differs slightly because the primary teaching focus shifts from the nurse to the dietician; however, the teaching/reinforcement remains a collaborative effort and so the instructions to the nurse follow in the unusual format.)

References for Nurse Preparation	Content	Teaching Aids	Guide Questions to Ask Patients
	celery, radish, cucumber, zucchini).	betes and high blood pressure and decreases life expectancy.	
	Avoid foods high in calories.	b. Look at eating habits or patterns to see times of increased caloric intake.	
	Limit portion sizes.	2. Diet Guidelines	
	With doctor's permission, increase exercise.	a. Limit eggs to 3 per week, including those in cooking.	
	For this part of teaching, emphasize what patient should remember for his/her diet.	b. Use cooking methods that help remove fat: baking, broiling, roasting, stewing.	
		c. Use polyunsaturated fats.	

References for Nurse Preparation	Content	Teaching Aids	Guide Questions to Ask Patients
		d. Use fish, poultry, veal for most meals; choose lean cuts of beef, lamb, pork. Trim visible fat before cooking.	

Note: Throughout the patient's hospitalization, the attitude should be to encourage some changes in dietary management and some modification in eating habits and patterns.

Sample Protocol: Cardiac Teaching Program

GOAL IV: The patient will be given information on physical activities so that he can choose a lifestyle that is suitable to his needs and will help him prevent further heart damage.

OBJECTIVE A: The patient will learn about the effects and benefits of exercise on the heart and will be given guidelines for resuming activities within the first two weeks at home.

References for Nurse Preparation	Content	Teaching Aids	Guide Questions to Ask Patients
	A. Regular exercise will:	Activity was restricted after heart attack (see E. under Content) in order to allow heart to heal (it takes 6–8 weeks for scar tissue to form). A gradual increase in activity can make the heart stronger than before the heart attack.	Did they get regular exercise before the heart attack? What activities do they enjoy?
	1. Help strengthen the heart muscle, thereby making it more efficient.		
	2. Increase heart rate.		
	3. Increase muscle tone; this aids in circulation.		
	4. Help to build collateral circulation around damaged area of the heart.		
	5. Help with weight loss and maintenance of of a desired weight.		
	6. Promote a general sense of well-being.		

References for Nurse Preparation	Content	Teaching Aids	Guide Questions to Ask Patients
	B. Guidelines for resuming activities in the first two weeks at home. *Avoid these things:* 1. Avoid exercise after eating; oxygen is being used for digestion. 2. Avoid extremes of hot and cold temperatures in surroundings. 3. Avoid pushing, pulling, lifting, and straining: Avoid moving heavy furniture/objects (pushing); avoid vacuuming, mopping (pulling); avoid carrying groceries, children (lifting); avoid constipation (straining) — if occurs, ask doctor for laxative.	Walking against the wind makes the heart work harder. These are general guidelines and the patient should discuss with her/his doctor the specifics of how far to walk, how many times a day, etc.	

Sample Protocol: Cardiac Teaching Program

GOAL IV: The patient will be given information on physical activities so that he can choose a lifestyle that is suitable to his needs and will help him prevent further heart damage.

OBJECTIVE: A (continued): The patient will learn about the effects and benefits of exercise on the heart and will be given guidelines for resuming activities within the first two weeks at home.

References for Nurse Preparation	Content	Teaching Aids	Guide Questions to Ask Patients
	4. Avoid reaching above your head for prolonged activity, e.g., painting, sawing tree limb, playing hard game of tennis.		
	5. Let someone else shovel the snow or carry a suitcase and mow the lawn.		
	6. Avoid climbing stairs briskly (if patient has stairs in home, advise sleeping downstairs first week; then go up once at night and come down once in the morning).		Ask the patient if she/he has stairs at home. Organize activities so patients only use stairs twice a day.
	C. Continue your activity and increase gradually.		

References for Nurse Preparation	Content	Teaching Aids	Guide Questions to Ask Patients
	1. Activity at home comparable to last day in the hospital.		
	2. Get up and dress each day.	The better they look, the higher their morale.	
	3. Schedule a walk each day.	Plan ahead—walk as much as in the hospital.	
	4. May do light housework (dusting, straightening a room) and simple cooking. May cook one meal a day; don't do dishes for same meal.		
	5. Enjoy quiet hobbies, e.g., sewing, photograph sorting, editing, reading, journals, planning projects, watering houseplants, playing cards, watching TV, writing letters, visit with friends (not more than 30 minutes).		Encourage patients to tell friends they have a 30-minute limit before the the visit.
	6. Space activities.		

87

Sample Protocol: Cardiac Teaching Program

GOAL IV: The patient will be given information on physical activities so that he can choose a lifestyle that is suitable to his needs and will help him prevent further heart damage.

OBJECTIVE A (*continued*): The patient will learn about the effects and benefits of excercise on the heart and will be given guidelines for resuming activities within the first two weeks at home.

References for Nurse Preparation	Content	Teaching Aids	Guide Questions to Ask Patients
	throughout day. Give heart a chance to rest. Don't push; dust, dishes, and TV all will be there to-morrow.		
	D. Be sure to get enough sleep and rest, includ-ing emotional rest.	Refer to section on stress for methods of reducing anxiety.	
	1. Anytime you get tired during an activ-ity, stop and rest 15–30 minutes.		
	2. Rest twice a day, morning and after-noon, 20–30 minutes.		
	3. If you plan to stay up late, take a nap.	Doesn't have to be in bed—chair will do nicely. En-joy yourself; relax.	

References for
Nurse Preparation

Content

Teaching Aids

Guide Questions
to Ask Patients

Get as much sleep after your heart attack as you did before (see next section)

E. The following list should help you determine which activities require the most energy. The "energy cost" is a relative measure established by equating the "basal oxygen consumption" (the amount of oxygen consumed at rest) with the level of 1.0 and comparing all other activities to this.

Bedrest:	1.0
Walking: 3:5 mph	5.6
2.5 mph	3.6
Sedentary	1.6
Mowing lawn	7.7
Housework:	
Sweeping	1.7
Ironing	4.2

Show AV cassette, "Signal for Action" (17 minutes). Produced by the American Heart Association, Dallas, Texas.

Sample Protocol: Cardiac Teaching Program

GOAL IV: The patient will be given information on physical activities so that he can choose a lifestyle that is suitable to his needs and will help him prevent further heart damage.

OBJECTIVE A (continued): The patient will learn about the effects and benefits of exercise on the heart and will be given guidelines for resuming activities within the first two weeks at home.

References for Nurse Preparation	Content		Teaching Aids	Guide Questions to Ask Patients
	Scrubbing floor	3.6		
	Sewing	1.5		
	Recreation:			
	Painting	2.0		
	Drawing	2.8		
	Bowling	4.4		
	Swimming	5.0		
	Walking dog	3.0		
	Bicycling (5mph)	4.5		
	Golfing	5.0		
	Dancing	5.5		
	Horseback Riding	8.0		

Sample Protocol: Cardiac Teaching Program

GOAL IV: The patient will be given information on physical activities so that he can choose a lifestyle that is suitable to his needs and will help him prevent further heart damage.

OBJECTIVE B: To present guidelines to help patients and their partners enjoy a satisfying sexual relationship while minimizing the workload of the patient's heart.

References for Nurse Preparation	Content	Teaching Aids	Guide Questions to Ask Patients
"All About Sex . . . After a Coronary." Puksta, N., B.S.N. *American Journal of Nursing*, April, 1977.	A. Before resuming sexual intercourse, the patient should discuss this with her/his physician. The decision as to when to begin is up to the doctor. Generally patients resume their previous sexual life about 4–8 weeks after their heart attack. For middle-aged men, the cardiovascular response evoked during sexual intercourse with spouse of many years is considered to be similar to response when climb-	The doctor will consider any complication, such as congestive heart failure, or arrythmias, in making a decision. Doctor may want to use a treadmill or Holter monitor to determine the patient's readiness. To overcome any fears the patient may have, discuss them with the doctor and spouse, so that misconceptions can be clarified from the very beginning.	Ask patient to articulate concerns about resuming sexual activity. Follow up with guidelines to help alleviate fear and anxieties.

Sample Protocol: Cardiac Teaching Program

GOAL IV: The patient will be given information on physical activities so that he can choose a lifestyle that is suitable to his needs and will help him prevent further heart damage.

OBJECTIVE B (continued): To present guidelines to help patients and their partners enjoy a satisfying sexual relationship while minimizing the workload of the patient's heart.

References for Nurse Preparation	Content	Teaching Aids	Guide Questions to Ask Patients
	ing stairs at a brisk pace. A common method of assessing a postcoronary patient's readiness to resume sexual relations is the two-flight stair climbing test. Climb two flights of stairs at a brisk rate, taking at least 20 steps in 10 seconds (2 steps per second). If climbing of stairs at this rate does not cause chest pain or abnormal heart rate, it is usually safe for him to resume sexual relations. (Patient's	A brief history may be obtained to identify the patient's particular needs and to individualize teaching. Review points include: 1. Time of meal and alcohol consumption. 2. Common time and amount of sleep and typical rest pattern. 3. Sexual activity prior to infarction. 4. Preferred time of day for sexual relations. 5. Previous episodes of chest pain during or after intercourse,	

References for Nurse Preparation	Content	Teaching Aids	Guide Questions to Ask Patients
	heart rate is said to be abnormal if it does not return to resting after 15 minutes and/or if patient experiences palpitations, irregularities, or arrhythmias.)	6. Episodes of sleeplessness after sex or extreme fatigue on the following day.	Assure patient that normal sexual intercourse is possible for most cardiac patients.
"The Joy of Sex After a Heart Attack." Moore, K., MSN, et al. *Nursing '77*, June, 1977.	B. After finding out when the patient can have sex again, the next concerns are usually how often, and what precautions are necessary, if any.	Commonly, the heart rate increases with sexual intercourse. This should not be viewed as too much strain on the heart. The doctor would not give permission to resume sex if he thought there was any real risk.	
	1. The frequency will be influenced by the couple's previous sexual pattern.		
	2. Unless they have had cardiac complications, such as congestive heart failure, or arrhythmias, they have no reason to modify their sexual habits.		

93

Sample Protocol: Cardiac Teaching Program

GOAL IV: The patient will be given information on physical activities so that he can choose a lifestyle that is suitable to his needs and will help him prevent further heart damage.

OBJECTIVE B (*continued*): To present guidelines to help patients and their partners enjoy a satisfying sexual relationship while minimizing the workload of the patient's heart.

References for Nurse Preparation	Content	Teaching Aids	Guide Questions to Ask Patients

Sex Can Save Your Heart and Your Life. Eugene Schieman, Stanford Hospital Pamphlet.	C. Guidelines for sexual activity, once patients have talked with doctor and have been given "green light."
	 1. Be relaxed.
	   a. Have the room a comfortable temperature. Extremes of hot or cold add to heart stress.
	   b. Intercourse should be resumed in familiar surroundings. A strange environment adds to stress.
	   c. Meditation, a warm bath or shower,		

Nurse Preparation References for	Content	Teaching Aids	Guide Questions to Ask Patients
	and music may encourage relaxation. 2. Foreplay is desirable, as it helps prepare the heart gradually for the activity of sex. 3. Position should be comfortable, and can include the following. a. Lying on back, with the person recovering from the heart attack on the bottom. b. Lying on side, with rear entry c. Lying on side, with front entry. d. Cardiac patient seated on a broad, armless chair, feet flat on the floor, and the partner on the lap.		

Sample Protocol: Cardiac Teaching Program

GOAL IV: The patient will be given information on physical activities so that he can choose a lifestyle that is suitable to his needs and will help him prevent further heart damage.

OBJECTIVE B (continued): To present guidelines to help patients and their partners enjoy a satisfying sexual relationship while minimizing the workload of the patient's heart.

References for Nurse Preparation	Content	Teaching Aids	Guide Questions to Ask Patients
	4. Oral-genital sex places no undue strain on the heart. Use of this depends only on partners' preference.		
	5. Rest is beneficial before intercourse. Partners may want to have sex in the morning after a good night's sleep.		
	6. Postpone intercourse 3 hours after eating a heavy meal and/or after alcohol intake.	Digestion requires increased oxygen; therefore, sex and other physical exercise should be delayed.	
	7. Extramarital sex may add increased stress		

References for Nurse Preparation	Content	Teaching Aids	Guide Questions to Ask Patients
	and should be discussed with doctor first. 8. Medications such as Isordil (isorbide, dinitrate) and nitroglycerin may be taken before intercourse to prevent chest pain. Again, ask doctor if it is needed. 9. Masturbation usually does not require more energy than intercourse, but should be discussed with doctor. 10. Anal intercourse does add more stress to your heart and should be avoided until your doctor okays it. 11. If there is stress or anxiety, especially between partners, wait until you both feel more relaxed.		

Sample Protocol: Cardiac Teaching Program

GOAL IV: The patient will be given information on physical activities so that he can choose a lifestyle that is suitable to his needs and will help him prevent further heart damage.

OBJECTIVE B (*continued*): To present guidelines to help patients and their partners enjoy a satisfying sexual relationship while minimizing the workload of the patient's heart.

References for Nurse Preparation	Content	Teaching Aids	Guide Questions to Ask Patients
	D. Warning signs of heart strain after intercourse include the following. 1. A rapid heart and respiratory rate for 15 minutes or longer after sex. 2. Chest pain during or after intercourse. 3. Palpitations that continue for 15 minutes or longer after sex. 4. Sleeplessness after sex. You should report any of these symptoms to your doctor immediately!	Emphasize that these are warning signals and the patient should alert his/her doctor of symptoms right away. Patient should avoid sexual relations if strenuous activity is planned after intercourse.	

References for Nurse Preparation	Content	Teaching Aids	Guide Questions to Ask Patients
	E. Drugs such as antihypertensives (reserpine, aldactone), tranquilizers, antidepressants, and hypnotics can cause these effects on sexual performance. 1. Impotence 2. Decreased libido 3. Impaired ejaculation 4. Menstrual irregularities 5. Gynecomastia in men If the patients experience these side effects, they should tell the doctor so alternates can be considered. If patients cannot return to the sex lives they enjoyed before their heart attack, they may need specialized counseling, i.e., sex therapist, marriage counselor, analyst, or psychiatrist.		

Sample Protocol: Cardiac Teaching Program

GOAL V: The patient will be given instructions on medication and will be able to apply to his own lifestyle the regimen set by him/her, the physician, and the nurse.

OBJECTIVE A: The patient will be able to name his/her medication, its purpose, and any pertinent information or adverse side effects.

References for Nurse Preparation	Content	Teaching Aids	Questions to Ask
A. Approach physician, at least 1–3 days prior to discharge, regarding medications patient is taking home. B. Check medication patient is on in hospital to see if it will be the same when at home.	Will be based on what medications patient is taking and those that will be given at discharge. Reinforce teaching about medications in hospital. Then selectively do teaching on 1. Digoxin 2. Hydrochlorothiazide 3. Isordil, Lasix 4. Nitroglycerin 5. Nitropaste 6. Procainamide 7. Propanolol 8. Potassium 9. Quinidine	Use medication cards from pharmacy for patient's permanent use. Give and go over general information card.	What medication the patient is taking?

GOAL V; OBJECTIVE B: The patient will be able to plot out a time schedule for each of his medications that will best suit her/his lifestyle.

Nurse Preparation
References for

Content	Teaching Aids	Questions to Ask
A. Teach patient to take her/his own pulse accurately (plus or minus 5 beats).		Ask the patient her/his daily routine and assist with medication program to suit her/his lifestyle.
B. Teach patient the importance of daily weighings.		a. Time she/he gets up
		b. Meal time
		c. Bedtime
C. Help the patient to plot out on the medication record her/his medications and the times she/he should take them.	Use the weekly medication record and give patient copies.	Use these as guides for specific times to take medication.

Questionnaires and Forms

When the protocol was developed, several questionnaires were planned for use as a pre–post measure of knowledge gained from the teaching program. In practice, however, the questionnaires are used only as a predischarge assessment of the patient's status.

Knowledge Assessment Questionnaire
(Covers Protocol Goals and Objectives)

1. The following are normal feelings for persons recovering from a heart attack. Circle the feelings you experienced while recovering from your heart attack. (You may choose more than one.)

   a. Anger   e. Denial
   b. Depression   f. Guilt
   c. Worry   g. Other (Specify) _____
   d. Fear

2. Circle the feelings your family experienced while you were recovering from your heart attack. (You may choose more than one.)

   a. Anger   e. Denial
   b. Depression   f. Guilt
   c. Worry   g. Other (Specify) _____
   d. Fear

3. Circle the letter of any definition that you feel describes what stress is. (You may chose more than one.)

   a. An emotional response to persistent, intense, and excessive demands
   b. A physical response to persistent, intense, and excessive demands on the body
   c. Something that can affect an individual's body
   d. Something that can be reduced through a change in response to the stress
   e. All of the above

4. List two situations that cause you to experience stress.

   a.
   b.

5. The heart is (you may choose more than one):

   a. A four-chambered, hollow organ.
   b. The organ that oxygenates the blood
   c. Located in the right side of the chest

    d. The organ that pumps oxygenated blood to the body.
6. How does the heart muscle get its bloody supply? (Choose one.)
    a. From the blood passing through the heart chambers
    b. From its own system of arteries and veins called the coronary circulation system
    c. From the pulmonary circulation in the lungs
7. Which of these are risk factors that influence heart disease? (You may choose more than one.)

a. Age	f. Anemia
b. Sex	g. Stress
c. Heredity	h. Smoking
d. Diabetes	i. Ulcers
e. High blood pressure	j. Being overweight

8. Which of the following statements about angina are true? (Circle the letter.)
    a. Angina is caused by a part of the heart muscle not getting enough oxygen-rich blood.
    b. Angina may occur while a person is resting or during exertion.
    c. Angina usually occurs when one of the coronary arteries becomes permanently blocked.
    d. Angina may be triggered by an experience which requires the heart to do more work.
9. Which of the following symptoms are "early warning signs" that usually occur with the pain of a heart attack?

a. Sweating	d. Feeling sick to the stomach
b. Faintness or dizziness	e. Shortness of breath
c. Spitting up of blood	f. Coughing

(For questions 10–13, you may use the back of this page.)
10. What medication(s) are you on?
11. What is(are) the purpose(s) of each medication you are on?
12. How often is each to be taken?
13. Which facts are important to know about each medication?

a. Time to be taken	d. Possible side effects
b. Dosage to be taken	e. Storage of medication
c. Name of the drug	f. All of the above

14. Circle foods which are high in sodium and should be avoided in a restricted-sodium diet.

a. Oranges	e. Salted peanuts
b. Potato chips	f. Smoked pork chops
c. Bouillon	g. Baked chicken
d. Canned green beans	

15. Which food items below can be included in a low-saturated-fat diet?
    a. Beef gravy   d. Spare ribs
    b. Broiled chicken   e. Avocados
    c. Baked salmon
16. Which foods should be limited in a diet for weight reduction?
    a. Green salad   d. Fresh fruit compote
    b. Alcoholic beverages   e. Bacon
    c. Pancakes and maple
       syrup
17. The effect of physical activity on the heart is to:
    a. Increase heart rate and decrease blood pressure
    b. Increase blood pressure and decrease the need for oxygen-rich blood to the heart muscle
    c. Increase heart rate and increase need for oxygen-rich blood to the heart muscle
18. Upon discharge from the hospital, which of the following symptoms are indications to stop physical activity and notify your doctor? (You may choose more than one.)
    a. Chest pain not relieved by nitroglycerin or rest
    b. Prolonged shortness of breath
    c. Weakness
    d. Dizziness
19. Criteria commonly used by doctors in advising resumption of sexual activity include:
    a. Negative treadmill or Holter tapes
    b. Freedom from chest pain and other complications
    c. Discharge from hospital

Physical Assessment Form

This is completed by the nurse and adds to the data base on the patient.
Name:
Diagnosis:
Employment:
Risk factors:
Enzymes and isoenzymes (chronologically):
Course in CCU:
    Atrial arrhythmias_____ Ventricular arrhythmias_____
    Heart block_____ Congestive failure_____ Shock_____

Pericarditis-rub_____ No rub_____
Treatment (Meds.):
Lidocaine_____ Pronestyl_____ Digoxin_____ Quinidine_____
Lasix_____ KCl_____ Nitropaste_____ Nipride_____
Dopamine_____ Isuprel_____ I.V. Antihypertensives_____
Morphine_____
Treatment (Procedures):
Swan-Ganz line_____ Arterial line_____ Pacemaker_____
Cath/Angio_____ Lung scan_____ Echocardiogram_____
Countershock (reason):_____
Pertinent family information:
Any other helpful information:

Psychological Survey Questionnaires

The next two questionnaires are used together to develop a sense of the patient's psychological well-being. The first is completed by the patient and the second by the nurse. Answers are compared and the data are used to individualize the protocol for the patient.
Date: _____ Patient's name:_____
Observer: _____ Location: (CCU, etc.) _____
Day:_____

Please indicate to what extent the following questions are true for you at this time. Rating Scale: 0—Almost never   1—Sometimes   2—Often   3—Almost always

1. I get in a state of tension or turmoil as I think over my current situation.
2. I feel like I am becoming upset easily.
3. I need to know how I am doing.
4. I let others know when I am uncomfortable or upset.
5. I try to ignore a crisis or difficulty.
6. I dislike some of the things that are being done to me.
7. I feel angry about what has happened to me.
8. I feel down (or blue).
9. I feel like I want to be by myself.
10. I feel like I would rather think about than talk about what's happened to me.
11. My future seems dark to me.
12. I am content and have faith in the future.
13. I feel like I might as well give up.

Patient's name:_____   Date:_____
Location: (CCU, etc.)_____   Observer:_____
Please indicate to what extent the following items are present in the
patient at this time. Rating Scale: 0—Almost never   1—Sometimes
2—Often   3—Almost always
   1. Anxiety
   2. Becomes upset easily
   3. Seeks reassurance from staff
   4. Complains
   5. Denying
   6. Objects to routine procedures
   7. Angry
   8. Depressed
   9. Withdrawn
  10. Quiet
  11. Talks of gloomy things
  12. Cheerful
  13. Hopeless
Comments:

Teaching Progress Sheet

The following progress sheet (see fig. 4–1) is completed as the ap-
propiate sections of the protocol have been completed. It is stamped
with the patient's identification data and becomes a permanent part
of the medical record.

Discussion of Sample Protocol

This sample protocol meets many of the criteria for an effective patient teaching tool. Individualized patient assessment tools are included. Specific written instructions are employed, along with appropriate visual and written tools. Internal evaluation is accomplished by means of the teaching progress notes that are included as part of the patient's permanent record (q.v.). Thus it is systematic, detailed, and, even more important, it is *written*.

A weakness of the protocol, however, is the lack of formalized systematic external program evaluation. To remedy this lack, patients might be asked at the first posthospitalization clinic visit to fill out the same assessment sheets found in the beginning of the protocol. In addition, the teaching progress sheets could be used as a guideline to measure the current status of the patient's knowledge and behavior change. When these data are collected from a number of patients, some measure of the protocol's success might be obtained; however, it is important to identify as many intervening variables in the patient's milieu as possible, in order to interpret the data in a more balanced way.

In summary, this chapter has highlighted some of the bridges and barriers to effective patient education. The role of the nurse as health educator has been described briefly. Methods to prepare and evaluate patient education protocols have been enumerated and a sample protocol has been presented.

Figure 4-1.

Topics With Patient's Expected Behavior

CHECK ☑ APPROPRIATE BOX

☐ Pacemaker   ☐ Coronary Artery Disease   ☐ Dx

INITIAL and DATE APPROPRIATE BOXES

	Initial Teaching	Follow-up Teaching	Poor Understanding	Understanding w/Feedback	Needs Rein-forcement
DISEASE PROCESS / **DISEASE PROCESS** / **DISEASE PROCESS**					
Explains function and purpose of heart. / Explains function and purpose of heart. / Explains function and purpose of heart.					
Identifies function and structure of cardiac conduction system. / Identifies which structure of heart is affected. / Identifies which structure of heart is affected.					
Explains his basic conduction problem, i.e., sick sinus syndrome, asystole, heart block and its effect on his heart function. / Explains process of coronary heart disease. / Describes blood circulation.					
Describes signs and symptoms caused by disease process. / Explains risk factors. / Explains disease process.					
IMPLANTATION OF PACEMAKER / Describes signs and symptoms caused by disease. / List causes.					
Describes operative procedure. / If MI — describes healing process. / Describes signs and symptoms caused by disease.					
Describes expectations immediately post-op. / Identifies which signs and symptoms are indications to call M.D. or to visit E.R. / Identifies which signs and symptoms are indications to call M.D. or to visit E.R.					
PACEMAKER FUNCTION / Relates anticipation of health situation following hospitalization. / Relates anticipation of health situation following hospitalization.					
Explains purpose. / **MEDICATIONS**					

Figure 4-1. (continued)

Describes parts of pacemaker and their function.	Lists all medications he is taking.	TREATMENT INCLUDING MEDICATIONS					
Identifies signs and symptoms indicating pacemaker failure and need to call M.D.	Identifies mode and frequency of administration.	Explains current treatment plan.					
Explains future battery changes.	Explains expected effects of each medication.	Lists all medications he is taking.					
Lists environmental hazards.	Identifies which side effects are indications to call M.D.	Explains expected effects of each medication.					
MEDICATIONS		Identifies which side effects are indications to call M.D.					
Lists all medications he is taking.	DIET	Explains purpose of daily weights.					
Identifies mode and frequency of administration.	Identifies type of diet prescribed and lists foods to avoid.	DIET					
Explains expected effects of each medication.	Explains reason for diet.	Identifies type of diet prescribed and lists foods to avoid.					
Identifies which side effects are indications to call M.D.		Explains reason for diet.					
DISCHARGE PLANS	ACTIVITY	ACTIVITY					
Demonstrates pulse taking.	Describes activity prescribed for: 1) Hospital 2) Home	Describes activity prescribed for: 1) Hospital 2) Home					
	Demonstrates exercises prescribed. Stage I Stage II Stage III	Demonstrates exercises prescribed. Stage I Stage II Stage III					
Has received medic-alert bracelet info.	States effect of exercise on heart.	States effect of exercise on heart.					
Describes activity prescribed for home.	Has discussed implications for sexual activity.						

109

Figure 4-1. (*continued*)

STANFORD UNIVERSITY HOSPITAL
Stanford University Medical Center
Stanford, California 94305

TEACHING PROGRESS SHEET
FOR W1B & CCU

☐ Pacemakers	☐ Coronary Artery Disease	☐ Dx
TEACHING TOOLS	TEACHING TOOLS	TEACHING TOOLS
☐ "Your Heart and How It Works"	☐ Exercise Booklet	☐ Exercise Booklet
☐ "Pacemakers"	☐ "How to Mend a Broken Heart"	☐ "Your Heart and How It Works"
☐ Heart Model	☐ "Your Heart Has Nine Lives"	☐ "About Your Heart and Blood-stream"
☐ CIBA Book Pictures	☐ "Your Heart and How It Works"	☐ "High Blood Pressure"
☐ Other	☐ "Heart Attack"	☐ "Facts about Congestive Heart Failure"
	☐ "If You Have Angina"	☐ Heart Model
	☐ CIBA Book Pictures	☐ CIBA Book Pictures
	☐ Heart Model	☐ Other _____
	☐ Diagram of Coronary Arteries	
	☐ "How To Reduce the Risks of Heart Attack"	
	☐ "Coronary Artery Disease"	
	☐ Other _____	

110

Figure 4-1. (*continued*)

ADDITIONAL COMMENTS

ADDITIONAL COMMENTS

ADDITIONAL COMMENTS

References

American Nurses' Association. *The professional nurse and health education.* Kansas City: American Nurses' Association, 1975.

Becker, M. H. The health belief model and sick role behavior. *Nursing Digest,* 1978, *6,* 35–40.

Green, H. W., & Figa-Talamanca, I. Suggested design for evaluation of patient education programs. *Health Education Monographs,* 1974, *2,* 54–71.

Hockey, L. The future nurse: Selection and training; autonomy; should her health care role be modified for future patient demands. *Journal of Advanced Nursing,* 1978, *3,* 571–582.

Horn, D. A model for the study of personal choice health behavior. *International Journal of Health Education,* 1976, *19,* 89–98.

Jenny, J. A strategy for patient teaching. *Journal of Advanced Nursing,* 1978, *3,* 341–348.

Norris, C. Self care. *American Journal of Nursing,* 1979, *79,* 486-489.

Pohl, M. Teaching activities of the nursing practitioner. *Nursing Research,* 1975, *14,* 4–11.

Redman, B. *The process of patient teaching in nursing.* St. Louis: Mosby, 1972.

Steuart, G. Planning and evaluation in health education. *International Journal of Health Education,* 1969, *12,* 65–76.

Streeter, V. The nurse's responsibility for teaching patients. *American Journal of Nursing,* 1953, *53,* 818–820.

Winslow, E. The role of the nurse in patient education. *Nursing Clinics of North America,* 1976, *11,* 213–222.

5

Considerations on the Use of
Media in Patient Education

Robert Hecht

The use of media in helping patients to learn about their
health care has become an increasingly widespread phenomenon in
recent years (Allan, 1978a). Though significant variations exist in the
comprehensiveness, sophistication, and quality of such efforts using
media, it is becoming widely recognized that media can enhance and
complement the overall goals of institutional patient education programs (Lane, 1978).

The health care patient represents a very specialized audience
for media materials. The patient's entry-level knowledge and attitudes and the learning environment itself pose unique considerations
in the design and implementation of media programs. These characteristics bear examining here, as do basic principles of media design,
production, and critiquing. A complete concept of patient education
should include, of course, the education of potential patients—the general public—and efforts are being made to reach this audience via
the mass media (Farquhar, J., Wood, P. D., Breightrose, H., Haskell,
W. L., et at., 1977). Although much of what is covered in this chapter
is pertinent to such public health education efforts, the primary focus
is on educational media programs for people who are already patients
in health care facilities.

General Considerations

Why Media?

Great increases in the utilization of educational media have occurred,
particularly so in the health care field. A primary cause of this media

explosion in the health field is the amount of information that has itself exploded—such a quantity that it is no longer considered viable to deliver it all by traditional methods (*American Medical News*, 1972). Thus, sheer volume of information is no big reason for growth in the use of media. Another is cost; in many cases, a media program can reach more learners at less cost than the traditional instructional methods (Knopke & Diekelmann, 1978). There is also growing awareness among educators of the importance of self-paced, individualized learning experiences, which media can facilitate (Foster, 1970). Hence many teachers are using media to deliver material that normally would be presented repetitively via "live" presentations to class after class, year after year, thus freeing them in some cases to do more small-group and individualized teaching.

Motivating for Change

The delivery of cognitive material is not all that media can do, however, nor even what it can necessarily do best. Media can be highly effective in teaching physical skills and, perhaps most relevant to patient education, can be highly effective in motivating attitudinal and behavioral changes (R. B. Johnson & S. R. Johnson, 1971).

Here is where a problem sometimes arises insofar as patient education is concerned. In the author's experience some instructional media programs have been successful in increasing the learner's knowledge significantly but have not brought about the desired behavioral changes. As a result of such programs there are well-informed patients who have not been sufficiently motivated to implement the changes in their lives that they know would benefit them. This is a perplexing situation, but perhaps too much is being expected of media. Despite the oft-touted merits of self-instructional technology, one must not forget the need for the human ingredient in education and particularly in patient education. Clearly the motivational level of the medical student working through a self-instructional computer program is far greater than that of a passive, sometimes frightened sufferer of ill health. For this special audience the need for human interaction in educational efforts seems critical (Squyres, 1979).

A media program alone is not necessarily patient education. To be held responsible for more than just added factual knowledge, patients require not only well-designed, motivational media programs but personal follow-up by health educators and opportunities to question and discuss ideas, to share experiences, to give and get feedback. Generally the more interaction (and not just an interaction between a patient and a projector, videotape machine, or computer) in the educational experience, the better the results (R. B. Johnson & S. R. Johnson, 1971). The role of the patient tends to be a passive one anyway; we do not need to compound this by presenting more passive educational experiences. The more interactive our efforts are, the more likely it will be that patients will truly incorporate learning into their lives.

Education versus Information

A related question is that of information versus education. "Informational" media programs abound; true "educational" programs, unfortunately, are not as common in our patient education efforts as we might sometimes like to believe. The former class of program is usually fairly general in nature, its purpose primarily to give an overview or to create interest; and the audience is not held responsible for measurable performance. In the true educational program the subject is more specific and proof of learning is required (Anderson, 1976).

Being aware of this distinction is important as our patient education efforts evolve. Many programs seem to be developing despite a lack of great commitment on the parts of hospital administrators and physicians, and of necessity these pilot programs must be palatable to all decision makers concerned. This leads to a preponderance of diluted media programming, a lot of "This Is Your Hospital," "Welcome to the O.R.," and "Learning about Your Body" kinds of programs. This type of programming has a place in our patient education efforts, but we should recognize that it really isn't patient education in the truest sense. We should also make our administrators and physicians aware that it isn't really patient education. Thus, gradually we will be able to introduce more and more genuine educational programs.

Delivery Systems

Some of this has bearing on the types of media delivery systems used for patient education. In many cases closed-circuit television systems are the first employed in the hospital setting, and often these systems are technically limited in that they transmit to an entire hospital patient population, providing little or no capability for screening the audience. Naturally, the programming allowed on such systems has to meet stringent criteria of acceptability to the general patient population. Disease-specific teaching programs—the patients' highest expressed need in many instances—are a rare event on such systems.

Flexible media delivery systems are needed in patient education programs. Don't get locked into inappropriate technology. If the capability of reaching selected patients with specific educational programs is needed, then our delivery systems must be portable so we can take that slide program or videotape to the patient's bedside. Study centers for ambulatory patients can provide a monitored environment conducive to individualized learning (Allan, 1978b).

Evaluation

Another general consideration is evaluation of instructional programs. Unfortunately, this is a neglected area; lots of people know about evaluation but few seem to be practicing it. Many people, in the author's experience, expend great effort, time, and money to produce a media program but refuse to take the final step to evaluate the results. Some are afraid of evaluation as something too complex and too time consuming. The most elaborate, scientific evaluation scheme is not necessarily required to find out quite a bit about whether your program works or not; a small-scale, short-term assessment can often give you the fundamental feedback you need.

There is no mystery about evaluation. It can be made a very complex art and science, but basically it is all about having clear objectives, knowing where your audience is, and simply assessing the changes your program makes. The literature abounds with good references on specific evaluation techniques (Webster, 1976). The main thing, really, is this: What's the point of designing and implementing a program if you can not prove that it works? More and more, too, you will have to validate your program efforts in order to be cost accountable. Do not be afraid of evaluation, make it work for you.

Self-evaluation

Evaluation leads to a related topic: self-evaluation. When one talks about improving patient education using media, one usually talks about providing better films or tapes or printed handouts, and sometimes it seems we neglect looking at our personal teaching efforts or those of our colleagues. Yet if we are to incorporate significant human interaction in our educational programs, it is imperative that we look at our own performance as teachers; and there is a media tool that can help in this endeavor: videotape.

One of the most powerful attributes of the video medium is its usefulness for self-evaluation. In no other way can one receive such an objective look at oneself and one's interaction with others, immediately following the actual event. Seeing oneself performing a teaching activity can allow increased awareness of how one comes across to others, enabling one to better see strengths as well as where skills may need improving (Bedics, 1970). A "guided" self-evaluation with videotape is possible with a basic set of criteria for assessing one's performance (Foley, R., Smilansky, J., Brighman, E., Sagid, A., 1976). This can be enhanced by additional feedback from a colleague or student.

An additional aspect of using video for self-evaluation is the work being done with patients. In psychotherapy particularly, video is being used with often remarkable results (Whittaker & Whittaker, 1978). There are numerous reported cases of patients gaining important insights into their behavior as a result of seeing themselves on video, and the use of it in this context is growing rapidly.

Resource Sharing

One final point under the heading of general considerations: In the author's view, those involved in patient education are not doing an adequate job of sharing resources. There is an enormous amount of duplication of media production efforts—waste—occurring across the country. Consortia and other mechanisms for sharing programs and resources need to be established. Let each other know what is available in your neck of the woods and don't produce it if you can get it elsewhere for less cost.

Principles of Media Use

Planning

Frequently people approach media specialists with project ideas and say things like, "We want to do a videotape on such and such." They have already, in many cases, selected a delivery medium for a program, the objectives of which are as yet unknown. Good planning permits no such assumptions. One must progress step by step in analyzing the problem, setting measurable objectives, choosing a medium, planning a budget, and so forth (Green, Kreuter, Partridge, & Deeds, 1979).

The first and most important step is to define the problem. Clear objectives emerge from clear problem definition. Determine what needs to be changed in the learners' knowledge, attitudes or behavior (Mager, 1975). During this process consider your audience carefully. Consider age, sex, race, cultural background, occupation, knowledge, and attitudes. Involve members of your intended audience in defining learner needs or problems.

When this fundamental needs assessment has been accomplished, you should be able to outline the desired educational changes. State these as clearly as possible in behavioral terms; state what the learner should be able to know, do, or feel as a result of your program (Mager, 1975). There are many good works that can help you become skillful in setting objectives in behavioral terms.

Once you have completed these tasks consider how you feel about what you are trying to achieve. Is it clear? Is it reasonable for a single program? Ideally, packaged instructional programs should not be longer than 15 or 20 minutes. Will your program idea fit into this ideal length? If not, consider focusing it further or dividing it into more than one unit.

Look for it first. Again, a reminder: Do not produce it if it already exists. Fnd out whether a similar educational program is available. Search current catalogs of leading media distributors, contact a media librarian to help with the search, or call other health care facilities and inquire about available programs. There is obviously no point in duplicating someone else's effort if it will meet your needs. Very importantly, even if it doesn't fit your goals exactly, it may give you some good ideas on how or how not to produce your program.

Production

If no existing program fits your needs, it is time to proceed with the production phase and the development of a program script. But first a few general thoughts about production.

If you have access to a person or department with media expertise, use that resource if at all possible rather than trying to do it all yourself. Many health educators have considerable skill in instructional development and feel perhaps that they should therefore be able to do the whole production job themselves. If you try this, however, you may find that you spend so much time just acquiring the necessary expertise that the project winds up costing more than it would have if you had used a production specialist. By using an expert you will also be more likely to ensure the desired level of production quality.

Related to that last thought is this: Beware the amateurish production. Most people in this media age have very sophisticated standards for production quality, mainly as a result of decades of exposure to TV and the movies. Even though most people are not consciously aware of having these discriminating standards, they will often reject a "home-movie" kind of production as lacking in professional credibility. "Quick and dirty" videotapes, for example, may be okay for in-service lectures and other utilitarian purposes, but for most patient education programming a professional production standard should be sought.

On the other hand, do not overproduce. A polished, professional treatment is recommended but not necessarily that given to a Hollywood extravaganza. Make it good but unless you are planning on international distribution or widespread TV broadcast, do not try to make "Star Wards." There is just no point, with the relatively short-lived, ever-changing nature of today's health care knowledge, in spending huge amounts of money on the production of educational materials.

Contracting

Some suggestions on contracting with a media specialist, script writer, graphic artist, photographer, video producer, or media department: First, and foremost, clarify your production budget and get any cost estimates down in writing. Be sure you know what you are going to get for how much. If possible, budget some contingency amount (10–15%) in case of inflation, changes in program content, and so forth. Do not contract with someone just because the price seems right. Be sure you see samples of the person's previous work and that you have final say on such things as scripting and graphics. Many times clients seek out media professionals after an unsatisfactory experience with an inexpensive free-lancer, asking the professional to correct mistakes or generally improve on inferior work. This some-

times costs the client more than it would have to go to a qualified
individual in the first place.

Choosing the Medium

Which medium is best? is a question posed often to media specialists
by unknowing clients. The answer, of course, is For what? Do not
decide on your medium until you have accomplished your needs assessment and set your objectives. Only then can you intelligently determine the most appropriate medium for your goals (Kemp, 1971).
Of course budget constraints may dictate the choice of medium in
some cases, but nonetheless you should have a clear idea of how
best to do the job. Ask yourself the following questions:

> Must the program use a predominantly visual medium or could
> it achieve the same goals in a printed format or an audio tape?
> If it does require heavy use of visual materials, is motion essen-
> tial to get across the most important ideas? If so, film or video-
> tape would be indicated; if not, a slide program may be more
> appropriate.
> Would slow motion enhance learning significantly? If so, film
> or video would be necessary, depending on available facilities.
> Will the program need frequent content changes to update it?
> This can definitely affect the choice of medium; for example,
> slide programs are easier and less expensive to revise than
> either films or videotapes.
> Will the program be used primarily by individuals, small groups,
> or large groups? If the answer is large groups and the program
> requires a motion medium, film may be more appropriate
> than video in some instances, depending on the availability
> of appropriate video equipment. (Film still has the edge over
> video in resolution capability, especially for large-group view-
> ings.)

Costs

Insofar as production costs of the primary audiovisual media formats
are concerned, film is typically the most expensive and requires the
longest production time; video is less expensive and usually faster
to produce; and the slide-tape format is least expensive and often

fastest to produce. These are broad cost guidelines; cost information on all media formats is obviously not included here, nor are hardware costs. Actual production costs cannot be generalized and need to be estimated on a per-project basis. Consult with a media specialist for this information.

If you need to justify thoroughly the expense of creating or purchasing a media program, look first at the present cost of delivering that same information or instruction. In so doing, analyze all of the present staff time and materials involved annually, and present this information to your administrator with your program proposal. Nothing is as convincing these days as cost savings, and all too often people forget about this advantage of using the media.

Style

What style of program is most appropriate? If your primary program goals are in the cognitive area of learning, the emphasis should be on the clarity of the information presented. If you want to change specific behaviors, present the learner with specific steps. If you want to arouse interest or change attitudes, present an attractive and emotionally appealing program (S. R. Johnson & R. B. Johnson, 1970).

The most successful patient education programs tend to accentuate the positive. This means showing the patient as an active, informed participant in the health care process, reflecting wellness rather than illness, and generally presenting a patient-oriented image rather than merely a disease-oriented one.

One kind of program that is especially viable for changing attitudes is the so-called trigger film or tape. This is usually a 1- or 2-minute program that caricatures a fairly common occurrence. It normally covers only a segment of a larger series of related events and is aimed at provoking a strong reaction in order to stimulate discussion. Sometimes, in aiming for a laugh or an angry reaction, this type of program purposely presents an overstated situation. Triggers can be highly effective with either patients or professional staff in eliciting attitudes and feelings; and because of their brevity, they can be very cost effective to produce.

Scripting

The ability to write a good script is not easily acquired; it is often the result of years of work and study. Some basic suggestions are offered here, and many informative works are available on the subject.

To begin your script, analyze the objectives of your program and outline all the major points to be covered. Organize these in the sequence that is most logical for the topic. This may be a chronological sequence for a certain topic; an analytical one for another. In any case it is usually best to proceed from the general to the specific and from the simple to the complex.

Once your outline is complete, start filling in each section with a rough draft of the narrative. You might preface your script with a paragraph that provides motivation for the learner. Explain what is to be learned and why it is important. There is an old maxim, often applied to program development, which states: Tell them what you're going to tell them; tell them; then tell them what you've told them.

Try to write in a conversational manner. There is an obvious difference between the spoken word and the style one would use in a book or journal article. In addition, the visual component, when developed, will convey a lot of the total information, so your narrative should be as succinct as possible. Use a personal approach and speak to just one learner.

When you shift from one major section to another in your script, provide the audience with a clear transition or bridging statement. They will be able to stay with you best if you signal your turns.

You can stimulate active participation by inserting questions and problems into the script if it is appropriate for your program. These can be purely rhetorical, followed by a brief pause; or they can require a definite response, such as a written answer or choice of multiple answers. This type of self-testing should provide immediate feedback to the learner on whether the answers are correct (S. R. Johnson & R. B. Johnson, 1970). A supplementary workbook with your program can be a good format for this type of self-testing or as a means of providing the learner with practice exercises.

Last, when you have finished your first draft, go back to the beginning of the script and begin to indicate some visual ideas. A media specialist or graphic designer can help you to clarify and finalize these ideas, but it is a good idea to identify at least the basic visual concepts for each part of the script. The format called a *storyboard* is excellent for this, allowing you to arrange your text and visual ideas together. As you match your visuals and text, you will also have an opportunity to polish the first draft of your narrative.

It is important that your visual ideas always correlate closely with the narrative and not distract attention from it (Anderson,

1976). Visual pacing is crucial; changes in visuals should occur frequently enough to prevent learners from becoming bored. (The actual rate of change varies from program to program, depending on the nature of its visual content.) Keep visuals simple if at all possible; it is better to use a series of simple visuals to express a complex concept rather than to use a single complex visual.

When you have completed your script to this point, you might ask yourself the following questions. If you do not feel comfortable with your answers to those questions that are most applicable to your program, some revision or consultation with a media specialist would be indicated.

Have you made clear to the learner what he or she should know or be able to do as a result of the program?

Have you motivated the learners by letting them know why it is important to learn the material?

Have you planned any opportunities for the learner to practice the activity or apply the knowledge?

Have you given the learner any feedback on how well the material has been learned?

Is the narrative clear and succinct?

Are the visual ideas simple and understandable?

Does the narrative always correlate well with the visuals?

Is the content organized in the most logical progression?

Are transitions signaled clearly?

Is the program well paced, with visual changes occurring frequently enough to prevent boredom?

Does the program content correspond with your original goals?

Have you planned a means of evaluation to determine how well the material has been learned?

Program Critiquing

Those involved in reviewing materials need to know what to look for and why some programs are better than others. Many of the above criteria for assessing a script are pertinent to the review of program materials; in addition, a number of considerations emerge.

First, try to put yourself in the place of the intended learner when you review programs, rather than trying to assume the posture of a detached, all-knowing critic. On a basic gut level, try to evaluate whether the program lets you know why you should bother watching it and what you should get out of it. Also, try to be aware of whether the program feels boring. Many programs that may be quite instructionally sound may also be seriously boring, which can defeat the whole purpose when presented to patients.

One other, rather subtle, thing to be aware of is whether a program talks down to the learner. Although most programs need to be aimed at an average level of audience knowledge, some achieve much better than others a feeling of directness and a style that is free of any feeling of condescension toward the audience. Be sensitive to this issue, as it is one of the fastest ways to turn off your audience. At the other extreme, beware of the program that is aimed too high for your audience or that is full of unexplained terminology. In short, be conscious of a program's compatibility with your audience, in terms of race, age, knowledge, and attitudes. Obviously if your learners can not identify with the program, they will be much less apt to accept it.

Of the most typical shortcomings one sees in educational media programs, the lack of clear objectives is perhaps the most common and most serious. What should the learner know or be able to do as a result? Why is it important? If there is any doubt about the answers to these basic questions, then the program will usually be less than effective with the intended audience.

When reviewing programs keep in mind, as noted earlier, that fairly short programs are usually most effective in keeping viewer attention high. This is especially true of educational programs as opposed to informational ones. The more to the point, the more limited to a single concept an educational program is, the better it will usually be.

It should go without saying that one of the most important considerations is whether the information in a program is accurate and up to date. It may not be as obvious that the content, to be acceptable in your institution, should also be in keeping with that institution's medical practice and should be compatible with other patient education efforts there by physicians, nurses or other health educators.

Insofar as "technical" critiquing goes, there are a few basics to keep in mind. Take a critical look at the use of visuals in a program to see that they are clearly legible and correlate with the spoken word. Is the picture sharp where it should be sharp? Is the color accurate? Is the sound clear and the narrative understandable? Is the film free of distracting, jumpy splices or is the videotape electronically stable? Overall, is the production quality of a professional level? Beyond this point technical critiquing becomes a great deal more sophisticated and involves more complex directorial, editing, and scripting techniques. If interested in these aspects in greater depth, there are a number of works that deal with the intricacies of media production.

Summary

Media usage in patient education is growing rapidly owing to the overall information explosion, the cost benefits of media versus traditional methods, and the greater appreciation of alternative teaching techniques.

Patients are a specialized audience with specialized needs. Successful programs tend to emphasize wellness rather than illness and accentuate the positive wherever possible.

Increased learner knowledge may not by itself bring about desired behavioral changes.

Media programs should be as interactive as possible, and not just with hardware. Human follow-up may maximize the chance of learners effecting behavioral changes.

Informational programs are general and demand no proof of learning; educational programs are specific and require demonstrable proof of learning and of overall program effectiveness.

When planning media systems, keep them flexible.

A small-scale, short-term evaluation of program effectiveness may not tell you everything, but it is a lot better than no evaluation at all.

Self-evaluation using videotape is a powerful tool for improving teaching and, in some cases, for aiding patient self-understanding.

Sharing existing resources and materials should be a high priority.

Do not produce it if you can get it elsewhere for less cost.

Defining the problem is the first and most important step in planning a media program.

Consider your intended audience carefully and involve members of the audience in defining the problem.

Set measurable objectives, with an evaluation plan.

Do not preconceive your choice of medium.

Use media expertise and resources whenever possible to save time and money and to ensure program quality.

Avoid amateurish production quality if possible.

Do not overproduce; few extravaganzas are actually needed.

When contracting for production, do so in writing and know for sure what you are getting for how much.

Keep program scripts clear and succinct and be sure visuals correlate well with narrative.

Design learner feedback and practice exercises where appropriate.

In critiquing programs, put yourself in the place of the learner and see if you can identify with the program.

Validate your programs.

References

Allan, F. D. Hospital inpatient education. *Journal of Biocommunication,* March 1978, *5*:1, p. 14. (a)

Allan, F. D. Patient Education: Recommendation for the establishment of a program. *Journal of Biocommunication,* March 1978, *5*:1, pp. 16–17. (b)

American Medical News, As science progresses, how can MOs keep up? September 1972, p. 11.

Anderson, R. H. *Selecting and developing media for instruction.* New York: Van Nostrand Reinhold, 1976.

Bedics, R. A. *A study of self-evaluations of student-teachers through the use of videotape.* Unpublished doctoral dissertation, University of Alabama, 1970.

Farquhar, J., Wood, P. D., Breightrose, H., Haskell, W. L., et al. Community education for cardiovascular health. *Lancet,* June 4, 1977, *1*, pp. 1192–1195.

Foley, R., Smilansky, J., Brighman, E., Sagid, A., et al. *Improving Lecture skills.* Instruction booklet accompanying videotape. Chicago, Ill.: Center for Educational Development, University of Illinois Medical Center, 1976.

Foster, J. E. Individualized instruction for the college curriculum. *Medical and Biological Illustration,* September 1970, pp. 89–90.

Green, L. W., Kreuter, M., Partridge, K. B., & Deeds, S. G. *Health education planning: A diagnostic approach.* Palo Alto: Mayfield, 1979.

Johnson, R. B., & Johnson, S. R. *Assuring learning with self-instructional packages.* Chapel Hill, N.C.: Self-Instructional Packages, 1971.

Johnson, S. R., & Johnson, R. B. *Developing individualized instructional material.* Sunnyvale, Calif.: Westinghouse Learning, 1970.

Kemp, J. E., Which medium? *Audiovisual Instruction,* December, 1971, p. 14.

Knopke, H. J., & Diekelmann, N. L. *Approaches to teaching in the health sciences.* Reading, Mass.: Addison-Wesley, 1978.

Lane, D. S. Patient education in the community hospital. *Journal of Biocommunication,* March 1978, p. 10.

Mager, R. F. *Preparing instructional objectives.* Belmont, Calif.: Fearon, 1975.

Squyres, W. D. Using media in hospitals. In P. Lazes (Ed.), *Consumer health education handbook.* Aspen Press, 1979. pp. 133–162.

Webster, W. J. *The evaluation of instructional materials.* Washington, D.C.: Association for Educational Communications and Technology, 1976.

Whittaker, R. & Whittaker, S. Professional video and psychiatry. *Video Systems,* May 1978, pp. 28–31.

6

The Return on Investment Model

Dorothy Joan del Bueno

There is no single absolutely perfect program or approach to patient education. In the past few years many techniques and systems have been developed to help patients and their families learn about their health problems. Each of these techniques and systems has disadvantages and advantages. This article describes a unique model for patient education—the return on investment model—that evolved because of the recent emphasis on cost effectiveness in the health care industry. Although it too has disadvantages, it provides a logical framework for decision makers who must choose among options for development and implementation of patient education programs.

Conceptual Basis of the Model

The return on investment (ROI) model is conceptual rather than tactical. It is based on economic principles and uses the terminology of two disciplines, education and economics. The assumptions on which the ROI model is based are:

Resources are finite (limited).
Values affect the allocation of limited resources.
It is easier to quantify and measure *costs* of education than to quantify and measure outcomes of education.
Education can benefit some people more than others.

In classic economics, efficiency is highly valued. *Efficiency* is defined as using available resources in a combination that achieves an optimum and steady flow of income or benefits. In the ROI model, return on investment is described as a relationship between costs and outcomes, or to use a term very popular today, *cost effectiveness.*

Economic purists would argue that there is a difference between consumption costs and investment costs. Inasmuch as we are concerned with people, or human capital, I have decided to impose a bias on this model that all costs related to improving the health status of people will be considered investment costs.

In this ROI model, evaluation of outcomes will be made in *relation* to investment costs. In other words, the outcomes themselves are not as significant as the amount and allocation of scarce resources required to achieve such outcomes. The questions asked in this model are:

Could the same benefits or outcomes have been achieved at a lower cost?

or

Could greater benefits or outcomes have been achieved at the same cost?

Did the outcomes justify the expenditure of resources?

Outcomes of Patient Education

As indicated this model relates outcomes (benefits) to costs. What are the potential benefits or outcomes of patient education programs? Outcomes may be described both quantitatively and qualitatively. Quantitative outcomes are easier to measure than are qualitative outcomes.

The potential quantitative outcomes derived from patient education are:

1. *Awareness.* This outcome can be measured by a simple tally of the number of educational programs given or the number of participants. If this number is compared with the potential audience for any given program, some evaluation can be made about the impact of the program on the awareness of individuals. For example, if in a particular hospital there are 1,000 new diabetics admitted each year and 500 of these at-

tended an education program on their health problem, an impact has been made on the awareness of 50 percent of the potential audience.

Attendance at programs does not quarantee increased awareness. A survey tool would have to be used to measure whether or not the individuals were indeed any more aware of their health problem than previous to the program. Evidence of increased awareness does not equate with change in behavior, the usual definition of learning. However, increasing an individual's awareness is a desirable outcome for education programs.

2. *Increase in knowledge or skill.* This outcome can be measured by pre- and posttesting of cognitive and psychomotor objectives. Using the same example of the 1,000 new diabetic patients, materials could be used for teaching these individuals facts about their health problem and how-to skills such as giving insulin and doing foot care. Gain in knowledge of the facts or ability to perform the skills is evaluated by the pre- and posttests.

Studies have demonstrated that acquisition of knowledge does not automatically transfer into changed behavior. However, without the knowledge it is unlikely that the individual can change behavior. Thus acquisition of knowledge or skills is also a desirable outcome for education programs.

3. *Adherence to medical regimen.* This outcome is more difficult to measure because it requires follow-up over time. Also, unless it is possible to observe the individual continuously, the tools used for measurement, such as self-reporting, are subjective and therefore not reliable. For example, this same diabetic population may report compliance with diet restrictions but may indeed only comply the day or two before the visit to the physician or nurse so that urine and blood tests are acceptable. Compliance, a most desirable outcome, is also difficult to achieve because of the complexity of variables that affect a person's consistent behavior.

4. *Decrease in morbidity or mortality.* This outcome can be measured by reviewing charts and statistical reports. It is difficult to determine with certainty whether or not the decrease was the result of the education program. Because of all the intervening variables, cause-and-effect relationships are extremely difficult to demonstrate. The outcome is highly desirable, however.

Qualitative outcomes are difficult to measure objectively and reliably. Qualitative outcomes include:

1. *Quality of life.* Does the individual feel his or her life is just as satisfying or more so than prior to the health problem? Is he or she happier or just as happy? Perception of the quality of one's life is extremely individual and related to cultural background, religious values, philosophy of life, and other circumstantial variables.

2. *Participant satisfaction.* Did the learner find the educational experience worthwhile, useful, or gratifying? Satisfaction is highly perceptual and subject to change from day to day. What is satisfactory to one group of learners may be unsatisfactory to another. The reliability of such outcome measures is doubtful.

3. *Ability to cope.* This outcome may result from the acquisition and practice of new skills and knowledge. Ability to cope is generally valued in our society. However, some people may not value or get satisfaction from coping.

4. *Self-determination.* This outcome is related to the individual's ability to determine her or his own definition of health and to decide what actions she or he will take to actualize that definition. Self-determination, like coping, is generally valued in our society. Like coping, however, there may be people who do not desire self-determination.

    Both of these latter outcomes, coping and self-determination, also require a nontraditional approach to educational programming. The learning strategies that must be used may be difficult for patient educators to learn and practice. Also, both of these outcomes require longitudinal follow-up.

Costs of Patient Education

What are the costs of patient education? The traditional costs are:

1. Hours of staff time devoted to the educational programming
2. Materials developed for acquisition of knowledge and skills
3. Indirect costs such as overhead of facilities and administrative activities
4. Hours spent in evaluation, follow-up, and reinforcement-reward strategies

5. Out-of-pocket expenses reimbursed to patients or staff for classroom or follow-up activities

These line-item costs are relatively simple to measure reliably. The total of these costs can then be compared to the level of outcomes or benefits achieved. The result of this comparison of costs to benefits or outcomes can be used to evaluate the questions previously asked:

Could we have achieved these outcomes at smaller cost?
Could we have achieved higher level outcomes at the same cost?
Did the outcomes justify the expenditure of resources?

There should be some relationship between costs and benefits achieved.

Case Examples

The following hypothetical examples compare two patient education efforts that achieved different outcomes at different costs. The dollar amounts used are gross estimates only.

Hospital A has developed a highly formalized program of patient education for new diabetics and their families. There are twenty hours of lecture, and discussion classes given by a registered nurse clinical specialist on a weekly basis. Patients and families are referred to the classes by the physician and the nursing staff. A pharmacist also gives one of the two-hour classes on insulin and oral hypoglycemic medications. Objective paper-and-pencil tests are used for measuring knowledge increase. Return demonstrations by patients and or families are also evaluated.

YEARLY COSTS

Salary of nurse (half time)	$12,000
Teaching time of pharmacist	800
Clerical salary (prepare materials)	1,500
Overhead (office, classroom)	1,000
Audiovisual materials (amortized)	500
Equipment (syringes, etc.)	250
Total	$16,050

OUTCOMES ACHIEVED FOR 500 PATIENTS

Impact on potential audience (1,000) is 50 percent.

Objective testing results: Acquisition of knowledge and skills achieved by 75 percent of the participants.

Follow-up is limited to informal solicitation of information from physicians and clinic staff. No reliable data on morbidity, mortality, or compliance.

Clinic B has developed a formal program of patient education for hypertensive high-risk patients. The two nurse practitioners in this clinic have completed training courses in behavior modification and adult learning theory. The hospital has also used a training consultant to develop a set of self-directed learning packages on hypertension. The nurse practitioners assess the knowledge and readiness level of each new patient, assign the patient to use the appropriate learning materials, evaluate the achievement of the learning objectives, and also develop a learning contract with each patient that includes health goals, action plan, and evaluation methods. Patients are followed by the nurses by return appointments, telephone, and occasional home visits.

YEARLY COSTS

Salary of two nurses (50 percent of time spent on these activities)	$24,000
Amortized cost of teaching materials and audiovisual equipment	1,000
Clerical salary (record keeping)	500
Follow-up evaluation costs	5,000
Total	$30,500

OUTCOMES ACHIEVED FOR 500 PATIENTS

Impact on potential audience (600) is 83 percent.

Objective testing results: Acquisition of knowledge and skills by 90 percent of the participants.

Follow-up evaluation by using both subjective and objective measures (self-reporting, observation, blood pressure measurements, pill counts) indicate 75 percent of patients are maintaining acceptable blood pressure levels.

80 percent of the patients achieve the goals identified in their learning contracts.

Comparing these two examples, it is evident that the second program was almost twice as costly as the first in dollar amounts. It is also evident that the outcomes achieved by the second program were of a higher magnitude in relation to actual change in behavior and subsequent health status. Therefore, using the criteria of the ROI model, we could conclude that the second program was most cost effective, and therefore a better investment of resources.

There is an additional cost that needs to be considered in making decisions about allocation of scarce resources. That cost is called *lost opportunity cost*. Lost opportunity cost relates to what else could have been done with these same resources. Has a golden opportunity been lost to achieve even more meaningful or important benefits or outcomes? This is, of course, a hypothetical question, for we can never know what might have been. This question of lost opportunity may also have moral and ethical implications. Lost opportunity decisions certainly are related to philosophical values.

Summary

Patient education raises the issue or the degree to which we value and choose to invest in human capital. The ROI model can be useful in making decisions among options both in regard to how we will allocate resources and what we can reasonably expect as a result of such investment. This model can also be used by an individual patient to determine whether his or her own "investment" of time, energy, pain, pleasure, and dollars are equal to the benefits experienced as a result of new health behaviors. There may be tactics and methods other than education that would result in the same outcomes. The individual may even decide that the outcomes are not worth the investment or cost.

There is no question that patient education is an important activity for health professionals. Time, energy, money, and motivation are limited resources for both agencies and people. Consideration of the relationship between what can be achieved and at what cost, may help avoid disappointment and disillusionment with patient education programs.

Bibliography

Bera, I. *Education and jobs: The great training robbery.* New York: Praeger, 1970.

Blaug, M. (Ed.). *Economics of education,* Baltimore, Md.: Penguin, 1968.

del Bueno, D. Evaluation of patient education. *The Diabetes Educator,* Winter 1975, pp. 21, 22.

del Bueno, D. Patient education: Planning for success. *Journal of Nursing Administration,* June 1978, pp. 5–7.

Schultz, T. W. *The economic value of education.* New York: Columbia University Press, 1967.

7

What Is Quality in Patient Education and How Do We Assess It?*

Lawrence W. Green

My purpose is to define and describe quality in patient education and to suggest some measures and examples of quality assessment. This task has some inherent limitations. The definition will not be precise. Quality is an elusive thing, as it should be, especially in things educational. There is no hope that we could define it in such a way as to capture it for all time with any specificity.

A second limitation is that the description of quality is necessarily limited to the standards, data, and documentation available. Those have been limited in this field. I sometimes feel that attempting to draw standards out of the data available on patient education is like making concrete out of fluff.

Although we cannot presume a static definition or description of what quality is, ex cathedra, we can supply ways of measuring it. The first step in doing that is to define patient education in some way that allows us to isolate it and count it. It will be a moving target, but the movement can be known and understood if it can be detected when it occurs and distinguished from related activities that masquerade as patient education.

*Preparation of this manuscript was supported by grants HL07180 and HL22934 from the U.S. Department of Health, Education, and Welfare.

Definitions of Quality

What Quality Isn't

So first to the definitional issue: What is quality? I have first to
say what it isn't. I do this because there are three widespread misconceptions revealed by my friends when I asked them what they
thought quality was. They commonly cited three things that I
thought it wasn't, so I feel obliged to deal with those first. It is not
the opposite of quantity. One of the first misperceptions about quality is that it is intangible. If the components of quality can be defined
and isolated, they can be measured. If it can be defined, it can be
counted. Quality is quantifiable.

The second misconception is that it is equated necessarily with
feelings or affect. Quality is not the opposite of science or technology.
There is a tendency to think of quality as the opposite of technique
or technology, but most of us would rather have a competent technician who is not too warm treat us medically than an incompetent
humanist. Literary comment has so concentrated on the dehumaniz-
ing aspects of modern medicine that we are inclined to assume quality is the art rather than the science side of medicine or professional practice.

Novelists, playwrights, and philosophers, when we turn to the
humanities for definitions of art and quality, provide us with a variety
of accounts of science and technology carried to extremes: Orwell's
1984, H. G. Wells's *Time Machine*, Crichton's *Andromeda Strain*
and *Terminal Man*. What is not found in the literature so clearly
are parallel accounts or dramatizations of what it would be like if
scientists, technicians, or health professionals carried their artistic
side to extremes, at the expense of their science, technology, or professional discipline. Without claiming a thorough review of the literature, I found only one study that fit my rigorous criteria of a prosaic
dramatization of how it might be if health professionals were over-
zealous in their concern for their art. In *Without Feathers*, Woody
Allen (1976) presents us with a brilliant counterposition of the artist
as a dentist (what could be more technical than dentistry?), and
the artist he picks is Vincent van Gogh (what could be more artistic
than the impressionist?). In this chapter of the book he places Vincent van Gogh in the splattered white coat of the dentist. Now to
understand Professor Allen's selection of van Gogh as his illustrative
dentist carrying art to excess, it might be worth recalling that the

real van Gogh of the nineteenth century was dismissed as an incompetent from his first job, then failed theological school in Amsterdam, then lost his faith trying unsuccessfully to communicate his religious convictions to miners, finding art as some, I fear, have found patient education. Meanwhile his younger brother, Theo, was succeeding in the art dealership where Vincent had failed. To add insult to injury, Theo ends up supporting Vincent. Here is Vincent as a dentist writing to his brother:

> Dear Theo,
> Will life never treat me decently? I am wracked by despair! My head is pounding! Mrs. Sol Schwimmer is suing me because I made her bridge as I felt it and not to fit her ridiculous mouth! That's right! I can't work to order like a common tradesman. I decided her bridge should be enormous and billowing, with wild explosive teeth flaring up in every direction like fire! Now she's upset because it won't fit in her mouth! She is so bourgeois and stupid, I want to smash her! I tried forcing the false plate in but it sticks out like a star burst chandelier. Still, I find it beautiful. She claims she can't chew! What do I care whether she can chew or not! Theo, I can't go on like this much longer! I asked Cezanne if he would share an office with me, but he is old and infirm and unable to hold the instruments and they must be tied to his wrists, but then he lacks accuracy and once inside the mouth, he knocks out more teeth than he saves. What to do?
>
> Vincent[1]

If quality is not the opposite of quantity and if it's not to be equated with feeling or affect, what is it in relation to outcomes? That is the third thing I have to distinguish it from. Quality is not equivalent to outcome, though it may be based on previous experiences with outcomes.

If outcomes are such things as decreased mortality and reduced morbidity, we can identify the factors that determine those outcomes, such as environmental, technological, organizational, and behavioral factors (Fig. 7-1). The inputs of health education, then, are those qualities of practice that are directed in patient education primarily at behavioral determinants and organizational factors. It is necessary to acknowledge also that other determinants of both the inputs and the outcomes of patient education are biological, genetic, political, economic, and cultural factors. But the important thing to emphasize

[1]From Woody Allen, *Without Feathers,* Copyright 1976 by Warner Books, Inc. Reprinted by permission of Mr. Allen.

here is that outcomes are health benefits that we measure in evaluation, or at least in terms of impact on behavioral changes or knowledge and attitude changes.

Figure 7-1.
Levels of concern and levels of evaluation in the causal chain influenced by patient education.

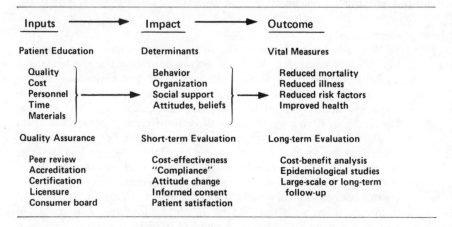

Quality has to do primarily with inputs. It is that distinction that I want to have you bear in mind as I proceed.

Five Approaches to Defining Quality

There are at least five alternative or complementary approaches to defining quality. There is, first, the *exclusionary approach* in which we define health education restrictively and then rule out everything that violates this definition. The definition that I prefer, for example, is that patient education is "any combination of learning experiences designed to facilitate voluntary adaptation of behavior conducive to health" (Green, 1978). If we define health education in that way, it becomes possible to exclude specific technologies, techniques, or inputs of health education practice when they violate the definition. Motivational techniques, patient counseling, mass communications through pamphlets and so forth, and behavior modification will fit this definition under some conditions and will not qualify as patient education under other conditions. By this exclusionary approach to quality we can identify those areas of motivational techniques, for example, that fail the definition of voluntary behavior change because they arouse excessive fear. Behavior modification techniques would qualify as appropriate patient education when the goals for the behavior to be modified are set by the patient. If the patient educator sets the goal for behavioral change without the informed consent of the patient, then behavior modification techniques would violate the condition of *"voluntary* adaptation of behavior" in the definition. Communications media are outside that definition of health education when they are used for commercial promotion. Patient counseling falls outside that definition when the patient is too emotionally distressed to make voluntary changes. This approach to defining quality, the exclusionary approach, leaves us without a sufficient specification of what to look for. We know what to rule out, but what do we consider appropriate qualities of patient education?

The second approach to a patient education definition of quality is the *problem checklist approach* in which we identify all the barriers to effective practice and then try to analyze each case of practice as to whether it makes these errors or deals with those barriers. This still leaves us without a clue of what quality education should be other than free of these problems.

The third approach to defining quality is the *prescriptive,* procedural, or less flatteringly, the cookbook approach. In this approach we identify the steps to be taken in most situations and then we require justification for departing from those steps. This approach is illustrated by the prescriptive suggestions offered by Richard Podell in his *Physicians' Guide to Compliance in Hypertension* (Podell, 1975). Podell's list is eminently reasonable, and I think this approach to defining quality is particularly appropriate for people who are not likely to have the background in either the technique or the science of education. If we can develop algorithms or protocols and standards that can be applied in different situations or if the range of patient characteristics and problems is sufficiently restricted, this approach to defining quality is most appropriate (Green & Brooks-Bertram, 1978). Unfortunately, this tends to restrict and constrain the self-respecting professional health educator and will stifle innovation and experimentation.

The fourth approach to defining quality is the *general principles,* or *process, approach.* In this approach we identify the essential characteristics of an educational process or of instructional programs, and we look for evidence in a given practice of patient education of these processes being adhered to or being implemented. Neufeld, in the first edition of Sackett and Haynes's *Compliance with Therapeutic*

Regimens, reviewed the literature on compliance studies where an educational strategy was being tested experimentally (Neufeld, 1976). He evoked five principles of learning: individualization, feedback, relevance, objectives, and motivation. He used these principles as criteria for judging the adequacy or, if you will, the quality of the patient education in each of these situations. He concluded that most of the sixteen studies reviewed lacked most of the criteria that one would apply in judging the quality of patient education. He found that the total scores out of a possible 10 on a scale for each criterion from 0 to 2, poor to good, were predominantly in the 3 and 4 range and none were greater than 6. Few studies provided sufficient individualization, for example. They came up even worse on some of the other four criteria. Most studies received scores of 0 or 1 on their application of most learning principles. D'Onofrio and one of her doctoral students have recently reviewed the same patient education studies and will be coming forth with a study that reanalyzes the research literature from a different perspective. The only drawback of this approach is that it often fails to make distinctions among the principles as to their relative importance in different situations, so that quality becomes dogma or religion. We develop schools of health education thought so that patient education becomes ritualized by the principles different people think are more or less important. Again, I would recommend this approach for noneducational specialists, but I would be cautious in applying it too rigorously to professionals, who ought to be able to make more critical judgments about the relative importance of these principles and exclude some of them sometimes if they are convinced they can get a more cost-effective outcome without compromising ethical principles.

The fifth approach—the one that I am most inclined to recommend—is the *diagnostic-experimenting approach* to health education (Green, Kreuter, Partridge, & Deeds, 1979; Green, Wang, Deeds et al., 1976). In this we prescribed a diagnostic procedure that assumes no particular characteristics of the educational content or methodology, but it does assume a scientific body of knowledge and a theoretical background available to assess the needed characteristics of the educational content depending on the goals and the circumstances in the situation. It starts with a body of systematized and specialized knowledge out of theory that enables a professional person to infer probable causes of the behavioral problem for a patient or clinical population. The concepts of education are then used to plan a series of actions relevant to the causes in a specific situation. The selection and application of specific methods and activities depends on the diagnosis of causes and the matching of methods appropriate to the factors extant in that patient or population. Philosophy also influences the practitioner, and documented practice helps to develop a philosophy for a discipline or a profession. Also, the practice, when it is experimentally and systematically pursued, contributes to the scientific base, which verifies, elaborates, and feeds back into this body of theoretical knowledge. The behavioral and biomedical sciences contribute to the practitioner's practice in the circular feedback cycle depicted in figure 7-2. It is this model of developing the

Figure 7-2.
The diagnostic-experimenting approach to quality in patient education.

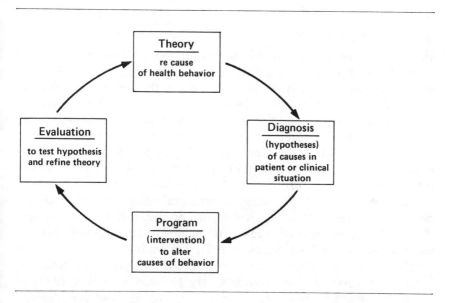

field of patient education that I would hope the next few years will allow us to pursue. More than anything else, this approach encourages making our assumption explicit, explaining why do we do what we do. Second, it encourages experimentation, and third, it encourages documentation.

In a particular model applying this approach (figure 7-3), the suggestion is that one first identify health outcomes and the risk factors that determine or represent those outcomes. Those risk factors become the medical control that is sought in self-care or medical practice. Second, one must identify the patient behaviors that contribute to those risk factors—the behavioral outcomes that will be sought in the evaluation of health education. Third, not necessarily in the categories shown in figure 7-3, one analyzes the factors that

Figure 7-3.
A diagnostic model for patient education (arrows indicate cause; numbers indicate diagnostic steps).

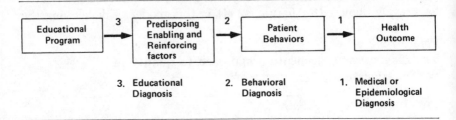

affect the behavior. I grouped them into these three categories for convenience. Predisposing factors refer to the availability and accessibility of resources and skills to carry out the behavior; and reinforcing factors refer to the things that determine whether or not the behavior will adhere once it is tried, depending on how much we support it or the reward it receives in the social environment.

This approach is problem-oriented; it identifies major determinants of health behavior; and it groups them according to the major strategies we use in health education practice to influence health behavior: (1) We employ communication directly with patients to influence their motivation or predisposition. (2) We employ training, community organization, and organizational development as educational strategies to influence enabling factors. (3) We employ indirect communications directed at parents, teachers, spouses, relatives, and employers to try to build a socially reinforcing environment for the behavior. By including all three strategies in a patient education program, we are more likely to be assured of affecting the behavior than if we include only one. So the third quality of this approach is that it emphasizes or at least draws attention to the need for directing patient education programs at multiple targets rather than at the patients alone.

Now let me suggest some definitions that I think grow out of this approach to quality assessment in patient education. I define *quality* as the appropriateness of a specific set of professional activities as performed in relation to the objectives they are intended to serve. I define *quality assurance* as long-range accountability for professional activities whereby consumers can know that they are appropriately performed. I define *quality control,* for these purposes, as the surveillance mechanism or procedure for producing evidence of quality.

Standards

Definitions

Standards are the minimum acceptable levels of performance used to judge the quality of professional preparation or practice. There are three types of standards that I think we implicitly use, if not explicity, and I think we ought to try harder to make them explicit. There are, first, *historical standards.* That is what we use implicitly when we ask how does our practice now compare with practices in the past. For this we lean on experience and evaluative evidence of appropriate practices in the past.

The second type of standard used in judging quality is a *normative standard.* Looking around the country or your region at the practice of your peers, you may well ask "Is my practice as good as theirs?" or "Am I doing all the things that my colleagues believe to be appropriate in the practice of patient education?" One approach to this at an institutional level is the survey conducted by Lee and her colleagues at the American Hospital Association, in which the norms of the mid-seventies for hospital-based patient education around the country are described statistically (American Hospital Association, 1977).

The third standard implicitly utilized in defining quality is a *theoretical standard.* This is the standard we apply when we suggest how it ought to be done if we were really applying what we understand today from theory and from previous research about what ought to work in patient education.

Applying Standards to Quality Control

Quality control in patient education can be illustrated by contrasting two of the models for defining quality that were presented before: the prescriptive approach and the diagnostic-experimenting approach.

In the prescriptive approach there are four problems. First of all, the lists become tediously long and too detailed for most practitioners. If we try to be thorough and specific about what people ought to do in different situations, the lists become multiple, overly detailed, cumbersome, and less likely to be used.

The second problem is that the prescriptive approach tends to ignore the motivational aspect of the professional's effort. McQueen analyzed what happens in the diffusion of a new practice among physicians or health professionals, noting particularly the importance of the motivational and attitudinal factors at several points: the acceptance of risk factors or the importance of the specific health behavior in question, belief in his or her ability to alter the risk factors or the behavior, desire to alter, communication of strong messages in his or her or patient education, and then finally diffusion to the community of other physicians (McQueen, 1975). Prescription is not enough. Along with prescription for patient education has to go a great deal of professional motivation to use the instructions or guidelines, particularly if the prescriptions for practice are going to be complex and directed at busy, overworked, or skeptical practitioners.

The third problem with the prescriptive approach in quality control in the practice of patient education is that it tends to get translated too literally and perfunctorily into information for patients. The most salient example of this is the patient package insert that has been besieged by every type of health professional who wants to get her or his message about a given drug into the patient package insert. These are now mandated by law. They will be included in all packages of estrogen dispensed to patients. Doctors, lawyers, and nurses, and many professional associations are trying to get their message into these patient package inserts, with the consequence that people are unable to read them or, if they do, they are frightened to death by all of the information on possible side effects. Prescribing educational content on a mass scale results in information that is too unintelligible for half the population and too boring or too frightening for the other half.

The fourth problem with the prescriptive approach is that the objectives of professionals keep changing. They make prescribed procedures obsolete rather fast. Unless you have a team of monks and scribes constantly revising these prescriptive approaches, they quickly fall out of date; and practitioners either apply them ritualistically or they abandon them.

The diagnostic-experimental approach, on the other hand, develops a model of the behavior more explicitly and then sets patient education aims in relation to the model or hypothesized cause-and-effect relationships. Ideally, though not essentially in all cases, the diagnosis consists of some kind of survey. From the diagnostic baseline survey, an inventory of behavioral problems for the patient population is generated. Out of that, measurable objectives can be established, and from that we get program planning, program implementation, and then a resurvey with the results of the resurvey providing evaluation that goes back into a redefinition of the inventory of problems.

This is an idealistic model of the diagnostic-experimenting approach. It is not always critical that a survey be done or even that measurements take place. One can approach the same kind of problem diagnostically, but rather than having data per se, a qualitative or logical analysis of the situation can be just as helpful. For example when we were trying to solve the problem of broken appointments in the Johns Hopkins outpatient clinics, we looked at the broken appointment problem as a cycle where broken appointments resulted in inefficient use of staff time, which resulted in overscheduling of appointments, which resulted in increased waiting time, which resulted in patient dissatisfaction, and thereby more broken appointments and inadequate care. Figure 7-4 shows the direct cycle as well

Figure 7-4.
The broken appointment cycle.

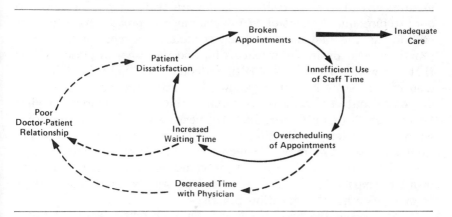

as some indirect spinoffs that have particular relevance for patient education. The overscheduling of appointments, besides resulting in increased waiting time, also resulted in decreased time with the physician so that the patient's brief encounter with the physician became even briefer. That resulted in a poor patient-doctor relationship, which resulted in more patient dissatisfaction and more broken appointments. The overscheduling of appointments also, through increased waiting time, resulted in an irate patient whose interaction with the doctor then went badly. The doctor reacted and the exchange resulted in further deterioration of the doctor-patient relationship, more patient dissatisfaction, and more broken appointments. This kind of diagnostic approach makes the behavioral model explicit, and then out of that explicit model one can design interventions. Watching those interventions in relationship to the explicit organizational and behavioral points enables one over time to adapt practice and improve on it (Green, Levine, Wolle, & Deeds, 1979).

In short, the prescriptive approach imposes predefined standards of practice on a situation in which they may not be wholly appropriate to the circumstances and the population in which patient education is being planned or practiced. The diagnostic approach formulates new standards as hypotheses to be tested experimentally and refined or adapted systematically.

Measuring Quality

Now I venture some approaches to measurement of quality, quality assurance, and quality control. There are three steps, I believe, to approaching quality control as a developmental process over the next decade. As the first step we need to determine which professional practices yield desirable outcomes for specific types of patients. For that we want to evaluate health outcomes and behavioral impact. You can consider impact on knowledge, attitudes, and behavior as outcomes, but the medical community thinks of outcomes in vital terms such as reduced mortality. To measure mortality or morbidity we need long-term evaluation or very large samples. For those patient education programs in which the epidemiologic or medical evidence linking behavior to health outcomes is firm, it is sufficient to evaluate impact in terms of increased patient behavior that results from specific health education practices.

We need as the first step in developing quality assurance to fill the gaps in the literature with clinical trials of health education or patient education in order to develop better knowledge of what educational practices influence behavior in the ways that we intend. Cost-effectiveness analysis is one type of such evaluation. As a second step we then need to define quality in terms of those practices known to yield the best results. Those will become our standards. That is what is commonly called process as opposed to outcome. Professional practice is the best indicator of process. Quality assurance is the mechanism we use to evaluate it, and peer review is one example of an approach to doing so (see fig. 7-1). After we define quality in terms of practices known to yield the best results, we need to set up procedures to monitor the quality of patient education practice in terms of the standard set in step two. We can do this through peer review, record audit, and staff conferences.

We have accumulated already a very substantial body of literature that addresses step one, determining which professional practices yield desirable behavior or outcomes to specific types of patients. Hulka, for example, recently showed that communication, however it is measured, correlates with three types of patient errors in taking their medication: errors of omission, errors of commission, and errors of scheduling. All three are more extensive when the communication is low than when it is high (Hulka, Kupper, Cassel et al., 1975). That is the most obvious and simplistic statement of what I mean by step one. If we can then concretize what we operationally define as communication for specific types of patients, we will have taken a large step toward quality assurance and quality control.

A series of studies in hypertension have gone through this kind of process, however unintentionally. Williamson (Williamson, Aronovich, & Simonson, 1975) developed an approach to quality assurance in medical practice in which he and his colleagues first got together a group of doctors who practiced together and set priorities with them. They conducted initial outcome assessments in relation to those priorities, and then they obtained a definitive assessment of their practice. They then conducted continuing education for the physicians; then looked again at the outcomes. He calls this "health accounting," which is a quality assurance process in practice.

Williamson got the physicians to estimate what they expected if they were practicing correctly, if they were doing good patient education, and they agreed they should get no more than 5 percent who could not achieve blood pressure control. When they did the baseline assessment, they found that 36 percent of their patients were not under blood pressure control. They then conducted the continuing education directed at the physicians' patient education skills that reduced to 19 percent the patients who were not under blood pressure control. In a second round of studies he did the same thing, but he added a patient educator with minimum educational background but trained specifically to deal with hypertension patients. He obtained an even better improvement in blood pressure among those educated by the patient educator (Williamson et al., 1975).

Inui followed Williamson's approach but directed his efforts at tutorials for the physicians to improve their patient education practices. He set certain criteria about what should constitute quality patient education practice. One of his criteria was that physicians ought to be more realistic as to how extensive the patient compliance problem is. They ought to be able to make more realistic assessments of how many of their patients are not taking their pills, not adhering to their diets, and not keeping their appointments. As a result of his tutorial approach, educating the physician, he did achieve a significant improvement in the percentage of physicians who more correctly estimated that their patients were not taking their pills, not adhering to their diets, and not keeping their appointments (Inui, Yourtee, & Williamson, 1976).

The second standard or criterion that Inui used to test physician behaviors in the quality of patient education practice was that they would dedicate more of their time, proportionally, to educating the patient as opposed to physical examination and interim history taking. Now this, of course, applies to a patient population that previously has had rather thorough physical examinations and histories so that interim history taking is really just a medical ritual that avoids talking to the patient. He got a very significant improvement in the percentage of the time spent on patient education in the experimental group of physicians compared with control, at the expense of time taken in histories and physical examinations.

The third standard or criterion of quality control that Inui employed was that the physicians should make more chart notations about patient education and about behavior. Again, significant improvement was obtained through his educational process in the percentage of charts on which physicians noted dietary recommendations, patient compliance, patient understanding of hypertension, and patient education. There was also significant improvement in the percentage of physicians who were making notes about patient education in the charts.

Another criterion Inui used was that there should be some improvement in the patients' knowledge, attitudes, and beliefs. On a variety of different criteria of knowledge and attitudes, he obtained significant improvements in the patterns of the tutored physicians. Finally he thought that he should expect patient behavior to improve as a result of this educational program. Indeed it did, at least for taking the pills. It did improve between experimental and control groups significantly. It did not improve in relation to diet adherence and keeping appointments. The bottom line was that he achieved very substantial increases in blood pressure control as a result of this intervention. The patients whose physicians did receive the tutorials showed significantly greater improvements in blood pressure control. Thus, quality in patient education can be defined in measurable terms, can be improved measurably, and such improvements can have a significant influence on health outcomes (Inui et al., 1976).

We then followed this experience at Hopkins with another diagnostic-experimental approach to patient education. On the basis of a diagnostic-baseline survey with hypertension patients, we identified the sources of compliance problems that might be amenable to educational change. This baseline survey, conducted during the period that the National High Blood Pressure Program had been going on, found that while the Hopkins patients still had some misconceptions about hypertension, by and large they were much more knowledgeable about the disease in general, about the disease process, and about the sequelae of the disease; and the nursing and medical staff were more knowledgeable than they were when Inui conducted his study there eighteen months earlier. The patients already held positive attitudes and most of their beliefs and attitudes seemed to be in place. Side effects and costs, which we heard were big problems for hypertension patients, were not cited as major reasons for noncompliance by the patients themselves. There may be a denial process here, but we could not get them to admit that side effects or costs were a problem; none of them was correlated with compliance. We were left in a stalemate as to where to go from there.

Our revised plan, then, was not to go directly back to the medical staff with information from the baseline survey, because we did not know what we could tell them that would improve their practice (Green, Levine, & Deeds, 1975). Rather, we squeezed out of those data some hypotheses as to what might be the problem for these patients and then conducted a series of experimental interventions ourselves.

The first experimental intervention was the patient exit review, an interview in which we try to help patients clarify the specifics about their own regimens in relation to home environment. While the patients were highly knowledgeable about hypertension in general, they were confused about some of the specifics of their own regimen. This intervention took place immediately after patients had seen the doctor. We had the doctor just check on a small sheet what he or she had prescribed, and we went over that prescription with the patients in relation to their own home situations. We used clocks and calendars as visual aids to help the patients get their pill regimens straight in relation to their daily routine (Green, Levine, Wolle, & Deeds, 1979).

The second experimental intervention was a home visit in which we were trying to develop some kind of family support, some reinforcement in the home environment, by talking to a family member about the importance and problems of medication, diet, and appointment keeping for the patient, and ways the family member could help the patient with these things (Levine, Green, Chwalow et al., 1979). The third intervention was a series of small group meetings in which we were trying to develop a sense of confidence in the patients' ability to achieve blood pressure control.

The basis for these interventions was that (1) the patients were confused about their own regimens even though they were knowledgeable about the disease—hence the exit interview; (2) they did not feel that they had very much sympathy or encouragement or support from family or friends in taking pills—hence the home visit; and (3) they seemed to be frustrated by their efforts to adhere to their diets and their medication regimens, so we thought that we could work with them in small groups on developing a greater sense of control (Green, Levine, Wolle, & Deeds, 1979). The interventions achieved a substantial improvement in blood pressure control, comparing the control group with all the experimental groups. The experimental group who received the combination of an exit interview and a home visit had the best improvement in blood pressure control (Levine, Green, Chwalow et al., 1979).

Quality in this case was defined by the diagnostic-baseline survey, which allowed us to determine the most appropriate educational interventions for this specific patient population at this specific time. A diagnostic approach to patient education planning could assure quality more generally, even without universal standards of quality.

Self-care and Quality of Patient Education

One other dimension of quality in patient education relates not so much to practice as to the preparation and participation of the patient in the process of care. This relates to the self-care issues Levin discusses in chapter 11. The quality of patient education might be improved by stimulating or activating the patient to take more initiative in the clinical setting.

Roter (1977) carried out her dissertation research on education of the reticent patient to ask the questions he or she needs to ask in order to clarify the regimen or to reduce anxiety. Her hypothesis was that, if the patients asked more questions, they would get more answers and that the doctor is more likely to initiate information that he or she knows the patient wants to have. Roter carried out an educational diagnosis to identify the determinants of question asking. The predisposing factors she identified included belief in the acceptability of asking questions, the value placed on health, the salience of the question, and the expectations for information. The enabling factors she identified were their ability to articulate questions and their ability to recall questions in the presence of the provider. Feedback from the question-asking process was expected to result in some reinforcement such as encouragement by the doctor to ask questions, receiving answers, reduced anxiety from the increased information, and increased satisfaction from the information.

Roter then designed a patient education intervention in the waiting room where she talked with individual patients, drawing out their problems and questions they were not likely to ask unless the doctor were to evoke them. She wrote the questions down for them and she tried to convince them that it was very acceptable for them to ask these questions. The patients then went into the examining room with the physician, and the result was that a statistically significant improvement in the percentage of questions was achieved. Now the one problem here is that we are in a transition period of history with this kind of quality assurance method. If we are going to create assertive patients, we have to expect some blacklash. In fact Roter found that, while patient question asking increased, patient satisfaction did not increase. The patients came out somewhat atremble. She tape-recorded the sessions with the doctors' and patients' permission; with a content analysis of the interaction in the sessions, she found that the patients who had received the experimental treatment were involved in somewhat more acrimonious exchange with the physician. On the other hand she did improve the behavioral outcome of appointment keeping. The experimental group patients were more likely to come back for the next appointment than the control group who asked fewer questions (Roter, 1977).

Summary

The foregoing definitions and series of examples suggest an approach to the development of quality assurance over time. We cannot expect to impose standards based on the current inadequate coordination of the limited information available upon compulsory quality assurance mechanisms in patient education. But we can expect, I think, to develop over time some estimates of what kinds of practices do work best, to develop standards out of those practices, and ultimately to apply quality assurance mechanisms using these standards to the process of diagnosing patient education needs and planning patient education programs.

The practitioner will be concerned with the availability of standardized measurement tools. There are some available, but not as many as there should be. We need to develop the instrumentation in this area. If a review of the literature fails to turn up an appropriate measurement tool for the given practice situation, improvisation is in order.

In conclusion I have suggested that quality can be defined in a general framework of appropriateness of patient education practice in relation to the objectives to be served. This allows for a variable standard or range of expectations to be applied to different types of practitioners according to the role they can best play in patient education with their position in medical care and with their own professional and technical knowledge. I have also suggested that quality can be measured, and thereby controlled or assured, in questionnaires, record keeping, audits, and ultimately, we might hope, in peer review.

However primitive our own theories and measurement tools may be, a concern with quality in patient education can only grow because it is becoming more and more central to medical care. As patient education becomes less peripheral, it will become an integral part of quality assurance of medical care so that, if we are not ready with the standards and criteria for patient education, somebody else will define them for us and their standards rather than ours will be built into quality assurance mechanisms. The need for evaluation of patient education methods and strategies is therefore more urgent as the pressure for standards and quality assurance increases.

References

Allen, W. *Without feathers.* New York: Warner Books, 1976.

American Hospital Association. *Hospital inpatient education: Survey findings and analyses, 1975.* Atlanta: U.S. Public Health Service Center for Disease Control, Bureau of Health Education, 1977.

Green, L. W. Determining the impact and effectiveness of health education as it relates to federal policy. *Health Education Monographs,* 1978, *6* (Suppl.) 28, 66.

Green, L. W. Health education policy and the placement of responsibility for personal health care. *Family and Community Health,* Vol. II(3): Fall, 1979.

Green, L. W., & Brooks-Bertram, P. Peer review and quality control in health education. *Health Values,* 1978, *2,* 191, 197.

Green, L. W., Kreuter, M. W., Partridge, K. B., & Deeds, S. G. *Health education planning: A diagnostic approach.* Palo Alto: Mayfield, 1979.

Green, L. W., Levine, D. M., & Deeds, S. G. Clinical trials of health education for hypertensive outpatients. *Preventive Medicine,* 1975, *4,* 417, 425.

Green, L. W., Levine, D. M., Wolle, J., & Deeds, S. The development of randomized patient education experiments with urban poor hypertensives. *Patient Counseling and Health Education,* 1979, *1,* 106, 111.

Green, L. W., Wang, V. L., Deeds, S., et al. *Guidelines for health education components of maternal and child health programs* (Prepared under Grant No. MCT-001032-01 from the Bureau of Community Health Services, USDHEW, Rockville, Md., 1976.

Hulka, B. S., Kupper, L. L., Cassel, J. C., et al. Doctor patient communication and outcomes among diabetic patients. *Journal of Community Health,* 1975, *1,* 15, 27.

Inui, T. S., Yourtee, E. L., Williamson, J. W. Improved outcomes in hypertension and physician tutorials: A controlled trial. *Annals of Internal Medicine,* 1976, *84,* 646.

Levine, D. M., Green, L. W., Chwalow, A. J., et al. Clinical and behavioral effects of randomized health education trials with hypertensive patients. *Journal of American Medical Association,* 1979, *214(16),* 1700, 1703.

McQueen, D. V. Diffusion of heart disease risk factors to health professionals. In H. Enelow & J. B. Henderson (Eds.), *Applying behavioral science to cardiovascular risk.* New York: American Heart Association, 1975.

Neufeld, V. R. Patient education: A critique. In D. E. Sackett & R. B. Haynes (Eds.), *Compliance with therapeutic regimens.* Baltimore: Johns Hopkins University Press, 1976.

Podell, R. N. *Physicians' guide to compliance in hypertension.* Rahway, N. J.: Merck, 1975.

Roter, D. L. Patient participation in the patient-provider interaction. *Health Education Monograph,* 1977, *5,* 281, 315.

Williamson, J. W., Aronovich, S. and Simonson, L. Health accounting: An outcome-based system of quality assurance. *Bulletin New York Academy of Medicine,* 1975, *51,* 727.

8

Evaluating Patient Education: Purposes, Politics, and a Proposal for Practitioners

Carol N. D'Onofrio

Pressures to evaluate patient education are increasing apace with rapid expansion of the field itself. As with any social phenomenon that captures the attention of people who play widely diverse roles in different institutions, patient education promises to meet many needs. The arguments are now familiar: Through education, patients will make more timely and appropriate use of health resources, assume more responsibility for the management of disease, and adopt health practices that protect health and avoid preventable illness or complications. These changes, in turn, are expected to result in increased patient satisfaction, better use of provider time, fewer hospital admissions, and shorter hospital stays, thereby helping to control rising health care costs. Evaluation is required to determine whether, in fact, patient education leads to these results.

To the extent that patient education can be shown to produce desired outcomes, more support for programs can be expected. On the other hand failure to find positive evidence leads to further questions: Is the fundamental rationale for patient education wrong? Were the techniques of evaluation at fault, or was the evaluated program itself somehow flawed? Further evaluation is indicated, although clearly it must focus on the validity of program assumption and the nature of educational inputs as well as effects. What was the basis for predicting that certain interventions would produce particular results? Was the educational problem analyzed adequately in terms of patient needs and characteristics? Did the combination of educational messages, methods, and communicators reach the intended audience in a way conducive to learning and change? Did experiences with health care delivery and other factors in the system contribute to or detract from the achievement of educational goals?

Such evaluation, of course, need not wait for the program to be terminated. Questions about the effectiveness of educational inputs can—and should—be asked during the formulation of an educational plan and throughout its implementation, in order to correct incipient problems before they irrevocably damage chances of program success. Formative or progress evaluation is particularly important in education where so many variables influence learner response and where so much insight can be gained through teacher-learner interaction in the educational process. In this respect, patient education shares an essential characteristic of all direct health care, that is, patient reactions must be monitored continuously throughout the treatment process so that adjustments can be made as necessary to assure the best possible outcomes.

Evaluation thus may address a variety of questions and it may be applied at various points in time (Roberts, 1962). Exactly which questions we ask and the methods we use will depend on our reasons for undertaking evaluation at all. Similarly our purposes will influence our selection of evaluation criteria and the standards we set for success. In initiating evaluation, then, our first task is to clarify what it is that we wish to evaluate—and why.

Here we may hypothesize that reasons for concern with the evaluation of patient education differ according to responsibilities within the health care system (Van Maanen, 1973; Weiss, 1972) and that as a consequence certain issues have emerged that must be resolved if the field as a whole is to progress. With few exceptions the current push for evaluation has come not from patient education practitioners but rather from administrators, legislators, and third-party payers, as well as from faculty in academic institutions. Both the need for evaluative data and the methodologies through which such data should be obtained have been heavily emphasized, but the purposes to be served by evaluation seldom have been discussed.

Textbooks, of course, point out that the purpose of program evaluation is to contribute to decision making (Van Maanen, 1973), but when practitioners have not participated in identifying the decisions to be made, they can only speculate about the alternatives being considered and ways in which evaluative data will be used. Resulting ambiguities are compounded by awareness of the political dynamics permeating health care delivery and the tenuous toehold of patient education in the system.

In the face of such uncertainties some practitioners have found their own reasons for undertaking program evaluation. Others, however, have resisted externally imposed demands, citing both methodological and political reasons. Methodological issues have been addressed in detail (Green 1974, 1975, 1977; Green & Figa-Talamanca, 1974); hence this chapter explores the political problem, considering in particular the major evaluative question being asked about patient education to date.

Can Patient Education Help to Control Health Care Costs?

This question is paramount for anyone concerned with health care financing, including health agency administrators, hospital trustees, third-party payers, and legislators. Indeed the potential of patient education for controlling costs has been largely responsible for generating such widespread interest in the subject.

The need to demonstrate both the cost benefits and the cost effectiveness of patient education has been stated frequently. Unfortunately these terms are often used interchangeably, adding to the confusion resulting from different technical approaches to each type of evaluation and certain elements that they have in common. In either case, estimating the costs of program inputs is essential. In cost-benefit evaluation, these costs (often plus the costs of foregone opportunities to which program resources might have been directed) are compared with the economic value of program effects. Cost-effectiveness evaluation does not place a dollar value on program outcomes but rather simply estimates the cost of achieving a given effect. This assists decision makers by indicating the returns they can expect from a certain investment of resources, especially when cost-effectiveness data are available for alternative possibilities. Ultimately, however, the use of cost-effectiveness evaluation in decision making about resource allocation also requires reaching a quantitative judgment about how much anticipated program outcomes are worth (Andrieu, 1977).

A growing number of studies evidence that patient education can lead to improved patient recovery, reductions in hospital days, lowered hospital readmission rates, and fewer visits to emergency rooms and outpatient facilities (e.g., Avery, Green, & Kreider, 1972; Egbert, Battit, Welch, & Bartlett, 1964; Healy, 1968; Levine & Britten, 1973; Lindeman & Van Aernam, 1971; Miller & Goldstein, 1972; Rosenberg, 1971). If cost control is our central concern in evaluating patient education, these findings are impressive. Nevertheless, in most reports the costs of educational intervention have not been assessed and so both cost benefits and cost effectiveness must be inferred. In addition, more evaluations are needed to determine whether the results can be replicated with different patients, with different conditions, and in different settings. Systematic variations in educational approach are also needed to discover whether alternative methods can achieve similar or better outcomes with a smaller investment of resources—a question relating to cost-efficiency.

Further, a good deal of evaluative work is needed to test the extent to which patient education may achieve other effects with cost-savings potential. Drawing together evidence from many sources, Green (1976) has suggested that patient education can help to control costs through bringing about more appropriate utilization of health care resources in a variety of ways. These include not only reducing emergency room visits, hospital stays, and readmission rates, but increasing the capacity of patients for self-care, improving and speeding diagnosis, and reducing broken appointment rates. Further cost-controlling potentials of patient education discussed by Green are reductions in unpaid bills and malpractice suits, and increased community support for hospital programs. To these may be added more efficient use of provider time, lowered staff turnover rates resulting from improved morale, and more effective coordination and utilization of community resources.

In his suggestion that the cost benefits of patient education be compared with alternative health services, Green identified yet another approach to evaluation:

> . . . when the choice is between investing marginal capital in expanded pulmonary surgical facilities and investing in smoking cessation clinics, the cost benefits are compelling. Even if the success rate in smoking cessation clinics is "only" 20 percent, it compares very favorably with lung surgery success rates of less than 10 percent; the costs are lower per case, and the long-term economic benefits are far greater for the younger smoker who quits than for the older lung cancer victim whose lung is successfully removed. (Green, 1976)

A more recent example of such cost-comparative evaluation concerns kidney dialysis: In home dialysis where the well-trained patient essentially treats himself, the cost of one treatment is approximately

$43, while the average hospital treatment costs about $159. Over the period of a year, expenditures for three weekly dialysis maintenance treatments would amount to just under $7,000 in the home and $24,700 in the hospital ("Dialysis Is Cheaper at Home," 1977). The difference clearly provides a generous margin within which to provide kidney patients with the training necessary to perform home dialysis while still demonstrating substantial cost savings.

Now obviously these possibilities for evaluation of patient education have differing degrees of appeal for different providers, depending on anticipated economic consequences. Thus while third-party payers may be enthusiastic about lowering hospital utilization rates, it is not at all clear that this would be to the advantage of hospitals whose budgets are based on bed occupancy rates. Similarly, investment in smoking cessation clinics rather than expanded surgical facilities may be cost beneficial to the insurer and the insured, but it is likely to be detrimental to the hospital whose financial structure depends on attracting surgeons and their patients to the operating suite. By considering what is at stake for the physician in private practice, we may also anticipate receptivity to patient education aimed at reducing broken appointments but possible resistance to an educational program in self-care.

Assessing the cost benefits of patient education therefore involves much more than application of a simple formula, for each of the potential outcomes we have discussed will have different costs for different actors in the health care system, and these will influence the value each attributes to effects. The equation is further complicated in that values other than dollars enter in, including concern with quality of care and patient rights.

Why Evaluate the Costs of Patient Education?

The predominant emphasis on the need to evaluate the cost benefits and cost effectiveness of patient education has overshadowed concern with other evaluative questions that might be asked about the role of education in health care delivery. Similarly, although the major literature on methods for evaluating patient education (Green, 1974, 1975, 1977; Green & Figa-Talamanca, 1974) clearly recognizes that a variety of outcomes may be measured, the economic orientation of this work implicitly defines costs as the primary issue.

Because this focus suggests that patient education must be justified in terms of its ability to effect cost savings, this thrust has evoked a cool, if not outspokenly critical, response from those who see the need to educate patients for other reasons. Thus health professionals who regard education as both a fundamental patient right and an essential dimension of quality care view the costs of patient education as a secondary concern. Their interests in the outcomes of the education also differ. Accordingly they ask why should reductions in the use of health care services be the criterion? Why not rather evaluate the extent to which education improves understanding of health status, leads to more timely diagnosis and treatment of disease, contributes to informed decisions in selecting from health care options, reduces pain and anxiety surrounding illness, teaches patients the skills they need to participate in the treatment process, and organizes family and community resources to these ends?

By stressing the need to demonstrate the economic advantages of patient education, advocates of cost-benefit and cost-effectiveness evaluation have tended to slight these humanistic issues. This inevitably has given rise to speculation about their motives, regardless of how humanistic these actually may be. Suspicions have been heightened by the observation that demands to evaluate the costs of patient education have not been accompanied by pressures for similar scrutiny of other aspects of health care. Why should this be so?

As Knutson (1959) observed two decades ago, values influence evaluation in many ways, including our selection of what is to be evaluated and our motives in undertaking evaluation at all. More recently Fein (1975) pointed out that "economics and public policy are not merely technical affairs, but relate to values." Similarly Van Maanen (1973) has observed that "the system for attaching values to facts is, fundamentally, a political one and it is inherently a part of any program evaluation environment." Accordingly we may ask what values and motives underly the current emphasis on the need to evaluate the costs of patient education. What different purposes might this serve? Four alternatives come to mind:

1. *Determining whether to support patient education programs.* The problems of health care financing cannot be avoided. In an economy of scarce dollars and escalating health care expenditures, competition for resources is great. Those charged with resource allocation therefore need some basis for determining which programs to initiate, expand, curtail, or cancel. In addition those responsible for cash flow and balancing the books must know not only what savings might accrue through patient education, but also what investments this will require.

Moreover as taxpayers and purchasers of health insurance, it behooves us all to seek reasonable justification for spending on medical care. Public demand for fiscal responsibility has accelerated with rising expenditures, resulting in a general increase in emphasis on program evaluation and accountability. Pressures to evaluate patient education can be understood partially in this context. Additionally, as Thorner (1971) has discussed, program evaluation becomes of special interest when change is introduced, and certainly the organization of patient education programs involves changes of many types and levels.

Demands for cost-effectiveness evaluation therefore do not necessarily reflect a crass preoccupation with dollars at the expense of human values. Likewise, cost-benefit evaluation can be an important tool for coming to grips with some of society's most pressing problems. Even those most deeply dedicated to social improvements must find ways to implement their vision or else remain but dreamers. This requires considering money.

Given the paucity of existing data on both the costs and the effects of patient education, more evaluation clearly is required, but this of course cannot be accomplished unless there are more programs to evaluate. The operational dilemma thus becomes how to obtain support for such programs if funding sources require more evaluative data first. Such a dead-center situation suggests a second purpose that demands for evaluating patient education may serve.

2. *Delaying development of patient education programs.* Education has long been recognized as a source of power, for knowledge is power, as is the ability and confidence to apply it in problem solving. Fulfilling the promise of patient education therefore would have a profound impact on the present health care system. Small-scale shifts in power are already becoming apparent in new provider relationships with patients who are "activated" and aware of their rights, as opposed to passively dependent in the sick role (Reeder, 1972).

Larger, less predictable changes can be expected as patients who are prepared to take increased responsibility for their own health begin to raise fundamental questions about the ways in which health care institutions are organized and governed, and to challenge existing patterns of health care delivery (Johnson, 1972). In addition, reductions in hospital days and other potential effects of patient education would drastically alter requirements for primary and acute care facilities, specialized types of health-care providers, and health insurance coverage, thus shaking existing centers of political, economic, and academic power.

Those who stand to lose by these changes therefore may be threatened by accelerating interest in patient education. If so, one strategy for hindering the development of patient education programs without revealing vested interests is to endorse the concept in principle, while apologetically stating that economic pressures are too severe to justify the investment of resources in such endeavors until further evidence of cost benefits and cost effectiveness has been provided. This is particularly clever because the potential scope of patient education and the limited data now available make it possible to identify more needs for evaluation than can be met for years to come. Further, as stated in the Fogarty Task Force Report on Health Promotion and Consumer Health Education (*Preventive Medicine U.S.A.*, 1976), "there will never be a time when 'all the data are in,' since the whole context of American society is constantly in flux."

Viewing the demands for evaluation of patient education so cynically suggests yet another purpose that emphasis on its economic aspects may serve.

3. *Diverting attention from other issues.* As expressed succinctly in a popular cliché, the health care system is in crisis. Pressures for change are coming from multiple directions. As stated in the Fogarty Task Force Report:

> . . . the widespread evidence of patient noncompliance with prescribed regimens; the growing evidence of unnecessary surgery and overmedication; the increasing realization that technical virtuosity is not necessarily synonymous with effective care; the repeated exposés of miserable care in many nursing homes now expensively reimbursed under Medicare and Medicaid; the growing public demand for more attention to the humanities and amenities of death and dying and the renewed interest in euthanasia . . . all indicate the public's growing impatience with overemphasis on the technology of medicine and neglect of the patient as a responsible agent in the treatment of his or her own illness. (*Preventive Medicine U.S.A.*, 1976)

The ferment generated by these events is stirred to still greater proportions by the spector of national health insurance, increasing regulatory requirements, the trend toward litigation to resolve disputes, and many other factors. Clearly the crisis in health is moving us toward major social change. Resistance and counterpressures are inevitable.

One form that resistance may take is the creation of a red herring to divert attention away from the central issues. Patient education can serve this fishy purpose well, for the concept is quickly recognized as worthy and deserving of support. At the same time, there is much misunderstanding and confusion about the term, many disciplines and territories are involved, and a sufficiently wide range of goals and philosophies is represented to generate a lot of hot discussion.

Given these elements, diversionary tactics are relatively simple: Spend a few dollars on small-scale projects to create the illusion of change (Geiger, 1975), while hinting at the possibility of major, long-term funding. The resulting scramble for elusive resources will in itself successfully distract a number of change agents from the central issues; however, as Knutson (1959) has pointed out, evaluation can also be used for this purpose. Therefore the powerful can further concentrate and sustain activity around the side issue of patient education by requiring evidence of cost savings as a condition for making good on promises of support. Concern with the economics of patient education not only adds credibility to expressions of interest but effectively buys time. Thus the appearance of serious intent can be maintained indefinitely with only token investments pending the results of evaluative studies.

A complementary strategy for rechanneling energies aimed at reform is to inflate the potential impact of patient education and to nourish the unrealistic expectation that herein lies the panacea for all the system's ills. By forcing premature and rigorous evaluation, it then can be concluded that patient education is neither a miracle cure nor even a readily applied technological solution. Should positive findings emerge despite unfavorable circumstances, the need for more sweeping changes and bolder solutions can always be dramatized. On this cue, patient education can be relegated to the ranks of unsuccessful experiments, and a new diversionary tactic can then be introduced with appropriate fervor and fanfare.

To participate in the evaluation of patient education within this context is to offer it up as a sacrificial lamb, or in Somer's (1975) words, "to commit statistical harakiri." Whether evaluation would indeed have this effect or would result in greater support for patient education programs is a source of contention among those sincerely dedicated to meeting patients' educational needs. While the question is real, the debate can be destructive in that it adds fuel to the fire of a side issue.

4. *Learning and change.* A fourth purpose to be served by evaluating patient education is that of learning and change. Thus by analyzing the results of their efforts, health professionals can gain new insights leading to continued improvement of their performance.

In discussing various reasons for evaluating health education, Roberts (1962) gave priority to evaluation for this purpose, suggesting that "we evaluate primarily to study the effects of practice so that we can turn our findings back into practice and improve it and, at the same time, strengthen the scientific basis of practice."

Certainly those committed to fostering education in health, including patient education practitioners, have a special obligation to engage in evaluation of this type, which is itself educational. Nevertheless because such evaluation is intended to assess and improve the quality of professional intervention, it may not be readily apparent how this can be achieved through investigations of cost-benefit and cost-effectiveness relationships. Although data on the effects of patient education clearly are essential to identify areas of practice needing improvement, as previously pointed out, not all outcomes of patient education can—or should—be evaluated in terms of the costs required to achieve them. Moreover, evaluating the costs of education provides few clues for increasing educational effectiveness. Rather what is needed is information about the patient's learning needs and variables in the educational process so that judgments about the appropriateness and adequacy of intervention can be made.

In addition, one must question whether an emphasis on cost-effectiveness evaluation, with the inherent implications that results will be used to determine program funding, is compatible with the supportive climate under which open and honest evaluations of professional performance can best be conducted. This, of course, is related to the larger issue of whether cost-effectiveness evaluation undertaken for purposes of improving patient education would, in fact, be used to undermine it.

Evaluating the cost benefits and the cost effectiveness of patient education therefore would appear to be of limited value in fostering professional growth and change. At the same time, other purposes that such evaluation may serve implicitly question the need for education as an integral part of quality health care. As a consequence practitioners would seem to have little incentive for engaging in cost-related studies.

Despite these problems, to ignore or resist demands for cost-effectiveness data places patient educators on the defensive—hardly an advantageous position from which to win the support of administrators, legislators, and third-party payers. Being on the defensive also affords little power to counter moves of those who would make patient education but a pawn in the struggle for control over health care delivery.

These essentially political observations give rise to an intriguing question: Might supporters of patient education gain more power if they were to unite in a commitment to cost-effectiveness evaluation? Given current skepticism about the purposes such evaluation may serve, this proposal may seem radical indeed. As Goodenough (1963) has pointed out, however, change agents may do better in the long run to ride with a social movement rather than to resist it. Further reflection suggests that adopting a positive stance toward cost-effectiveness evaluation could be instrumental in advancing the development of patient education programs. Applying well-grounded principles of health education, let us see how this might work.

Cost-effectiveness Evaluation as a Strategy for Change

Regardless of underlying motives, interest in evaluating the cost-savings potential of patient education is high in many quarters. By taking a community development approach to the health care system, this widespread expression of "felt need" can be considered a positive sign. Herein lies the possibility for agreement on common goals, and hence an opportunity to initiate the process of planned social change.

Inasmuch as there are straightforward purposes for wishing to learn more about the role of patient education in cost containment, support for evaluation can be expected from third-party payers, including government, as well as from other public and private sources. Indeed such support is already being provided in relatively modest amounts and should increase when project proposals include sound plans for evaluating the cost effectiveness of educational interventions. If more adequate funding fails to materialize when these conditions are met, then patient educators can publically remind those in charge of health care financing that they need to support the evaluation they themselves have claimed is crucial.

Now in order to evaluate patient education, some sort of program has to be in place. Because formal patient education programs are relatively scarce, funding for evaluation therefore necessarily must include provision for program development and implementation. Health care systems, such as prepaid group practice associations, whose economic conditions would be improved through more appropriate patient utilization and increased patient capacity for self-care may be especially receptive to the initiation of patient education programs when these include a strong evaluative component. In addition, other providers who are concerned with the quality of care and the assurance of patient rights are likely to initiate or expand organized education efforts when these can be supported through outside funds. Thus an emphasis on evaluation may well be an effective strategy to bring about the extension of patient education programs.

By role-modeling readiness to engage in the evaluation of the patient education programs in which we ourselves are involved, practitioners also earn the right to inquire about the cost effectiveness of other educational approaches. Thus in the face of glittering promises used to market commercially developed educational packages, we can demand to see the data supporting such claims and help other providers learn to do the same before making expensive investments in hardware and software. Naturally measurements of outcomes should be based on methodologically sound studies of patient groups with characteristics similar to those for whom canned programs are intended, while cost figures must include operating, maintenance, and replacement needs as well as the initial development and purchase price.

Our commitment to evaluating the cost effectiveness of patient education must also include assessment of existing programs and activities. Therefore whether working within a single institution or on a broader scale, we might logically inquire about the extent to which such evaluations of on-going programs have been conducted. This clearly requires the prior step of identifying these programs. In the case of institutions and services that have a legislative or professional mandate for patient education, survey results permit evaluation at another level: To what extent are mandated responsibilities for patient education being fulfilled?

Consider the nation's hospitals as one example. The obligation of hospitals and other health care institutions "to promote, organize, implement, and evaluate health education programs, not only for patients and their families, but also for personnel, including employees, medical staff, volunteers, and trustees, and for the community at large" was formally recognized in a 1975 policy statement by the American Hospital Association (1975). Nevertheless the Fogarty Task Force on Health Promotion and Consumer Health Education reported in that same year that "only a handful of the nation's 7,000 hospitals maintain even a token health education program" (*Preventive Medicine U.S.A.*, 1976).

Later in 1975, a survey of 5,770 U.S. community hospitals conducted by the American Hospital Association revealed growth in the number of hospitals with inpatient educational activities, but carefully planned and organized patient education programs were still scarce. Whereas 2,680 hospitals indicated that they had at least one program, less than half of these had designated specific line responsibility for coordination. Just 694 institutions reported that they had a specific patient education budget; only 329 had a written policy concerning inpatient education; and only 88 had organized a patient education committee. Fewer than 500 reported *any* committee with oversight responsibilities for patient education (AHA, 1977). Evaluating such data against the AHA's policy statement as a criterion clearly provides practitioners with yet another powerful tool to advance the development of patient education programs.

Beyond this, however, evaluating the cost effectiveness of existing hospital-based educational programs is critical. In view of the rapidity with which such programs are expanding, data are needed to indicate how well current activities are achieving their stated aims, both so that institutions already engaged in patient education can make the best use of their resources and so that other hospitals will know which models to follow. Not so incidentally, evaluating existing programs will also determine the extent to which some hospitals can remain complacent about patient education "because we're already doing it." As advocates of evaluation, we must regard such statements as rhetoric unless they are supported by objective measures of program effects.

This opens the way for patient educators to offer assistance to health care facilities in evaluating their current educational efforts. Such help is definitely needed according to a 1974 AHA survey of a selected sample of 113 hospitals identified as having patient education programs (Peters, 1975). The 67 hospitals responding identified as one of their greatest needs "adequate evaluative studies and how to use them." While some 73 percent of these hospitals indicated that they had a planned evaluation of their patient education program, only two of the five most common evaluation procedures suggested the measurement of educational effects: 48 percent of the respondents indicated follow-up of treatment regimen and 43 percent reported knowledge testing. Two additional evaluation procedures simply reported patient contacts, that is, records kept of patients receiving patient education, and telephone and home visits. The most common evaluation procedure, employed by 55 percent of the hospitals participating, was personal interview of patient by staff member.

Such methodology obviously must be strengthened in order to

meet the requirements of cost-effectiveness evaluation. Outcomes, in terms of expected effects, must be clearly specified and measured. Before this is done, however, the contributions of anticipated educational outcomes to improvements in health status should be questioned in order to assess the appropriateness of educational goals. According to Podell (cited in *Preventive Medicine U.S.A.*, 1976):

> Any assessment of the effectiveness of health education should be prefaced by assessment of the recommendations and practices of health scientists and physicians as to what constitutes behavior which promotes health. This is essential because these recommendations and practices usually determine the substantive goals of health education programs. . . . The commitment to adequate evaluation at the level of behavior change is inextricably linked to adequate evaluation at the level of health status results.

Rigor in evaluating the cost effectiveness of patient education, then, leads us directly into evaluating the scientific basis for medical advice—frequently an arena of much dispute. Therefore by dedicating ourselves to evaluation we circumvent the danger that patient education will be used to shroud larger issues. To the contrary, we confront such issues head on.

At the same time, meeting the requirements of cost-effectiveness evaluation necessitates precision in defining educational inputs, for only on this basis can the *costs* of patient education be determined. Although documenting the specifics of educational interventions may be regarded as a burdensome task, this can do a great deal to advance our knowledge of educational methodology. Creatively used, this can also became an opportunity to challenge the simplistic notion that "patient education" is a single variable.

By controlling what we document we can demonstrate that planned educational programs vary along multiple dimensions. These include the indications that are recognized for initiating education, the context in which it is provided, the specific content presented, the methods used, the time when the educational approach is made, the settings where this is done, the characteristics of the educators, the nature of their interactions with patients, and the number of educational encounters with each individual, as well as the total time and sequencing involved. Further variations within each of these broad categories can, of course, be identified.

When this information is made explicit we can undertake additional evaluations to assess the adequacy of our rationale for adopting a particular educational approach, the resources available for implementing it, and the skill with which it was applied. By sharing our findings with each other, among institutions and across disciplines, our insights into the process of patient education cannot help but grow. Moreover, through such documentation and review we will generate the case studies so often requested for training purposes, thereby enabling us to increase the numbers of health professionals prepared to conduct and support patient education programs. Within this framework, cost-effectiveness evaluation can serve the purposes of professional growth and change after all.

As we increase our own capabilities to facilitate patient learning, our programs should also progressively improve. This in turn should contribute to the mounting evidence that patient education is indeed cost effective and also should increase the consumer demand for education and professional understanding of education's indispensable role in the provision of quality health care. Through a commitment to evaluation, then, we may set in motion a series of forces that will gain significant new support for patient education and foster new alliances to advance program development, consequently tipping the present balance of power to make this possible.

Potential Risks and Sources of Resistance

No strategy of change is without its hazards, and so our proposal would be incomplete without an assessment of the risk its implementation may entail. This is essential in order to take preventive action wherever possible and to be prepared with adequate coping mechanisms in other cases. Perhaps even more important, a realistic appraisal of potential problems is necessary to win converts to the cause.

Ethical Concerns

The ethics of our proposal may be troublesome to some who doubt that evaluation should be used for political purposes. Therefore let us be very clear that we are *not* suggesting the introduction of deliberate bias into the design, methodology, or interpretation of evaluative studies. Quite the opposite. Our rationale requires dedication to objectivity and scientific rigor. Thus we find no quarrel with Green's (1975) view that "evaluation is a professional responsibility that distinguishes us from politicians and technicians." Rather we suggest that this professional responsibility can be a source of increased power for effecting planned social change.

We would argue further that power is necessary in order to bring about the changes necessary to integrate patient education into the health care system. Traditional hierarchies of relationships and patterns of communication must be altered to permit planned and coordinated educational approaches responsive to patient needs. Because effecting these changes will require institutional adjustments, they by definition involve social reform and the art of power politics (Kotler, 1969).

Power, however, need not be antithetical to the advancement of human values. To the contrary, Bennis (1969) has suggested that the most likely source of power for change agents lies in the values they hold "based on Western civilization's notion of a scientific humanism: concern for our fellow man, experimentalism, openness and honesty, flexibility, cooperation, democracy." Barnes (1969) additionally has pointed out that, regardless of the specific strategies used to effect organizational change, the most successful approaches studied to date do not attempt to establish new power concentrations, but, rather, attempt to bring about *power equalization* through shared decision making among the individuals concerned.

In this context, evaluation is clearly recognized in the literature as one of several data-based strategies of social intervention. Barnes (1969), in fact, has identified "data-discussion" as one of the more open and participative approaches to organizational change. Analyses by Hornstein, Bunker, Burke, Gindes, & Lewicki (1971) and Fairweather (1971) are particularly useful in suggesting specific evaluation approaches that may increase support for patient education programs while also relating these to broader human concerns.

In undertaking cost-effectiveness evaluation to further planned social change, we therefore can embody humanistic values both in purpose and in process. Indeed we can hardly do otherwise, for these are the very values on which patient education is based.

Methodological Concerns

A second source of resistance to our proposal may rest in the methodological difficulties involved in evaluating patient education. Thus participants in a recent patient education workshop cautioned against attempting to "prove education's effectiveness" with experimental studies in a practice setting, specifically pointing out that the assignment of patients on a random basis into experimental and control groups is exceedingly difficult when the number of patients available is small and the characteristics of the patients, the factors which influence the course of the illness condition, and the variations in patient management are numerous. (Bureau of Health Education, 1976)

Certainly the great number of variables involved in patient education itself also poses problems in adequately defining and measuring educational interventions. Additional complications are introduced by the likelihood that any one educational variable alone is not so important as the total mix of such variables in determining program effects. In other words it is not only what is said, but how, by whom, when, and where, that together influence behavioral response. Furthermore, holding some variables constant while experimentally manipulating others often violates the body of educational theory, research, and experience that indicates that education must be adjusted to the particular needs, motives, values, and understandings of individual patients. Thus, for example, the educational approach likely to be most effective with an unwed pregnant teenager might quickly alienate an expectant mother of four who is late in her child-bearing years.

Other dilemmas in evaluating health education are discussed in detail by Green (1977), who, however, also identifies various approaches for dealing with these constraints. In addition, cost-effectiveness studies of patient education already completed illustrate a variety of feasible evaluation designs, some of them relatively simple. Various texts on evaluation provide help with specific methodological problems, and advice from experienced evaluators also can be sought. Moreover we should remember, as Evans (1972) has pointed out, that

our task in evaluating social action programs in the real world is not to produce methodologically perfect studies, but rather to *improve decisions* by doing the best that can be done in a timely and relevant way. Evaluation, every bit as much as politics, is the art of the possible.

Methodological limitations therefore need not hold us back. Acceptable methodologies are available for evaluating patient education, and more can be developed with experience. In the meantime, inasmuch as methodological weaknesses seldom can be avoided completely, it should be a standard practice to acknowledge possible sources of bias when reporting evaluative findings and interpreting the results.

Fear of Negative Results

Quite possibly, however, our concerns about methodology are related to a deeper fear of the consequences should evaluation fail to demonstrate positive results. If this should happen, several alternative responses are possible. In some cases it might be best to accept the findings at face value and eliminate the educational program at stake. Certainly we should be prepared to weed out the ineffective, except perhaps where it is necessary to keep something in place in order to experiment with other approaches for meeting patients' educational needs.

In the latter situation we might point out that the lack of positive findings does not necessarily mean that the educational program is ineffective, for the problem may lie in the methods and techniques of evaluation. Similarly we could apply some basic statistics, pointing out the possibility of a Type II statistical error, that is, concluding that patient education makes no difference in patient behavior when, in fact, it does (Selltiz, Wrightsman, & Cook, 1976). Given the severe problems of health care financing and limited alternatives for cost containment, this is a mistake the health care system clearly cannot afford. Therefore rather than discontinue such a program, it should be evaluated once again.

While the preceding strategy may buy time, it will only perpetuate past problems unless steps are taken to identify and correct them. Therefore it should be coupled with a careful review of the educational approach used, considering both the adequacy of the theoretical framework to guide intervention and the skill with which this was applied. At the same time, the evaluation design should be studied in order to strengthen it wherever possible. This may include testing for program side effects, as well as for the achievement of educational objectives stated in terms of patient behavior. Surely such spillovers as improved staff morale and productivity, increased patient satisfaction, more efficient use of existing resources, and improved coordination with community agencies deserve to be considered in cost-effectiveness calculations.

Introducing more formative evaluation is another excellent way to increase the chances that summative evaluation will show patient education to be cost effective in comparison with other alternatives. Not only does this provide early and periodic indicators of program progress, it keeps open the question of the values to be applied in making final judgments. Thus obtaining measures of such "intermediate" objectives as gains in patient understanding and increased family support makes it more difficult to conclude that the only criterion of effectiveness should be the program's ability to save the system money.

Building formative evaluation into patient education programs has the additional advantage of fostering an experimental approach from the outset. This in Campbell's (1969/1972) view should characterize all attempts at social reform, for it avoids threats to the reform effort should a program fail. Thus he has recommended a political stance that emphasizes the *seriousness of the problem* rather than the efficacy of any given solution. From this perspective, the implementation of a particular program represents a policy decision to try one of several plausible alternatives for a specified period of time, after which another alternative will be tried should evaluation results fail to show significant improvement.

By adopting Campbell's experimental philosophy, patient educators can avoid the implication that evaluating the cost effectiveness of any one specific program constitutes an evaluation of patient education in general. Accordingly the task is not seen as "proving the worth of what you're doing," but rather as "keeping after the problem until something is found that works." This, then, should free us to experiment with many approaches for meeting patients' educational needs, to evaluate the outcomes honestly, and to use the results for improvement and change.

Nevertheless if our experiments are to advance the development of patient education programs, they must not be conducted in isolation. Involving those who hold the power to effect institutional change is fundamental to data-based strategies of social intervention. Therefore we should seek the active participation of administrators, physicians, patients, and other decision makers at every stage of educational evaluation. The specific techniques we apply to gain such collaboration will necessarily depend on our analysis of the situation, our relationship to the target system, and our skill as change agents. In general, however, our efforts should be directed toward creating meaningful opportunities for involvement from the initial selection of the questions to be addressed in evaluation through final determination of how findings will be used. Intermediate steps, of course, may include participation in collecting data about patients' educational problems, in designing relevant educational programs, and in testing their effects.

Through such involvement we can help others to understand the critical need for patient education, the dynamics of the educational process, and the difficulties of educational evaluation. In this way we can gradually build a team of decision makers willing to share responsibility in planning, implementing, and evaluating educational experiments. This, then, reduces the risk that failure to demonstrate cost-effective results will lead to the abandonment of planned educational approaches. At the same time, as Grossman (1961) observed some years ago, through such involvement we can make evaluation provide a supportive structure for introducing change, and evaluation itself can become a truly educational function.

The Risk of Change

The preceding discussion suggests a number of ways to overcome some of the more obvious hazards inherent in this proposal. Nevertheless in undertaking cost-effectiveness evaluation as a strategy for planned social change, we should not expect to avoid all risks. As Machiavelli (1940) said, there is

> nothing more difficult to carry out, nor more doubtful of success, nor more dangerous to handle, than to initiate a new order of things. For the reformer has enemies in all those who profit by the old order, and only lukewarm defenders in all those who would profit by the new order, this lukewarmness arising partly from fear of their adversaries, who have the laws in their favour; and partly from the incredulity of mankind, who do not truly believe in anything new until they have had actual experience of it.

Conclusion

In this chapter we have proposed that evaluation can be an effective strategy for providing decision makers with actual experience in patient education, thereby leading to a new order of things in health care delivery. If we are to implement this strategy, however, we must recognize that evaluation is political (Weiss, 1970). Moreover, we ourselves must change by gaining experience in evaluation and objectively examining the results of our educational efforts. To the extent that we are lukewarm about this idea, we would do well to reconsider our readiness to engage in social reform. Is our commitment to patient education sufficient to risk evaluation?

References

American Hospital Association. *Health education: Role and responsibility of health care institutions* (Policy statement). Chicago, 1975.

American Hospital Association. *Hospital inpatient education: Survey findings and analyses, 1975.* Atlanta: U.S. Public Health Service, Center for Disease Control, Bureau of Health Education, 1977.

Andrieu, M. Benefit cost evaluation. In L. Rutman (Ed.), *Evaluation research methods: A basic guide.* Beverly Hills, Calif.: Sage Publications, 1977, pp. 219–232.

Avery, C. H., Green L. W., & Kreider, S. *Reducing emergency visits of asthmatics: An experiment in health education.* Testimony presented to the President's Committee on Health Education, Pittsburgh, January 11, 1972.

Barnes, L. B. Approaches to organizational change. In W. G. Bennis, K. D. Benne, & R. Chin (Eds.), *The planning of change* (2nd ed.). New York: Holt, Rinehart and Winston, 1969, pp. 83–84.

Bennis, W. G. Theory and method in applying behavioral science to planned organizational change. In W. G. Bennis, K. D. Benne, & R. Chin (Eds.), *The planning of change* (2nd ed.). New York: Holt, Rinehart and Winston, 1969, p. 74.

Bureau of Health Education. *Patient education workshop: Summary report.* Atlanta: U.S. Public Health Service, Center for Disease Control, 1976, p. 8.

Campbell, D. T. Reforms as experiments. *American Psychologist,* April 1969, *24,* 409–429. Reprinted in A. Zaltman, P. Kotler, & I. Kauffman (Eds.), *Creating Social Change.* New York: Holt, Rinehart and Winston, 1972, pp. 640–664.

Dialysis is cheaper at home. *Public Health Reports,* March-April 1977, *92,* 188.

Egbert, L. D., Battit, G. E., Welch, C. E., & Bartlett, M. K. Reduction of postoperative pain by encouragement in instruction of patient. *New England Journal of Medicine,* April 16, 1964, *270,* 825–827.

Evans, J. W. Evaluating social action programs. In A. Zaltman, P. Kotler, & I. Kauffman (Eds.), *Creating social change.* New York: Holt, Rinehart and Winston, 1972, p. 637.

Fairweather, G. W. Experimental social intervention defined. In H. A. Hornstein, B. B. Bunker, W. W. Burke, M. Gindes, & R. J. Lewicki (Eds.), *Social intervention: A behavioral science approach.* New York: Free Press, 1971, pp. 330–341.

Fein, R. Some health policy issues: One economist's view. *Public Health Reports,* September-October 1975, *90,* 387–392.

Geiger, H. J. The illusion of change. *Social Policy,* November-December 1975, pp. 30–35.

Goodenough, W. H. *Cooperation in change.* New York: Russell Sage, 1963, p. 313.

Green, L. W. Toward cost-benefit evaluations of health education: Some concepts, methods, and examples. *Health Education Monographs,* May 1974, *2* (Suppl. 1), 34–65.

Green, L. W. Evaluation of patient education programs: Criteria and measurement techniques. In *Rx: Education for the patient.* Proceedings, Department of Health Education, Southern Illinois University, Carbondale, 1975, pp. 89–98.

Green, L. W. The potential of health education includes cost effectiveness. *Hospitals,* May 1, 1976, *50,* 57–61.

Green, L. W. Evaluation and measurement: Some dilemmas for health education. *American Journal of Public Health,* February 1977, *67,* 155–161.

Green, L. W., & Figa-Talamanca, I. Suggested designs for evaluation of patient education programs. *Health Education Monographs,* Spring 1974, *2,* 34–71.

Grossman, J. Overcoming barriers to effective evaluation of education in public health programs. *California's Health,* December 15, 1961, *19,* 81–83.

Healy, K. J. Does preoperative instruction really make a difference? *American Journal of Nursing,* January 1968, *68,* 62–67.

Hornstein, H. A., Bunker, B. B., Burke, W. W., Gindes, M., & Lewicki, R. J. Data-based strategies of social intervention. In H. A. Hornstein, B. B. Bunker, W. W. Burke, M. Gindes, & R. J. Lewicki (Eds.), *Social intervention: A behavioral science approach* (introduction to part three). New York: Free Press, 1971, pp. 255–269.

Johnson, R. L. Health education: ramifications and consequences. *Health Education Monographs,* 1972, 13–21.

Knutson, A. L. The influence of values on evaluation. *Health Education Monographs,* 1959, 25–31.

Kotler, P. The five C's: Cause, change agency, change target, channel, and change strategy. In W. G. Bennis, K. D. Benne, & R. Chin (Eds.), *The planning of change* (2nd ed.). New York: Holt, Rinehart and Winston, 1969. p. 74.

Levine, P., & Britten, A. F. Supervised patient-management of hemophilia. *Annals of Internal Medicine,* February 1973, *78,* 195–201.

Lindeman, C. A., & Van Aernam, B. Nursing intervention with the presurgical patient. *Nursing Research,* July-August 1971, *20,* 319–331.

Machiavelli, N. *The prince and The discourses.* New York: Modern Library, 1940.

Miller, L., & Goldstein, J. More efficient care of diabetic patients in a county hospital setting. *New England Journal of Medicine,* June 29, 1972, *286,* 1388–1391.

Peters, S. J. Health education in a hospital setting: Report of a status study. In *Rx: Education for the patient.* Proceedings, Department of Health Education, Southern Illinois University, Carbondale, 1975, pp. 79–88.

Preventive medicine U.S.A.: Health promotion and consumer health education (Task Force Rep. sponsored by the John E. Fogarty International Center for Advanced Study in the Health Sciences, National Institutes of Health, and the American College of Preventive Medicine). New York: Prodist, 1976, p. 5.

Reeder, L. G. The patient-client as a consumer: Some observations on the changing professional-client relationship. *Journal of Health and Social Behavior*, December 1972, *13*, 406–412.

Roberts, B. J. Concepts and methods of evaluation in health education. *International Journal of Health Education*, April-June 1962, *2*, 52–62.

Rosenberg, S. G. Patient education leads to better care for heart patients. *HSMHA Health Reports*, September 1971, *85*, 793–802.

Selltiz, C., Wrightsman, L. S., & Cook, S. W. *Research methods in social relations* (3rd ed.). New York: Holt, Rinehart and Winston, 1976, pp. 485–486.

Somers, A. R. Consumer health education: An idea whose time has come?" *Hospital Progress*, February 1975, pp. 10–11.

Thorner, R. M. Health program evaluation in relation to health programing. *HSMHA Health Reports.* June 1971, *86*, 525–532.

Van Maanen, J. *The process of program evaluation.* Washington, D.C.: National Training and Development Service Press, 1973.

Weiss, C. H. The politicization of evaluation research. *Journal of Social Issues*, Autumn 1970, *26*, 57–68.

Weiss, C. H. *Evaluation research: Methods for assessing program effectiveness.* New York: Prentice-Hall, 1972, pp. 14–15.

9

Working Through the Territorial Imperative in a Hospital Setting

Elizabeth Bernheimer

My first experience with territoriality occurred on either my first or second day on the job as coordinator of patient education in a large metropolitan hospital. Two nurses from the Nursing In-Service Department marched into my office that memorable day, sat down, and flatly stated, "You are on our turf." I was astounded and responded that I was not aware that they were involved in any patient education programs. They replied, "Patient education is a nursing function." And that is an example of territoriality.

Reflecting on that experience I have learned that that incident was not unique to me; and as I explored the subject, I discovered that territoriality is undoubtedly one of the biggest barriers to patient education. I want to share here some of my thinking on the subject. I contend that the boundaries of one's territory consist of one's concept of role, one's social status, and one's values—all of which are learned and can be changed.

This phenomenon of territoriality is not limited to the hospital or the medical care situation. Much work on territoriality has been done by biologists. Representative of one school of thought is Ardrey (1966), who states that the tendency among the animal world to possess a territory is an innate quality and that the need to defend it is also instinctive. However, he continues, the boundaries of one's territory must be learned.

One of the examples in his book that I'd like to relate is that of Arctic wolves. A group of wolves in the Arctic who had a hunting territory of about 100 square miles was studied. The boundaries were fairly precise, and periodically the adult wolves made the rounds, refreshing their markers as a warning against intrusion. The wolf marks his property with a squirt of urine, the fragrance of which is reinforced by the output of a special scent gland. By marking their boundaries wolves reduce the likelihood of conflict over property rights. Like the wolves, humans map out their territory; we, however, use different means for marking our boundaries.

Ardrey also discusses the work done by another biologist, Darling (1952), who describes the psychological functions of territoriality; it satisfies two needs: stimulation and security. To this, Ardrey adds a third need satisfied by territoriality: that of identity. In his description of the hierarchy of values for these three needs, identity is the most powerful and most pervasive among all species with very few exceptions. It is this aspect of territoriality that I am addressing here—the need for identity.

Let me apply this aspect of territoriality, the need for identity, to humans, and consider one of the forces that make up our identity —that of role. Arnold (1955) offers this definition of role: "A role can be considered as a set of behaviors consistent for an appropriate social position, that is perceptually shared in at least certain aspects for all persons in the social situation." This definition is consistent with other authors' (Parsons, 1964; Robischon & Scott, 1969; Sorbin, 1954) perception of role—that it encompasses the norms of social behaviors. People do not behave in a random fashion; their behavior is influenced to some extent by their own expectations and those of others in the group of which they are members. The role behavior of any person is related to his or her perception of the norms of the system, his or her relationship to the system, and expectations of the others in this system.

When our territory is invaded by someone who assumes a role we had perceived as ours, friction, often called "role conflict," develops. An article in the *San Francisco Chronicle* (1979) describing a sleuth of computer crime provides a good illustration. Having tracked down forty cases of electronic fraud as a consultant for Stanford Research Institute, this man submitted a proposal, based on his experience, to investigate "computer-related crime." It was rejected by law researchers who stated that he was unqualified to decide what constituted a crime. He then changed the title to "Anti-Social Use of Computers," with which he then managed to offend the sociologists. He finally received support with a new title, "Computer Abuse."

Role conflict can range from open confrontation with such statements as "You are on my turf," to passive aggression. When there are differences in expectations for a particular role, there is apt to be difficulty in effectively performing that role, and problems will arise. This is as true in the social context as in the professional one. Goldberg (1976) describes the dilemma of modern man in having to conform to the traditional expectations of masculine behavior (being the providers, the warriors, and the fearless ones), the role we expect them to play. In similar fashion we, too, in our professional roles may have difficulties in living up to the expectations we have learned in our training as well as the demands placed on us by society. These roles are learned, and they form the boundaries of our territory—that area of knowledge and expertise we have mapped out for ourselves.

This theoretical concept applies to patient education, too. The physician and nurse were once the primary care providers; as medical care has become more technical, new health professionals, such as dietitians, respiratory therapists, and clinical pharmacists have been trained to carry out this new technology. Each of these professionals and many more consider patient instruction to be an important facet of their patient care. All of these health professionals have expertise in their respective fields, but they are in fact impinging the traditional role of the nurse and the physician. As Kahn (1974) maintains, "Each has thus entered further into the domain of others or has entered into competition with others in previously uncharted territory" We have crossed the boundaries of roles and are in someone else's territory as they define it. This "professional territoriality" (Pluckham, 1972) is characterized by a zealous guarding of function and is endemic to our society, in which we have a profusion of overlapping interests and skills (Kane, 1975).

To illustrate this aspect of professional territoriality I designed an exercise on role conflict, which was completed by some of the participants attending the Second Annual Symposium on Patient Education in San Francisco. Forty-two nurses, eighteen health educators, six physicians, and nine other professionals completed the exercise (see fig. 9-1).

Although a complete analysis by each professional group is not feasible here, there were interesting responses to some of the questions. For instance the majority of health professionals in all categories stated that patients should be the ones determining the amount of information needed; yet all agreed that currently the physicians are the ones making that decision. Interestingly enough—although the nurse and the physician were named as having the responsibility in statements three, four, five, and six—other health professionals such

Figure 9-1.

Role conflict exercise in patient education.

Health Profession_____

Instructions:

Please identify yourself by listing your health profession.
Select only ONE of the following multiple choices for each square.
Please consider these statements in light of (a) <u>status quo</u> (the
way it is now) and (b) the way you think it <u>should be.</u> There are
NO right or wrong answers. Place the appropriate letter in each
square.

1. Determining the amount of information a patient needs about his/her
medical status is best done by

				a.	b.
a. clinical pharmacist	e. patient				
b. dietitian	f. physical therapist			☐	☐
c. health educator	g. physician				
d. nurse	h. social worker				
i. other_____					

2. Assessing possible obstacles to patient compliance in the home
environment is best done by

a. clinical pharmacist   e. patient
b. dietitian   f. physical therapist
c. health educator   g. physician   ☐ ☐
d. nurse   h. social worker
i. other_____

3. For patients with a chronic medical condition, assistance in
complying with the regimen is best provided by

a. clinical pharmacist   e. patient
b. dietitian   f. physical therapist
c. health educator   g. physician   ☐ ☐
d. nurse   h. social worker
i. other_____

4. Assessing the patient's "readiness to learn" is best done by

a. clinical pharmacist   e. patient
b. dietitian   f. physical therapist
c. health educator   g. physician   ☐ ☐
d. nurse   h. social worker
i. other_____

5. One to one counselling with the patient on the prescribed regimen
is best done by

				a.	b.
a. clinical pharmacist	e. patient				
b. dietitian	f. physical therapist			☐	☐
c. health educator	g. physician				
d. nurse	h. social worker				
i. other_____					

184

Figure 9-1. *(continued)*

6. Counselling a patient on his/her prescribed drug regimen (with attendant possible drug interactions and side effects) is best done by

    a. clinical pharmacist   e. patient
    b. dietitian   f. physical therapist
    c. health educator   g. physician
    d. nurse   h. social worker
    i. other_____

7. Helping arthritic patients incorporate a prescribed daily exercise plan in the home is best done by

    a. clinical pharmacist   e. patient
    b. dietitian   f. physical therapist
    c. health educator   g. physician
    d. nurse   h. social worker
    i. other_____

8. Helping a patient change his/her eating pattern is best done by

    a. clinical pharmacist   e. patient
    b. dietitian   f. physical therapist
    c. health educator   g. physician
    d. nurse   h. social worker
    i. other_____

Designed by E. Bernheimer, October 1978.

as health educators and patients (and clinical pharmacists for number six) were named as those that should have that responsibility.

One of the basic concepts in role theory is that roles complement each other. A role does not exist in isolation but is patterned to mesh with that of role partner (Hiltner, 1957). As we look at the new roles of health professionals in patient education, we must examine the other side of the coin and look at the patient. Just as we place the health professional in a new role, so we are also placing patients in a new role for which they often have no preparation. Whereas in the past we've assumed patients to be submissive and compliant, we now are asking that they take an active role in this learning process, that they make the major decisions about their care. This, too, can be threatening to the care givers. The patients are in fact invading our territory.

Another important aspect of territoriality is our sense of social structure. In most animal species each group develops a complex social organization based on territoriality and consisting of dominant and subordinate members, the so-called pecking order. The acceptance of this hierarchical order reduces fighting and other forms of social tensions, providing a stability that is beneficial to the whole group (Dubos, 1965). However, this pecking order is only valid for well-defined environmental conditions. For instance in an undisturbed organized flock of chickens, the individual animals peck each other less frequently, eat more, maintain weight better, and lay more eggs than chickens undergoing social reorganization through removal of some animals or addition of new ones. We in the medical field have similar social tensions. As new types of health professionals enter the medical field, the social organization gets somewhat shaken up and the problems with territoriality are exacerbated. This is not unique to the medical profession or even to humans.

Another factor of our boundaries are our differing values, which have a direct relationship to our behavior. A physician who believes that a little knowledge for the patient is a dangerous thing will be reluctant to have the patient exposed to patient education. Conversely a patient comfortable in the passive role will be reluctant to assume responsibility for her or his well-being and care.

A recent background document of the World Health Organization (1978) states: "The driving force in man which determines, shapes and reshapes his attitudes is his values. For it is man's values, not necessarily his needs that determine his behavior." Values underlie the behavior of individuals; dissimilar values may induce courses of action that are directly opposed, even when the motives are similar. Cultural values must be assessed with our professional colleagues as well as with our patient population (Susser & Watson, 1962). These differing sets of attitudes and values produce strikingly different perceptions and actions, and they require different approaches.

One of the techniques being used to assess values is *value clarification*. Simon (Simon, Howe, & Kirschenbaum, 1972) and Raths (Raths, Harmin, & Simon, 1966), concerned with the *process* of valuing, focused on how people come to hold certain beliefs and establish certain behavior patterns. Raths states that the process has three steps: (1) prizing one's beliefs and behaviors; (2) choosing (from alternatives), and (3) acting on one's beliefs. The value-clarification exercise is an application of this process. The aim is not to instill any particular set of values but to apply the processes to those beliefs already formed and to those still emerging. Participants discuss the pros and cons of each belief and how each of these attitudes or values will affect their behavior.

As a method for health professionals to use with their colleagues, the following value-clarification exercise was completed and discussed during the symposium on patient education. The participants completing this exercise were forty-eight nurses, eighteen health educators, six physicians, and nine other health professionals. The participants were asked to write whether they agreed, disagreed, or were undecided about each statement. They were then asked to share their responses with each other. The purpose of the discussion was to seek understanding of each other's views and values rather than to argue for or against a viewpoint. Although the large size of the groups, the poor accoustics, and the limited amount of time hampered the discussion portion of this exercise, a breakdown of the written responses may be seen in table 9-1.

Table 9-1.
Responses (in percentages) to a Values-clarification Exercise on Patient Education

Participants	Agree	Disagree	Undecided
Like other aspects of a patient's treatment, I believe patient education should be based on a physician's order.			
Nurses	10	88	2
Health educators	11	78	11
Physicians	50	50	0
Others[a]	11	89	0
I feel that, if a patient does not comply with his/her regimen, I have somehow failed.			
Nurses	14	81	5
Health educators	11	72	17
Physicians	17	50	33
Others[a]	11	89	0
I would keep information from a patient if I thought he/she could not handle the information constructively.			
Nurses	27	32	41
Health educators	33	29	38
Physicians	50	33	17
Others[a]	33	22	45
I believe that all medically oriented questions a patient asks should be referred to the physician.			
Nurses	10	83	7
Health educators	6	88	6
Physicians	17	83	0
Others[a]	0	100	0

Table 9-1. *(continued)*
Responses (in percentages) to a Values-clarification Exercise on
Patient Education

Participants	Agree	Disagree	Undecided

I think the hospital is an appropriate setting for patient education.

Nurses	55	32	13
Health educators	65	15	20
Physicians	100	0	0
Others[a]	22	67	11

Patients are more likely to accept medical advice when it comes from their doctor.

Nurses	39	44	17
Health educators	65	15	20
Physicians	83	0	17
Others[a]	22	67	11

Patient education and patient teaching are the same.

Nurses	20	65	15
Health educators	29	65	6
Physicians	17	83	0
Others[a]	0	78	22

To be an effective patient educator, it is more important to be an educator than a clinician.

Nurses	25	63	12
Health educators	61	33	6
Physicians	50	50	0
Others[a]	33	44	23

Most people will do what is good for their health if they know what it is they should be doing.

Nurses	42	55	3
Health educators	28	67	5
Physicians	33	67	0
Others[a]	44	33	23

[a]Medical librarians, dietitians, patient advocates, physical therapists, occupational therapists, and a respiratory therapist.

Although this was a skewed population (being given at a symposium on patient education for people primarily interested in or involved with the subject), the responses illustrated significant differences in values within each professional group as well as between groups. On the statement "Like other aspects of a patient's treatment, I believe patient education should be based on a physician's order," physicians were divided evenly on their responses in contrast to other health professionals, who disagreed with the statement. Although there was some indecision in the response to the statement "I feel that, if a patient does not comply with his/her regimen, I have somehow failed," most health professionals did not feel that they had failed if a patient did not comply. The discussion revealed some dissonance between what one should feel and what one actually felt. Nurses as a group were most in disagreement with the statement "To be an effective patient educator, it is more important to be an educator than a clinician," whereas the physicians were evenly divided. On the statement "Most people will do what is good for their health, if they know what it is they should be doing," responses were divided within each professional group. As one example of how these values will affect our behavior in patient education, the value that health professionals place on patient compliance will affect the number of options provided the patient and the opportunity the patient will be given to make an educated decision.

One approach to patient education that addresses the issues in territoriality is the team approach. Smoyak (1977) states that four conditions are necessary in order to achieve a good working relationship between professions:

1. Mutual agreement on a goal
2. Equality in status and personal interactions
3. A shared base of scientific and professional knowledge with complementary diversity in skills, expertise, and practices
4. Mutual trust and respect for each other's competencies

Let me share with you some of my experiences as a health educator selected to coordinate a team approach to patient education in a large metropolitan hospital (Bernheimer, 1977; Bernheimer & Clever, 1977) and the methods we used to defuse the situation. I was viewed as an interloper wherever I turned. I found every task that I attempted was an invasion of the domain of someone else. Much of my effort was expended initially in dispelling the fear of others that I would take over the direct teaching of their patients. I continually had to assure the other health professionals that that was not how I interpreted my role.

One of the ways I lessened this anxiety was to involve my colleagues in the process of defining our respective roles. Committees were formed to define specific educational objectives for the patient education program. The questions raised at these meetings were: What did we feel was essential for the patient to do? What did the patient need to know in order to do it? What did we need to know about the patient? Who would do what? These are a seemingly simple set of questions that actually required some complex thinking.

During this process, health professionals perceived the overlapping territories that already existed and had been creating problems. Each had been doing some patient education without any idea what the others were doing. This process served as the first step in breaking down communication barriers. It was also the first step in developing a team (Wise, Beckhard, Rubin, & Kyte, 1974) out of the group of health professionals directly involved in patient education: nurses, dietitians, a social worker, a pharmacist, and a health educator. The hypothesis was that a team was needed to achieve a consistency of messages and a continuity in the teaching of them in order to attain effective education. To function as a team, however, one of the basic requisites is that there be a commitment to the team concept. The first step for teams is that they define their respective roles. A group of health professionals can not function as a team unless there is a conviction that each member is vital to the whole and each contributes significantly to the overall task.

In our experience we found that the dietitians added immeasurably in providing information on the home environment of patients based on their assessment of the patient's food habits. Nurses were helpful in identifying the significant other to be included in formal instructions; social workers identified fears patients had regarding such things as injections or the disease itself, information essential for team members to utilize in their interactions with the patient. This overlapping of boundaries was viewed as positive reinforcement and provided assistance for all involved. The equal status on the team was achieved by two important factors: the recognition that each member had significant contributions to make in his or her own field even when it overlapped with the domain of another and that the health educator served as the group facilitator, not as a physician (Friedson, 1970).

During the first year the program was in operation, an attitudinal survey was undertaken with twenty-one of the hospital staff who were serving as team members at different times. The results revealed some major differences in values. In response to the question Who do you think should teach the patient in the hospital? 58 percent of the nurses interviewed felt that *only* nurses should be involved in patient education, whereas 17 percent responded that patient education should be a team effort. In contrast to the responses, the team approach was recommended by 40 percent of the dietitians, 100 percent of the pharmacists, and 50 percent of the social workers. The resistance we encountered with the nursing staff in that first year and the positive reaction of other departments reflected these values.

During the second year a second survey was completed. Major changes had taken place. To cite just two examples, staff nurses welcomed the help from other team members in teaching the patients; the pharmacists enjoyed the patient contact, and by having access to the patient's medical records, they were often able to suggest to the physician more appropriate drugs. In the process of defining roles and melding boundaries, the role of the health educator also became more explicit and led to a greater acceptance of that role and the program in general.

To summarize, we surround our territory with boundaries made up of our learned roles, our learned sets of values, and our learned position in the social structure. This results in our encountering different value hierarchies, different perspectives on people and their needs, different assessments of the significance of other interventions, and different ranks of prestige when we attempt to cross boundaries to effect interprofessional collaboration. I've attempted to examine these boundaries as they pertain to patient education and to offer several approaches that have been used successfully to overcome these traditional barriers to patient education. The examples used describe the process of defining roles, the attainment of equal status in the social organization, and the process of clarifying one's values.

References

Ardrey, R. *The territorial imperative.* New York: Dell, 1966.

Arnold, M. F. *A study of professional roles in a multi-disciplinary health setting.* Unpublished doctoral dissertation, University of California at Berkeley, 1965.

Bernheimer, E. Shared leadership—A new approach to patient care. Atlanta: U.S. Public Health Service, Center for Disease Control, Bureau of Health Education, 1977, 19 pp.

Bernheimer, E., & Clever, L. H. The team approach to patient education: One hospital's experience in diabetes. Atlanta: U.S. Public Health

Service, Center for Disease Control, Bureau of Health Education, 1977, 47 pp.

Darling, F. F. Social behavior and survival. *The Auk,* April 1952, *69*:2, p. 183.

Dubos, R. *Man adapting.* New Haven, Conn.: Yale University Press, 1965.

Friedson, E. *Professional dominance.* New York: Atherton, 1970.

Goldberg, H. *The hazards of being male.* New York: Nash, 1976.

Hiltner, S. Tension and mutual support among the helping profession. *Social Service Review,* 1957, *31*, 377–389.

Kahn, A. Institutional constraints to interprofessional practice. In H. Rehr (Ed.), Medicine and social work. New York: Prodist, 1974.

Kane, R. A. *Interprofessional teamwork.* Syracuse University School of Social Work, monograph, 1975, 86 pp.

Parsons, T. Social structure and personality. New York: Free Press, 1964.

Pluckham, M. Professional territoriality. *Nursing Forum,* 1972, *11*, 300–310.

Raths, L., Harmin, M. & Simon, S. *Values and teaching.* Columbus, Ohio: Charles E. Merrill, 1966.

Robischon, P., & Scott, D. Role theory and its application in family nursing. *Nursing Outlook,* July 1969, pp. 52–59.

San Francisco Chronicle. "The Sherlock Holmes of Computer Crime," March 31, 1979, p. 6.

Simon, S. B., Howe, L. W., & Kirschenbaum, H. *Values clarification.* New York: Hart, 1972.

Smoyak, S. A. Problems in interprofessional relations. *Bulletin of the New York Academy of Medicine,* 1977, *53*(1), 51–59.

Sorbin, T. R. Role theory. In Gardner Lindzey (Ed.), *Handbook of social psychology* (Vol. 1). Reading, Mass.: Addison-Wesley, 1954, p. 223.

Susser, M. W., & Watson, W. Sociology in medicine. London: Oxford University Press, 1962.

Wise, H., Beckhard, R., Rubin, & Kyte, A. *Making health teams work.* Cambridge, Mass.: Ballinger, 1974.

World Health Organization Regional Office for the Eastern Mediterranean. Health education with special reference to the primary health care approach. *International Journal of Health Education,* 1978, *21* (2, Suppl.).

10

The Course for
Activated Patients

Keith W. Sehnert

The interest in medical self-care and health promotion programs is rapidly increasing in the United States. The reasons for this are based on many economic, educational, social, and medical factors. A prime factor, though, because of spiraling medical and hospital bills, is cost containment. An equally important factor for many people is a noneconomic one: a desire to be more self-reliant combined with a do-it-yourself philosophy.

McNerney recently said, "We have come to expect too much of our healers and too little of ourselves." He made this statement as he noted that the nature of illness has shifted from infectious diseases as the major killers to a new Public Enemy Number 1: lifestyle diseases. Heart disease, cancer, stroke, and accidents are due in large part to abuse and neglect of our bodies, he noted, and he concluded by pointing out that "magic bullets" and "miracle injections" are not going to provide the solutions. (McNerney, 1978).

It is my thesis in this chapter that one of the solutions to be considered to help combat modern-day health problems is the Course for Activated Patients. The course also provides an educational forum to help consumers make more appropriate use of health care resources and personnel, improve communications with professionals, and lower medical and hospital costs.

The History of the Course for Activated Patients

In 1970 the first Course for Activated Patients (CAP) was started in Herndon, Virginia (Sehnert, 1972). Then, as now, a class of 25 to 35 participants had as their objectives to:

1. Accept more individual responsibility for their own care and that of their families
2. Learn skills of observation, description, and handling of common illnesses, injuries, and emergencies
3. Increase basic knowledge about health with an emphasis on wellness
4. Learn how to make appropriate and economical use of health care resources, personnel, services, insurance, and medications

The name chosen for this educational effort was based on a term first used by Vernon Wilson, vice chancellor for health affairs at Vanderbilt University, who said, "Activated patients are persons whose clinical skills and understanding of health are upgraded in order that they can become active participants in their own health care rather than assume the passive role traditionally assigned to them by health care professionals (Wilson, 1970).

Over the years since that first course, the experiences gained have been reported in the literature (Sehnert, 1977; Sehnert & Osterweis, 1974). A typical course consists of a series of weekly two-hour sessions held over a period of twelve to sixteen weeks. Participants meet for presentations such as Your Medicine Chest: Friend or Foe; Responsibility for Your Own Care; Talking with your Doctor—Better Communication Pays Off; The Dangers of Eating American Style; and Self-help Skills (taking blood pressure, pulse, and temperature, and becoming a better observer of common clinical events); and presentations on learning to use clinical algorithms (medical self-help guides that assist lay people in making more informed health care decisions) and a variety of other topics determined, in part, by the age and interests of the participants.

All sessions incorporate these elements in the presentations:

1. *Appropriate use of the health care system.* Topics deal with consumerism as it relates to the health care system, for example, better use of money for insurance and medications, avoiding rip-offs, or establishing more realistic ideas about what the system can deliver.

2. *Compliance-health partnership.* Presentations are made regarding medical regimens for some common chronic diseases such as diabetes, hypertension, and obesity and various acute problems. This is "patient education" with a difference: Instead of the traditional professional orientation, presentations emphasize people-oriented options and the health partnership necessary for long-term compliance.

3. *Observations and treatment methods.* These how-to sessions emphasize improved skills of observation about common ills and injuries (when? where? what?). Such observations require learning the use of medical equipment and gaining the skills needed to describe and record the vital signs and other clinical events. With this information in hand, treatment methods are applied.

4. *Decision making and increased individual responsibility.* All sessions emphasize increased individual responsibility for health care decisions and actions. The sessions use medical self-help guides to assist individuals, first with the simple and short-term health problems and later with more complex and chronic problems. Such a process helps participants move away from doctor dependence to greater reliance on themselves and their families for many health care decisions.

5. *Health promotion and self-regulation.* The end product of the above elements is what is termed *health promotion.* It involves both use of more positive health habits and self-regulation that achieves greater harmony between the body and its external and internal environments.

Interest in CAP spread to other health professionals, and in 1973 Georgetown University began a series of workshops about the curriculum and the educational methods used. Similar courses were then developed for various audiences: those that were elderly, indigent, handicapped, or in schools and colleges. They extended to participants well beyond the middle-class families and individuals for which CAP was originally developed.

A result of these workshops was the Health Activation Network. This loose association of health professionals and lay people helps individuals, groups, agencies, colleges, and universities that are interested in starting courses in their communities. The network publishes a newspaper (*Health Activation News*, Box 923, Vienna, Virginia 22180) and provides course guides and other educational materials. It has helped start programs in over forty states since its formation in 1975.

The Concepts

Medical Self-care

The concept of people helping themselves solve their own medical and health problems is not a new one. In ancient Greece there were well established self-help resources. Nearly every city had a people's corner in the agora, or market square, where families could bring their ailing and injured. There, other citizens who had knowledge and skills to treat a particular condition were legally required to help (Scarborough, 1976). Anyone who refused assistance was subject to high fines—even seizure of property—a far cry from today's Good Samaritan limitations.

Throughout most of our history, lay people have of necessity helped themselves. Several of America's founders, including Thomas Jefferson and Benjamin Franklin, took training as apothecaries, the equivalent of today's physician's assistant, so that they could learn to handle the common ills and injuries that afflicted themselves and their families (Weiss, 1977).

In more recent times most people fended for themselves when it came to health care needs. During the Depression years I clearly recall from personal experience there simply wasn't the money or transportation needed for professional help. Older, more experienced members of the family provided the necessary services—with an assist from the "doctor book" in the family bookcase.

Modern days, with better access to professional medical help through all-weather roads, good cars, more doctors, better hospitals, wider health insurance coverage, good telephone service, and so on, have tended to make many individuals become doctor dependent. With a wider variety of good treatment methods, improved diagnostic equipment, superior drugs, and vaccines, it was assumed by lay people that the doctor could and should be able to solve all the medical dilemmas they faced.

Then a shift of perceptions about medical care occurred in the 1960s. With the leadership of Ralph Nader, the consumer movement began. The war in Vietnam helped spur the counterculture revolution. This was in turn nurtured by the women's liberation movement that spread across the nation from its beginnings in Boston and Berkeley.

These movements in turn gave birth to free clinics; and the associated anti-establishment, anti-intellectual, do-it-yourself attitudes laid the framework for a rebirth of medical self-care.

The Wheel of Health

One of the major concepts in the Course for Activated Patients is that participants assume increased individual responsibility for handling certain common health problems. These have been classified in selected categories (Rushmer, 1974) and are shown in the upper part of figure 10-1. These problems (with some examples noted in parentheses in each category on fig. 10-1), my experience has shown, can be handled appropriately by most individuals who have taken the course. Despite the concerns voiced by Alexander Pope in the eighteenth century—"A little learning is a dangerous thing; drink deep or taste not the Pierian spring"—and by more recent skeptics, lay people with increased understanding and skills do not misuse this knowledge. After a decade of working with these medical self-help programs, no case of blatant misuse has been brought to my attention. I am still more concerned with dangerous ignorance than with dangerous learning.

Methods

Many of the educational methods used in the Course for Activated Patients have been described in my book and in the literature (Hentges, 1978; Sehnert, 1976; Sehnert & Eisenberg, 1975). Some additional details of methods used are presented here.

Educational Strategies

The overall session content has already been briefly discussed in this chapter. Each session has three elements: session topics, type of problem and presentation, and attitude of the participants. How these interact is depicted in figure 10-2. The educational strategy involved is to use each session as a carrier for exploring appropriate use of health care resources, services, medicine, or insurance; or for exploring the compliance-health partnership; or for exploring other elements described on the top of the box shown in figure 10-2. The attitudes

Figure 10-1.
The Wheel of Health.

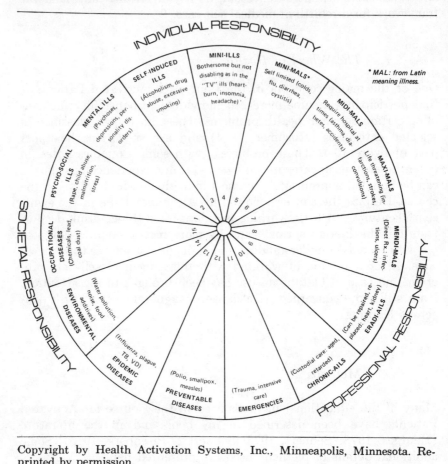

of participants (on the end of the box) indicate readiness for acceptance and educational impact.

The topics selected point out special interests of participants and vary with audience to some degree. For instance the session, "Up on Your Toes" emphasizes foot problems that are of great interest to a group of senior citizens but would provide little excitement for college students. Similarly, sessions emphasizing common pediatric problems could cause yawns for a class of senior citizens but be right on target in a class located in a suburban housing development with lots of young married couples in the course. The intensity and depth of the skills taught in the self-help sessions also vary: A participant with a spouse who has hypertension may want to become skilled in taking blood pressure; women with preschool children who have frequent earaches may want to gain some proficiency in using an otoscope; and so on.

Educational Tactics

THE ASK-THE-DOCTOR CHECKLIST. Several presentations in CAP emphasize the health partnership between professional and activated patient. Various educational tactics have been developed that provide participants with the communications skills and assertiveness training needed to establish the role of partner with the doctor. One such tactic is the Ask-the-Doctor Checklist. This checklist (see fig. 10-3) was developed after a 1972 American Academy of Family Physicians survey in which family doctors were asked, "What is the single most annoying thing that patients do?" The top choice was failing to follow instruction on diets, medication, bed rest, and so on.

My professional experience was that much so-called noncompliance was due in large measure to failure of communication. When a patient doesn't ask for explanation, the doctor usually fails to give it. The reasons that the patient is not more assertive are many, but a common explanation is "The doctor seemed too busy." Extensive use of the checklist over the last six years has shown that its use actually saves the busy doctor and other aides time by avoiding many unnecessary follow-up phone calls. The list has been found to be a convenience for both professional and patient.

The checklist is used in CAP through role playing by participants. Scenarios are developed featuring patients with common health problems, doctors who object to patients being "too inquisitive," and so on. (More details on its use can be found in *Family Health*, March 1976, pp. 10–11.)

THE MEDICINE CHEST: FRIEND OR FOE? Whenever a need assessment is conducted to determine which topics will be chosen for CAP, requests for information about medications, drug side effects, and consumer tips to use in pharmacies have high frequency. Because of this interest, one session —"Your Medicine Chest: Friend or Foe?" —provides consumer tips about the packaging, pricing, and labeling of medicines; increases awareness about both beneficial and adverse effects of medication; and provides interactive demonstrations built around the theme "Take the Chest Test," in which participants clean

Figure 10-2.
The elements of a health activation program

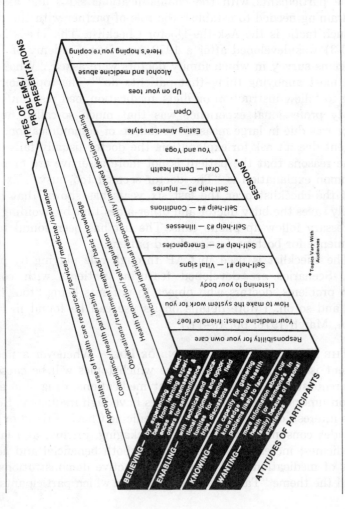

From K. W. Sehnert, "Background and Perspectives about Self-care/Self-help: Past, Present, Future." In Larry K. Y. Ng, M.D. and Devra Lee Davis, Ph.D. (eds.) *Public Health Strategies.* New York: Van Nostrand Reinhold, in press. Reprinted by permission.

Figure 10-3.
One of the CAP educational tactics is a checklist.

THE ASK-THE-DOCTOR LIST

BEFORE THE VISIT (complete this part yourself)

1. Why am I going to the doctor? (the main reason)_____

2. Is there anything else that worries me about my health?

   _____No

   _____Yes (please list)_____

3. What do I expect the doctor to do for me today? (in 10 words or less)

   _____

DURING THE VISIT (complete with help of doctor)

1. What is the diagnosis?_____

2. Why did I get it and how can I prevent it next time?_____

3. Are there any helpful patient education materials available for the

   condition? (describe)_____

4. Are there any medicines for me to take?

   _____No

   _____Yes (describe)_____

5. Are there any special instructions, concerns, or possible side effects I
   need to know about the medicine?

   _____No

   _____Yes (describe)_____

AFTER THE VISIT (complete with help of doctor)

1. Am I to return for another visit?

   _____No

   _____Yes (when)_____

2. What should I do at home?

   _____Activity_____

   _____Treatments _____

   _____Precautions_____

Figure 10-3. *(continued)*

---

3. Am I to phone in for lab reports?

_____No

_____Yes (when)_____

4. Should I report back to doctor by phone for any reason?

_____No

_____Yes (when)_____

---

the junk out of the family medicine chest and go on field trips to local pharmacies. (See "The Activated Patient," *Family Health*, August 1975.)

CLINICAL ALGORITHMS AND SELF-HELP MEDICAL GUIDES. Several sessions of CAP are used to provide participants with skills in using clinical algorithms (medical self-help guides). These algorithms are based on work done at Harvard, Dartmouth, Duke, and Georgetown and were initially designed to help nonphysicians make health care decisions. They were first used for triage by Red Cross volunteers to determine whether military personnel should be seen by a physician or a paramedic—and if the need for care was urgent or nonurgent. The algorithms came out of Project AMOS (Army Medical Outpatient System) at Ft. Belvoir, Virginia.

The algorithms used in CAP were then rewritten for civilian lay people and designed to cover the illnesses, injuries, and emergencies that are seen with highest frequency in private family practice clinics. Problems were chosen by the frequencies with which they would occur in a typical family. Participants in the course learned to use the algorithms by role playing, making clinical observations in the class, and practicing use of the algorithms when appropriate family health problems occurred.

RESULTS. A controlled study of the Course for Activated Patients has been done and its results summarized in Sehnert, 1977. A complete report is also available by writing the U.S. Department of

Commerce.[1] Briefly, Medicaid recipients and medicare beneficiaries showed distinct differences between those who took CAP (experimental) and those who didn't (control) in several ways:

1. Experimental groups used professional care services more appropriately a higher percentage of the time than did controls (experimental, 94.3%; control, 84.2%).
2. Those who took CAP had a higher percentage of appropriate self-care activities per person per year (experimental, 87.5%; control, 30.4%).
3. People in experimental groups were better able to perform clinical procedures and make better clinical observations (experimental, 69.1%; control, 49.3%).

In pre- and posttest evaluations of life-style activities (diet), knowledge about health and confidence, and knowledge about self-care, the experimental groups had scores that were higher at statistically significant levels.

In economic terms there were also several interesting results: In the Medicaid study the experimental groups showed lower drug and lab costs *after* the course than they averaged before and also had fewer primary care visits per personal year after CAP. Corresponding changes were not found in the Medicare groups because the posttest follow-up took place in the winter/spring season during which the participants experienced their usual higher incidence of primary care visits.

In situations that involved use of professional resources, the experimental groups for both the Medicare and Medicaid studies showed a greater willingness to use health care professionals (other than physicians) 30 percent of the time versus less than 6 percent for the controls. This was because paramedics, nurses, and other allied professionals helped teach CAP, so that participants better understood the roles of these professionals. A surprising but pleasing result (that should be an encouraging sign for clinicians who feel threatened by CAP and similar medical self-care courses) was the difference noted in patient satisfaction with professional services: 80 percent of the experimentals rated themselves "very satisfied or satisfied" compared to 63 percent of the controls.

[1] These reports were done at Georgetown University under contact HEW-100-75-0016 for the Office of Planning and Evaluation, U.S. Department of Health, Education, and Welfare, and the Technical Information Service, U.S. Department of Commerce, Springfield, Virginia 22761: *Report on Course and Evaluation of Course for Activated Patients* (PB-280-276); *Executive Summary* (PB-280-277); *Course Guide for Medicaid Citizens* (PB-267-282); and *Course Guide for Activated Seniors* (PB-267-588).

Conclusion

Experience since 1970 shows that CAP offers enough encouraging trends to warrant continued development and study. Settings that have a great potential for success include senior citizen living facilities, primary health care clinics, health maintenance organizations, and college health services. The benefits that can be expected for participants that take CAP include improved life-style health habits; savings in primary health care and medication costs; more appropriate health resource utilization; and increased self-reliance and skills among lay people in handling common illnesses, injuries, and emergencies that have usually been considered the province of professionals.

References

Hentges, K. Health activation education for self-care. *Health Education,* July-August 1978, pp. 31–32.

McNerney, W. J. Help yourself to better health. In Duane Carlson (Ed. Dir.), *Blueprint for health series* (Vol. 27, No. 1. Chicago: Blue Cross Association, 1978, pp. 1–7.

Rushmer, R. Design and analysis of primary care. In Kallstrom, M. & Yarnall, S. (Eds.), *Advances in Primary Care,* Seattle, Washington: Medical Computer Services Assoc., 1974, pp. 9–20.

Scarborough, J. Facets of Hellenic life. Boston: Houghton Mifflin, 1976, pp. 221-230.

Sehnert, K. W. The patient as a paramedical. *Virginia Medical Monthly,* April 1972, pp. 409–413.

Sehnert, K. W. Patient education: A new resource for family practice. *Delaware Medical Journal,* October 1976, pp. 587–599.

Sehnert, K. W. A course for activated patients. *Social Policy,* November-December, 1977, pp. 40–46.

Sehnert, K. W. Background and perspectives about self-care/self-help: Past, present, future. In Larry K. Y. Ng and Devra Lee Davis (Eds.), *Public Health Strategies.* New York: Von Nostrand Reinhold, in press.

Sehnert, K. W., & Eisenberg, H. How to be your own doctor . . . sometimes. New York: Grosset & Dunlap, 1975, pp. G1–G128.

Sehnert, K. W., & Osterweis, M. The activated patient: A concept for health education. *Continuing Education for the Family Physician,* October 19, 1974, pp. 53–56.

Weiss, E. *Who has been responsible for our health in the past?* Workshop of the Kentucky Bureau for Health Services, Lexington, March 22, 1977.

Wilson, V. E. Smith Memorial Lecture, Memorial Hospital, Rockford, Illinois, December 4, 1970.

11

Patient Education and Self-care: How Do They Differ?*

Lowell Stern Levin

The concept of patient education is readily understood by both health professionals and lay people. While the nuances of strategy and content may vary, the essential purpose remains: to teach patients those ideas and skills that will help them to cope with their immediate medical problems and even, perhaps, to maintain health and avoid disease. The precise boundaries of activities characterized as patient education, however, may be determined more by the realities of a particular institution than by definitions or the idealism of health education philosophers. Time, values, place, personalities, priorities, and sometimes the patients themselves profoundly influence what ultimately emerges in practice.

Thus if we set aside the accepted academic and professional criteria, we would probably discover that almost all inpatient and outpatient institutions could (using their *own* criteria) point to some form of activity they label as patient education. After all, patient education has by now achieved status to some degree akin to motherhood. Critics now limit their attacks to issues of for whom the service should be provided (issues of access), what should be taught (issues of patient privilege), who should teach it (issues of professional privilege), and the nature of evaluation (issues of process versus outcomes).

These are all serious concerns, but the fact remains that we have gone far beyond the earlier and more fundamental arguments of to be or not to be. That, I submit, given the snail's pace of changes in professional values and the rigidities of institutional habits, is not at all bad. After all, patient education as a purposeful, organized endeavor has been with us for less than one professional generation, and we have come to take its legitimacy, if not the nature of its impact, for granted. It is recognized by both the American Hospital Association and the Blue Cross Association, although reimbursement has yet to supplant rhetoric. It is now a matter of finding the right formula —one that will assure quality, equity, and accountability of educational services rendered.

A Matter of Motivation

The search for ways and means of financing patient education is, of course, heightened by the present institutional fiscal crisis. Hospital operators, both administrative and professional, are anxious at least to recover costs, even if to do so involves no more than parsing out the existing components of medical care and labeling some of them as "patient education." For, like it or not, patient education is becoming an attractive interest in terms of its income-producing potential and, even more significant, its potential for bending patient behavior to accommodate the needs of the system.

Now, some may say, what matters the motive so long as the programs continue and may be expanded? A moment's reflection reveals the problem: Interest in income-producing or efficiency-enhancing health services is in profound conflict with values of prevention, even more so with those of health promotion. To the degree that we concentrate on these financially or operationally beneficial services, we restrict our goals and strategies to ones that will not threaten long-range institutional or professional security or weaken the labor-intensive character of professional health care. Thus as long as patient education does not tamper with the control inherent in the care giver's role, it is a safe and appealing undertaking. We can comfortably offer patients those health care skills that are not competitive with professional services for various reasons, for instance, lack of professional interest or resources, as in the maintenance and management of people with arthritis or diabetes.

During most of the 1970s health educators have increasingly called for more emphasis on health education's "practical" contributions in systems and economic benefits. (Among the advantages cited have been such achievements as fewer broken appointments, increased bill payments, less likelihood of malpractice suits, more efficient use of professional resources, and an increase in patient compliance.) Many, indeed, have expressed the view that patient education cannot become a universal benefit until its contributions to the care system are demonstrated. One need not labor the painful irony of such an empty victory beyond pointing out the self-defeating "benefit" of equal access to the social control of the medical trust.

The Self-care Perspective

But enter now a new perspective on health education—the concept of self-care—which challenges both the economic and philosophic lifelines of professional health care services. This perspective is not always a welcome one, as exemplified by the reaction of one state hospital association committee as it considered the hospital's role in promoting self-care oriented health education. The committee asked, "Is it counterproductive, from a practical financial standpoint, for hospitals, which derive the greatest part of their resource from inpatient care, to urge courses of action for people which, if followed, may conceivably reduce hospital income?"

One must admire the honesty of the query, if not its insensitivity to the public good. It also demonstrates how some perceive the difference in economic terms between orthodox patient education and self-care education. But there are other, more substantive, differences that stand out clearly. Although I may exaggerate the distinctions for the sake of clarity, I believe the points are generally valid.

Sick Patient? Or Well Person?

The most obvious distinction between patient education and self-care education is captured clearly in the terms themselves. Patient education assigns a unique social role to the learner, that of a sick person under the care of another. Self-care education, in contrast, does not assume sickness, thereby assigning a generic meaning to care—that is, to look after, and in an autonomous way. Patient education goals are initiated in response to a state of disease; self-care educational goals are generally anticipatory of risk.

These are radically different starting points for formulating educational objectives, methods, and measurement of outcomes. Patient educators can use the same approach that the physician would in planning therapy: diagnose the needs, decide on acceptable outcomes, select a method appropriate to the patient's condition, administer the educational treatment, and observe results. Implicit in this approach is the professional's responsibility to help the patient achieve optimal compliance with professionally prescribed health behavior. Granted that some professional and patient goals may be identical, the fact is that professional regulation of the process and outcomes keeps the control in professional hands and does not transfer skills to the patient.

Phrased another way, the methods of patient education, aside from matters of content, are not usually directed toward reducing dependency. True, patient education algorithms, protocols, decision trees, and instruction tear sheets may be considerably more useful to patients than the virtual vacuum in doctor-patient communications that they fill. But these devices are the product of the professionals' construction of reality and thus are strategies that standardize and regulate the health behavior of the patient.

Beyond the direct political consequences of this regulation of behavior is the potentially serious iatrogenic effect of deprecating, reducing, or even shutting down the patient's autonomous healing capabilities. The result could be reinforcement of patient dependency with all of its counterproductive effects, among others, transforming the patient into a malleable component in the professional health care system—a minor stockholder in the complex firm of medical care.

Self-care education, however, derives its goals from the *learner's* perceived needs and preferences, regardless of whether or not they conform to professional perceptions of the learner's needs. It is the learner who determines the desired outcomes in accordance with his or her decision on which risks to avoid (or not to avoid); similarly, content is learner determined; learner preferences for education methods are honored; and evaluation is in terms of criteria proposed by the learner. Thus, both content and methods in self-care education help shift the control in health decision making and health care from the professional to the lay person.

This approach can not be labeled therapeutic in the sense that it modifies client behavior to improve health status (although clearly the health status can be expected to benefit—but on the learner's terms). Nor may the results always conform to professional values, particularly when the person opts for quality of life values in preference to quality of health values. But what we can expect from the self-care orientation is a lowering of dependency and its negative sequelae.

Content and Substance

Patient education and self-care education differ on substantive bases as well as educational strategy. The most signal difference has to do with the range of learner concerns that are perceived by the educator as legitimate or appropriate. When dealing with prevention and risk reduction, patient educators usually have in mind the insultive diseases and disabilities—the ones caused by biological, psychological, and environmental factors. There has been negligible interest, however, in the control of assaultive diseases, namely, those caused by the health care givers.

To be sure, there are patient education programs that include information on how to use the health care system. Criteria, guidelines, and information are offered regarding when to seek professional care, what services are available, and on what basis; in the case of inpatient education, there has been a good deal of emphasis on assisting the patient to make a good adjustment to the hospital, that is, to understand hospital routine. These how-to-use-the-system components of patient education may save some bruises, but by and large they reflect the expectation that the patient will adapt to the system. Few if any of these efforts encourage awareness of the hazards of medical care, of how to reduce the risk of iatrogenic illness, and of how to change the system to conform to patient needs and preferences.

Self-care education, often born out of people's desire to avoid or reduce iatrogenic illness (note self-care in the feminist clinics), puts special emphasis on lay skills in the management of the professional care system. The themes represented by such works as A. Levin's *Talk to Your Doctor* (1975) and Belsky and Gross's *How to Choose and Use Your Doctor* (1975) are central to self-care education. It is understandable that education for iatrogenic control is more feasible when undertaken in the nonstressful circumstances of people not already under care. Consider for instance the difficulties the institutionally based patient educator would have in cautioning the patient regarding the potential dangers of the institutional care she or he is receiving. Further, patients are often too sick, too frightened of retaliation, or too embarrassed to demand information or question authority.

Still another substantive distinction between patient education as now practiced and self-care education is that the former is often designed to impart new knowledge and skills in situations in which it is assumed that the patient has little or no previous experience, for instance, self-administration of insulin. But self-care education, with its more diffuse goals of promoting health and preventing, detecting, and treating disease at the primary care level, not only emphasizes the individual as decision maker but also relies heavily on knowledge and skills the patient already has—many of which are in the category of traditional family health practices or home remedies—and on autonomous self-healing capabilities.

Education in self-care assumes that most if not all of such practices are either appropriate and beneficial or at least not harmful. Studies in Britain and Denmark found that 90 percent of health practices undertaken by patients prior to seeking a medical contact were relevant (Eliott-Binns, 1973; Pedersen, 1976). Self-care builds on those current lay practices and supplements them with medical-technical concepts, strategies, and skills not previously in the domain of family remedies or, for that matter, of public health education.

Patient education usually refers to patients of allopathic care givers: those in professions we customarily think of as part of mainstream, Western medical culture. Self-care education, however, while largely focusing on the transfer of allopathic skills to lay use, does not exclude other healing strategies. This is particularly important with regard to strategies of health promotion and chronic disease management and the role of an individual's personal resources of mind and body in diagnosing, monitoring, and healing.

Enviropolitics

A fourth substantive distinction is the fact that self-care education relates personal health status to forces in the environment (Milio, 1977). Patient education in contrast generally focuses on a person's personal health behavior and the activities such as diet, life-style, or dental prophylaxis over which the person can exercise personal control. The latter is a valid focus, but as we awaken to the astonishing role environment appears to play in the etiology or exacerbation of many chronic diseases, it is necessary to consider skills that bring about social change as well as reduce personal risk.

Self-care education, therefore, attempts to place individual protection within the broader context of social protection. It tries to avoid the blaming-the-victim orientation of some preventive health education efforts and to help the learner identify those factors in society or the community that are complicit in disease production and for which solutions require social action. Thus, self-care education is concerned with strengthening the lay resource in health as a civil as well as a personal resource. Demystification of enviropolitics is as crucial as demystification of medical care practices.

Educational methods are another distinguishing factor. The patient educator uses the methods appropriate to teaching specific skills (hence, active learner trials under supervision) or strategies related to problem solving (skills in self-observation and knowledge of how to use resources effectively). Self-care educators, while employing similar techniques, go beyond them to include exercises designed to center health control in the individual.

The key strategy in self-care education is to encourage circumstances where problem-posing skills are acknowledged and supported. *That* is where the power of health control begins, not in the mechanics of problem solving per se. In defining the problem, the range of solutions is also defined. Freire in *Pedagogy of the Oppressed* (1973) elaborates some educational strategies conducive to shifting the locus of health control from professional to lay person. It is not enough to transfer skills or even concepts. The educational method itself must exemplify the experience of gaining fundamental control over one's health destiny.

Health and Social Values

I have contrasted self-care education with patient education in an effort to dramatize what appear to me to be the biggest differences and to help clarify the values we assign to all health education activity. Self-care education, it is clear, incorporates some goals, methods, and outcomes that may be at variance with counterpart aspects of patient education; but it is equally clear that it is dangerous to stereotype either one. There are instances where patient education is aggressively testing the margins of its orthodox traditions, and there are self-care education programs that timorously avoid incursions into the professional domain of skills.

Nevertheless I believe the previous characterization of at least the historical thrust of patient education and the current tenor of plans for promulgating self-care education to be reasonably accurate. Health educators, health planners, and health service administrators sense the difference between the two, although the whats and wherefores are elusive. Debate, even anger, has resulted, but these are wholesome indications of the growing acknowledgment of health education's crucial role in the next round of changes in health in our society.

Health education, generically speaking, is now entering a period of rapid transition as a result of forces beyond our control (Levin, Katz, & Holst, 1976). Changes in morbidity patterns (chronic dis- and significant potentials in society's mediating institutions (family, neighborhood, church, voluntary associations) are affecting not only health needs but preferences and priorities (Berger, 1977). Despite this, however, some professionals have come to accept certain values and beliefs about society's health care interests and intentions as im- mutable givens. Indeed when evidence is marshaled that threatens these assumptions, the reaction is predictably negative.

This is particularly true in relation to the possibility of one's own agency's culpability in causing or exacerbating the very needs or problems we seek to abate. Inpatient education is a case in point. The hospital environment itself may be hostile to the educational goal of reducing patient dependency; nurses dispensing medication by dose and physicians' refusal to provide medical records to patients are ex- amples. We don't always practice what we preach; indeed, we often send out double signals to our clients. Is it possible, or even moral, to attempt to reduce patient dependency through education when the very environment in which that education takes place tends to increase dependency?

The question now before us is: Should patient education adopt a stronger self-care orientation? Should it go beyond its present boundaries of service associated with an individual's patienthood? Some argue that it should and must (Simonds, 1977). Others point out the danger in further extending the influence of the health pro- fessions in our lives (Zola, 1977).

My own view is that we should not strive for synonymity among programs in self-care and patient education. Each has some unique, timely, and appropriate contributions to make. Thus I am not con- vinced that the hospital patient is in the best position to learn about issues of life-style, health promotion, and protection from iatrogenic assault. Conversely I need to be shown evidence that education re- garding the management of disease for which a healthy individual may some day be at potential risk is practical and lasting.

Components of a Whole

I would prefer that we recognize health education as a continuous process whereby organized programs for learning can be planned in a reasonably systematic way; where we respond without compromise or control to the learning needs of people for growth, fulfillment, freedom, and maximum self-sufficiency; and where each component of the health education enterprise consistently adheres to these values.

The growing demand for health education reflects, I believe, a general and broader interest by people today in gaining more self-control in an increasingly mass society. People are not waiting for health education planners to do much planning; in fact marketplace demand has encouraged the growth of a whole health education industry. In my view the impact of this phenomenon on self-care has been, on the whole, positive and relatively free of exploitation, although we must be exceedingly vigilant here.

Patient education, on the other hand, has not fared so well. Commercializing of patient education in predigested, prepackaged forms is an obvious money-maker. The ominous aspect of this trend is the nature of the intended use of these materials, one that casts suspicion on both their content and methods. One supplier of patient education materials, for example, promises that their approach will leave the patient "less frightened . . . more cooperative . . . less likely to sue" (*The Properly Informed Patient*, 1977). It sounds like a prefrontal lobotomy.

That brand of patient education in its extreme is easily recognized as inconsistent with self-care values. But it is the more subtle, repressive content in patient education that causes most of the trouble—for example, emphasis on the concepts of compliance and cooperation. These concepts are potentially hazardous to the patient's health; moreover they are not necessarily in the exclusive or even primary interest of the patient (Cousins, 1976). If we are to encourage patients to ask questions and make decisions, then we must anticipate and honor the potential benefits of their noncompliance with our regimens or their disobedience to our authority.

Mutual Aid Groups

As the self-care interest in society advances, we should be able to discern important changes in patterns of illness, if not disease. People's rejection of clinically defined and labeled deviance at the psychological, social, and economic levels will be their major interest. We see this already in the form of 500,000 mutual aid or self-help groups. Some 5 million people are turning to support groups as a resource to avoid or overcome the disabling effects of social, and professional labeling. Yet most members of categorical disease or disability groups remain in medical care contact.

These groups are an impressive resource in concert with patient education. Here is an area where patient educators can make a major contribution through referral, while at the same time forswearing the temptation to manage the group. Unfortunately, signs of this latter possibility already are present and ominous (Parsell & Tagliareni, 1974). Control of the mutual aid group would only serve to destroy the benefits of the lay initiative in self-determination in health and dilute the meaning of mutual aid.

On the other hand patient education programs can derive new perspectives and technology from the experience of the mutual aid group. Simond's concept of "hospital patient counseling" fits nicely with my view of patient education's bridging and continuing contribution to people in mutual support groups (Simonds, 1977, p. 43.) Patient education in this sense is a component in a system of health education. It is not necessary and may be counterproductive for patient education programs to attempt comprehensive, continuous coverage of the hospital discharge. We must identify the core expertise of patient education in concert with other community resources that provide a progressively client-controlled environment.

Education for the Care Givers

If the goal in patient education is to encourage the patient's self-sufficiency, then we must restrain our professional instincts to identify more needs and organize more educational care. The task, rather, is to hold to the minimal necessary professional inputs and to evaluate our success in terms of reduced client dependency on our services. That is a difficult perspective to achieve in the environment of this "serviced society" (Gorden, Bush, McKnight, Gilbred, et al., 1974), but it is the crux of the matter in drawing patient education closer to the self-care values with which society is now challenging us.

Patient education in the context of self-care values defines its goals in terms of reducing disability that develops not only as a sequel to disease but also as a sequel to professional help. To achieve the latter goal means that programs designed initially to help the patient must be broadened to include the care givers. An analysis of care-giver contributions to patient disability in the form of dependency-evoking activity should form the central curriculum for inservice education. Naturally such a program will call for extraordinary sensitivity and creativity in helping distinguish between activities stimulated by needs *of* patients and those stimulated by the need *for* patients. Perpetuation and expansion of services beyond the minimum that is needed in a given community may be of benefit to the provider but surely cause difficulties for the consumer (McKnight, 1976).

Unfortunately, motivation for minimizing unnecessary and counterproductive services, be they clinical or educational, confronts the fiscal pressures on institutions to maintain services. Here the recourse is to help in the phase-down period of institutional care (and later ambulatory care) services by assisting care givers to drop unproductive dependency-evoking procedures as a way of preparing for a more rational reduction of surplus services. In my view this will be an important new responsibility for patient educators as they define the total institutional environment as capable of making an important contribution to patient growth in self-sufficiency.

We are in an exciting era of transition in health and health care, a transition from a professionally dominated world of service to one of self-service. The process of demystifying medicine and demedicalizing society is just now rising in our consciousness as a profound turning point in the history of health. We must come to terms with changing patterns of morbidity, emerging pluralism in chronic disease care, less rigid and moralistic perspectives on avoidance of risk, recognition of iatrogenic effects, and appreciation of the lay resource as the primary and least dangerous health resource.

First Do No Harm

The integrity of patient education in enhancing the power of the individual to self-heal and self-regulate is at stake now. There are no signs that the social demand for more self-control in health will abate; indeed it becomes more clamorous with each passing day. Realities of demographic and epidemiologic changes and the diminishing utility of professional services and commodities within the context of those changes argue that health educators must examine the character of their allegiance and adjust their efforts accordingly.

Patient education must be defined in more limited and more precise terms, and the health educator must start with the caveat, *primum non nocere,* "first do no harm." During acute phases of illness, particularly those involving periods of institutional care or tight medical management on an ambulatory basis, patient education's role is centrally one of helping patients to maintain their integrity, to minimize the dependency-producing impact of medical care. Some may find this perspective on patient education too conservative, and it ease rising from 30 to 80 percent of all diseases in a forty-year period), demographic shifts, accelerated transport and communication, is conservative—intentionally so—in the sense that it implies prevention of unnecessary risk.

In a very practical and nonpolemical way, patient education and self-care education are advocacy strategies that can contribute to the public's health competence at different points on the same continuum. Now is the time to clarify the mutuality of their values and to identify their special contributions to health education, uncompromisingly operating in the public interest.

References

Belsky, M. S., & Gross, L. *Beyond the medical mystique: How to choose and use your doctor.* New York: Arbor House, 1975.

Berger, P. To Empower people. In P. Berger & R. Neuhaus (Eds.), *The role of mediating structures and public policy.* Washington, D.C.: American Enterprise Institute for Public Policy Research, 1977, p. 45.

Cousins, N. Anatomy of an illness (as perceived by the patient). *New England Journal of Medicine,* December 23, 1976, *295,* 1463.

Eliott-Binns, C. P. An analysis of lay medicine. *Journal of the Royal College of General Practitioners,* April 1973, *23,* 255–264.

Freire, P. *Pedagogy of the oppressed.* Harmondsworth, Eng.: Penguin, 1973.

Gordon, A. Bush, M., McKnight, J., Gilbred, L., et al. Beyond need: Toward a serviced society. Evanston, Ill.: Center for Urban Affairs, Northwestern University, 1974. (Mimeographed)

Levin, A. *Talk back to your doctor.* New York: Doubleday, 1975.

Levin, L. S., Katz, A. H., & Holst, E. *Self-care: Lay initiatives in health.* New York: Prodist, 1976.

McKnight, J. Professionalized service and disabling help. Evanston, Ill.: Center for Urban Affairs, Northwestern University, October 1976. (Mimeographed)

Milio, N. Self-care in urban settings. *Health Education Monographs,* Summer 1977, *5,* 136–144.

Parsell, S., & Tagliareni, E. M. Cancer patients help each other. *American Journal of Nursing,* April 1974, *74,* 650.

Pedersen, P. A. Varighed fra sygdoms begyndelse til henvendelse til praktiserende laege. *Ugeskr. Koeg.* August 1976, *138,* 1962–1966.

The properly informed patient. Santa Barbara, Calif.: Patient Audio Visual Information System (P.O. Box 30692), 1977.

Simonds, S. K. Hospital patient counseling problems, priorities and prospects. *Health Values: Achieving High Level Wellness,* January- February 1977, *1,* 41–49.

Zola, I. K. On the way to a healthist society. Waltham, Mass.: Department of Sociology, Brandeis University, 1977. (Mimeographed paper), 1977.

12

Self-Management Strategies

Linda Ormiston

Individual responsibility is a growing trend. In professional journals; in popular magazines; in educational opportunities provided by health organizations, communities, and commercial organizations; and in many other ways people are being exhorted to take charge of their own lives. Self-help and personal accountability are definitely ideas whose time has come.

Personal responsibility is an exciting and freeing notion; it can dramatically alter a person's perspectives and horizons. It can also be very threatening. However much a person may want to be and to feel in control of his or her own situation, it would be unusual for that person not to perceive as well the burden and the risk involved in the responsibility. People who have just nearly died from heart attacks are usually very motivated to make changes in their life-styles. They are also very frightened. Telling them to take charge of their lives and to make changes such as stopping smoking is not enough. Telling them *what* to do without telling them *how* to do it can threaten them so much they will not even venture to change. In fact a large number of patients who have had heart attacks do continue to smoke. Undoubtedly they know they should stop smoking; many have probably tried more than once to stop. Wanting to change and knowing how to change are two different issues.

Those of us who are involved in encouraging people to take charge of particular aspects of their lives need to be very sensitive to the fears as well as to the hopes of our clients and students. Individual responsibility and accountability involve skills that need to be taught systematically in conjunction with any behavior change program or course. Before people can begin to learn these skills, we must provide a setting in which they can have enough confidence in themselves and the program we are offering that they are willing to risk trying to make changes and to take charge. In an effective program the participants are totally responsible from the very beginning for any changes they make; thus they can take complete credit for their successes. However, the changes they are asked to make or choose to make are always very small. Over time they amount to substantial changes in life-style, but at any given moment the personal risks are minimized.

Personality Trait Theory

How has the growing emphasis on personal responsibility and self-management evolved? In the past, personal change was viewed from the perspective of personality trait theory. This model maintains that certain kinds of personality traits lead to certain kinds of behaviors, which in turn lead to certain consequences. Traits by definition are assumed to be relatively stable and difficult, if not impossible, to change. Willpower was considered one of those personality traits. According to this model some people have willpower and others simply do not, or at least, not very much. By the very nature of the programs we teach, all of the people we deal with, and frequently we ourselves, fall into the category of those who have none or not much willpower. There is a terrible burden of guilt in being labeled by yourself or by others as having little or no willpower. The question that automatically arises is Why not? Why don't I have much willpower? What is wrong with me? If we or the people we teach are operating from a personality model, it is almost impossible to affect life-style changes. Used in this context, the model is very pessimistic, for it presupposes that change is difficult if not impossible; a person cannot help being compulsive, impulsive, or weak willed. That burden of guilt (added to the guilt that is often already present from previous failures at change efforts) adds to the problem.

Behavior Modification

Behavior modification brought a much more productive and optimistic model according to which certain kinds of signals—people, places, and events—in the external environment trigger specific behaviors. The behaviors are in turn maintained by certain results or consequences.

$$\text{Signals} \longrightarrow \text{Behavior} \longrightarrow \text{Consequences}$$

The response to each set of signals is learned, and alternative responses can be learned.

For example a person walking past a bakery smells brownies baking. The enticing aroma induces him or her to enter the store, purchase and eat a couple of brownies. The immediate consequence is that they taste good; the long-term one is that the person may gain some weight. Any behavior pattern is made of a chain of such sequences in which the behavior or the consequences or both become the signals for a new behavior.

When signals automatically trigger a behavior, that behavior becomes a habit. A person may not be aware which specific signal is triggering a particular behavior. Thus signal control is important for eliminating inappropriate behavior. New behaviors that a person is attempting to learn, on the other hand, are not at first automatically triggered by specific signals; they have yet to become habits. Thus providing positive consequences—rewards—for new behaviors that are being learned is very important.

Within this framework, willpower is defined as a set of skills, skills that enable a person to manage the signals in different ways and use the consequences most effectively to support her or his efforts. Willpower is a set of skills anyone can learn, not an ingrained personality trait. If a person has trouble doing a particular thing, it is not because there is something wrong with that person but rather because he or she has never acquired the necessary skills. When one says this to some students one can sometimes hear an audible sigh of relief as if a tremendous burden of guilt were being liften. When people have difficulty managing a particular problem such as smoking or overeating, they often have a strong feeling of personal blame, of feeling something is terrible wrong with them. I have found from my experience with weight management that self-blame is one of the greatest obstacles to being able to risk trying to change. The combination of a more workable and positive definition of willpower and specifying other skills for managing the external environment made the earlier behavioral approaches much more optimistic and productive than the personality trait theory approach. Within the behavior modification framework, there was an obvious potential for change.

Yet because the behavioral approaches dealt with external signals and consequences, they imposed on themselves a limit to the amount of change that was possible.

Behavioral Self-management or
Cognitive Behavior Modification

In recent years the behavioral approaches have been extended to include thoughts and emotions within the definitions of both signals and consequences. There is a growing body of literature that suggests that this extended behavioral model—known as cognitive behavioral modification, behavior therapy, or behavioral self-management—is an effective model for life-style changes. The theoretical basis for the growing emphasis on self-management comes primarily from the work of Bandura in his book *Social Learning Theory* (1977b) and an article "Efficacy expectancies: Toward a unifying theory of behavior change" (1977a). Two other books have also contributed significantly to the theoretical development: *Cognition and Behavior Modification* by Mahoney (1974) and *Cognitive-Behavior Modification: An Integrative Approach* by Meichenbaum (1977). Instead of focusing on a single personality trait, the model developed through the theoretical work cited above focuses on a set of learnable skills or processes, brought together to influence a specific behavior. The model is based on a continual interaction between personal, behavioral, and environmental factors. Expanding on the work of Bandura (1977a), Coates and Thoresen (in press) have proposed a reciprocal interaction model that describes the ongoing interactions among

1. the *person:* individual goals and objectives, perception of self and environment, and subjective expectations, emotions, and evaluations
2. the *environment:* influences from peer group and family, physical settings, social customs, and standards for judging performances
3. *behavior:* actions the person takes to attain certain goals or change certain behaviors

Coates and Thoresen make the important distinction between learning (what skills the person has acquired) and performance (whether a person will apply those skills in a specific situation), the same distinction that social learning theorists have made previously in connection with other types of learning.

The reciprocal interaction model provides a means for developing life-style change programs by conceptualizing the factors that influence the performance of newly acquired skills. It makes clear what most health educators have found through experience, that an effective program must not only help the person acquire the necessary skills for making changes in behavioral patterns but also provide the necessary conditions for helping the person use newly acquired skills when they are needed (Coates & Thoresen, in press; Squyres, 1979). Ultimately the program must go on to help the person identify and structure those conditions that promote performance of her or his skills.

The interaction inherent in the behavioral self-management model can also be expressed by extending the model presented for behavior modification to include internal signals and consequences, that is, thoughts and feelings:

Internal	Internal	Internal
	(Thoughts and feelings)	
Signal $\longrightarrow$	Behavior $\longrightarrow$	Consequences
External	External	External
	(Actions)	

If one keeps in mind that behaviors recur in chains, one has another way of conceptualizing the interaction of personal, environmental, and behavioral factors. All of these conceptualizations firmly acknowledge the person—the person's thoughts, goals, feelings, perceptions, and expectations—as a significant factor.

A Model of a Behavioral
Self-management Program

I am using here as a model of a behavioral self-management program the weight management program described in the recent book *Taking Charge of Your Weight and Well-Being* (Nash & Ormiston Long, 1978a, 1978b). This eighteen-week program was developed between 1975 and 1978 at the Stanford Heart Disease Prevention Program. The Taking Charge program teaches weight management in the larger

context of learning general self-management skills. It has proved to
be a very effective weight-loss program. Participants in the program
were adults from the communities surrounding Stanford University.
They lost an average of 16.5 pounds during the program. The weight
was lost at a rate of approximately 1 pound per week (Nash & Ormiston, 1977). A six-month follow-up showed that 34 percent of the
participants (N = 60) had maintained the weight they had lost
during the program or had lost more weight. An additional 35 percent
of the participants still benefited from the program in that at the
six-month follow-up they weighed less than they did at the beginning of the program. They had regained some but not all of the weight
they had lost during the eighteen weeks of the program (Nash &
Ormiston Long, 1979). Participants themselves reported in both their
written evaluations and in the quantitative follow-up data that the
program was much more than a weight management program. The
more successful participants were in the program, the more they
agreed with the statement that the program had contributed to
specific improvements in other areas of their lives (Nash & Ormiston
Long, 1979). The more effectively participants were able to grasp and
apply the behavioral self-management strategies taught in the weight
management program, the more successful they were in directly applying these skills to other areas of their lives.

Principles Underlying the Program

The principles underlying the Taking Charge approach have seemed
radical at first to both some participants and some professionals who
have been previously involved in teaching or encouraging life-style
changes. Nonetheless they are typical of many of the programs developed within the context of behavioral self-management with its
emphasis on personal responsibility.

   The principles upon which the Taking Charge program is based
   include:
   1.   Each person is personally responsible for devising his own
        weight-management program and following through with it. In
        other words, each person has the choice to take charge of his
        weight problem. This includes choosing from the wide array
        of strategies that are presented throughout the programs—those
        strategies that are best for him. Probably none of the strategies
        will work for every person. But some of the strategies *will* suit
        each person.

2. Regular and consistent record-keeping is an *essential* part of the Taking Charge program. Records are necessary to establish where the person is starting from, to assess what changes have been made, and to determine what problems still exist. Without records, it is virtually impossible to put into practice the other aspects of the program.

3. Each person also has maximum choice in how he decides to handle the situations he encounters. He can choose to set certain limits or adopt specific tactics. Those tactics can be *reasonably* stringent, moderately stringent, or relatively lax. If the limits are broad, he may choose to compensate in some appropriate way. He can also choose not to set limits or adopt any strategies if the situation seems important enough to him. Any of these choices is okay. The important thing is to make a choice.

4. Making choices implies planning ahead for situations. Once a person is face to face with a situation it is much more difficult to cope with it. Planning ahead can take many forms. All of the forms help prevent being caught off-guard.

5. Progress is made in small steps by shaping. Patterns and habits can only be changed gradually. Even taking charge can be done gradually. The program makes people aware of many problems, besides eating, in other parts of their lives. Knowing about these does not imply that *all* of them should be tackled at the same time. That is a sure way to invite failure. Instead the person needs to set priorities and address each problem in its turn.

6. The Taking Charge approach is guilt-free. Making choices, planning ahead, and shaping, help the person put this perspective into practice. Success is not viewed as "all or nothing" but rather as progress in the desired direction. Failures are viewed as learning experiences. Each person is encouraged to ask, "Why did that happen and how can I avoid it happening again?"

7. The Taking Charge approach is positive. People should be encouraged to emphasize their successes and the progress they have made. Doing so has a large impact on their self-esteem and, in time, their self-image. They begin to develop a new self-definition.

8. The program also allows for imperfection. Self-management skills take time to learn, just like playing the piano or tennis. Each person should be encouraged to accept the fact that making mistakes is inevitable. Expecting perfection is a sure way to set yourself up for failure.

9. There are times when staying put or even slipping backwards a bit can be considered progress. When evaluating the effective-

ness of the program, a leader has to use absolute measures. The individual, however, does not have to be so absolute and should not be. For him success is relative. He needs to ask himself, How does how he handled a particular situation now compare with how he used to handle the situation? What changes has he made? He isn't in perfect control yet, but what progress has he made?

10. People need to develop measures of change and success that focus on behavior, rather than on the scales.[1]

Elements of the Program

How are the conceptual model and the principles just described translated into a definite program? The following outline of the elements in the Taking Charge program encompasses those elements that should be in any program designed to teach self-management skills whether it be specifically for weight management or for some other problem.

ELEMENTS OF A BEHAVIORAL SELF-MANAGEMENT PROGRAM

     I.   Self-screening: develop commitment and positive expectations
    II.   Defining the problem in behavioral terms
   III.   Self-observation: record keeping
   IV.   Analyzing the problem
    V.   Setting reasonable goals
   VI.   Adopting tactics for change
       A.   Managing the external environment
       B.   Developing positive alternatives to present coping methods
       C.   Changing self-perceptions and thoughts
       D.   Developing social support
          1.   From within the group
          2.   From family and friends
       E.   Using self-reward
   VII.   Evaluating progress
  VIII.   Planning for maintenance

---

[1]Used by permission from *Taking Charge of Your Weight and Well-Being,* 1978, Palo Alto, Calif., Bull Publishing Co.

SELF-SCREENING. The first step for any person undertaking a behavior change program is to establish a commitment to the program. In order to do this a person needs to have realistic expectations about the nature of the program, the time, and energy commitment involved, and the types of changes that can reasonably be expected. In addition, an expectation of success is essential. It may also be necessary to screen for medical problems in certain programs.

By their very nature, behavioral self-management programs are concerned with behavior patterns that exist now and with strategies for changing those patterns or for establishing new patterns. Many students enter programs with the expectation that they will achieve insight into how or why a particular pattern developed. Such insights although very interesting do not often produce behavior changes. The conditions that instigated a particular behavior pattern may no longer exist even though the pattern itself persists.

Behavioral self-management programs also involve a considerable time investment for each participant. The only way to determine what the behavior patterns are and then later what changes have occurred is to keep daily records of the target behaviors. Depending on the problem area involved, the time investment amounts to approximately a half an hour per day for record keeping.

The commitment of energy devoted to the program is often even more important than the commitment of time. Because people are aware of a problem and troubled by it, they often feel a need to deal with it immediately. However, if they are burdened with other major concerns such as a job change, family or marital problems, or illness, the present may not be the best time to try to make major changes in their life-styles; there are already enough life pressures or crises. Each participant needs to be able to make the program a major concern until new self-management strategies are established. It is perfectly legitimate, in fact desirable, for a person to decide that now is not the best time to undertake major changes and hence to decide to wait for a freer opportunity to devote the time and energy needed.

Ethically speaking, I have very strong reservations about telling students just to sit through the program and, if it doesn't work out, take it over again. Their chances of doing well the next time are less than they would be if they had just waited for a more opportune time. If a person is not willing to make the commitment to regular group attendance, to about a half hour per day of record keeping, and to really devote the time and energy necessary to the course right now, it is better to wait.

Each participant also needs to have realistic expectations about the types of changes that can be expected and how quickly some of these changes may take place. These expectations are a particular problem with weight management. People frequently enter a program expecting to lose a great deal of weight and to lose it very quickly. The first expectation is a by-product of behavior change (when the habits are changed the weight will take care of itself), and the second expectation is definitely counter to the goals of a weight management program. It is difficult, but essential, for people to realize that behavior patterns and habits take a lifetime to acquire. These habits can be changed, but not usually in a matter of days. In fact making changes too rapidly usually results in people sooner or later feeling overwhelmed by the changes and the extreme motivation necessary to maintain them when they should rather have sought gradually to incorporate the changes into their life-styles.

DEFINING THE PROBLEM IN BEHAVIORAL TERMS. The problem needs to be defined in terms of behaviors before self-management strategies are applicable. For example, stating that you need to lose weight is not specifying a behavioral problem; the only behavior involved is stepping on the scales. However stating that you need to eat less or exercise more is specifying two behavioral areas. Another example is the person who complains of being too anxious and under too much stress. What is causing the anxiety? Is the person managing time inefficiently? Is she or he causing some of the anxiety by making frequent negative self-evaluations in her or his thoughts? Inefficiently budgeting time or negative self-talk are behaviors than can cause both stress and anxiety.

SELF-OBSERVATION. The purpose of self-observation through record keeping is to obtain factual information about the signals, both internal and external, that are triggering problem behaviors and also about the consequences these behaviors receive. Introspection or discussing the problem behaviors with another person will not suffice. There is no substitute for records that are completed at the time of the behavior.

Initially these records provide baseline information, that is, information about the behavior patterns before any attempt is made to make changes. Students are often frustrated about the need for baseline data. They are excited about beginning a new program and want to *begin* immediately, not mark time. One of my students, referred to the Taking Charge program by a family doctor, illustrates the need for baseline data. This doctor regularly asked his patients to keep food diaries; however, he gave them the eating plan he wanted them to use at the same time that he gave them the food diaries they were to keep. Thus the completed forms they returned to him were records of their attempts to use his food plan. Looking very sheepish this particular student returned to my class with a week's worth of baseline data. Her comment was, "You know, I was really giving my kids a hard time about how fast the cookie jar was going down around our house, and I found out who the cookie monster is."

Regular records also provide a way to measure change in the frequency of the problem behaviors after various self-management strategies are implemented. It is important with any problem area to have a means of assessing progress in behavioral terms. This is especially true with weight management where people typically measure their progress with the scales.

The important questions to include on a self-observation form include:

Under what circumstances does the behavior occur?
What exactly was the behavior?
What were you thinking and feeling at that time?
What happened as a result of the behavior?

Figures 12-1a, 12-1b, 12-2, and 12-3 are examples of self-observation forms. Note how each of these forms adapts the general questions listed above to a specific problem area. These forms provide models for forms that could be developed for other problem areas.

Record keeping as a means of self-observation is a skill that needs to be learned. Many students will have a fear of judgment by the group leader, which will need to be dispelled. In practice, students often have more difficulties with their own judgments of themselves. It is difficult for them at first to view the records as facts about

Figure 12-1a.
The Daily Behavior Record.

1200 CALORIE FOOD EXCHANGE PLAN

	6 Meat *	3 Fat *	4 Bread *	2 Milk *	5 Veg.	3 Fruit	1 Misc. **
Morning Meal	☐	☐	☐	☐		☐	☐
Mid-morning Snack							
Afternoon Meal	☐		☐		☐	☐	
Mid-afternoon Snack	☐	☐	☐	☐	☐ ☐		
Evening Meal	☐ ☐ ☐		☐		☐		
Evening Snack				☐	☐	☐	
Extras							

Food Plan Calories _____ +Extras _____ = Total Calories Today

*Adjust for Fat Exchange where applicable.
**Optional

Fill out one of these forms each day

MEAT EXCHANGE: 1 Exchange = 55 calories

Lean Meat: 1 oz.
All poultry (without skin) chicken, turkey, cornish hen — Fresh, frozen or canned fish; Dried peas or beans (omit 1 Bread Exchange), 1/2 cup; Cheese (5% fat); Cottage cheese (dry or 2%), 1/4 cup

Medium-fat Meat: 1 oz. (Omit 1/2 Fat Exchange)
Ground beef (15% fat), round, pork tenderloin, butt, picnic, Canadian bacon, boiled ham — Liver, heart, kidney, sweetbreads; Cottage cheese (creamed), 1/4 cup; Peanut butter (omit 2 Fat Exchanges), 2 T.; Cheese: Mozzarella, ricotta, farmers, neufchatel; Parmesan cheese, 3 T.; Egg, 1

High-fat Meat: 1 oz. (Omit 1 Fat Exchange)
Ground beef (20% fat), chuck, rib roasts, steaks, lamb breast — Pork spareribs, loin, ground country style ham, veal breast, capon, duck, goose; Cheese: Cheddar and Swiss types; Cold cuts, 4-1/2" x 1/8" slice; Frankfurter, 1 small

FAT EXCHANGE: 1 Exchange = 45 calories
Butter, margarine, mayonnaise, oil lard, bacon fat, 1 t.; Margarine, diet, 2 t.; Avocado (4" diameter), 1/8; Olives, 5 small — Almonds, 10 whole; Peanuts, Spanish, 20 whole; Peanuts, Virginia, 10 whole; Walnuts and other nuts, 6 small; Bacon, crisp, 1 strip; Cream, light or sour, 2 T.; Cream cheese and heavy cream, 1 T.; French and Italian dressing, 1 T.; Mayonnaise, imitation or diet, 2 t.; Diet salad dressing, 2 t.

BREAD EXCHANGE: 1 Exchange = 70 calories
Bread, 1 slice; Roll, 1/2; Tortilla, 1; Pita bread, 1/2 — Cereal, dry, 3/4 cup; Cereal, cooked, 1/2; Pasta, 1/2 cup; Crackers, see expanded list in manual; Legumes, 1/2 cup; Starchy vegetables, see expanded list; Prepared foods, see expanded list and adjust for Fat Exchange

MILK EXCHANGE: 1 Exchange = 80 calories
Nonfat, 1 cup; See expanded list — Low fat (omit 1 Fat Exchange), 1 cup; Whole (omit 2 Fat Exchanges), 1 cup

VEGETABLE EXCHANGE: 1 Exchange = 25 calories
See expanded list — Group A, 1/2 cup serving; Group B, up to the serving indicated on expanded list

FRUIT EXCHANGE: 1 Exchange = 40 calories. See expanded list for serving size.

MISCELLANEOUS EXCHANGE: (optional) 1 Exchange = 50 calories
Hard candy or caramel, 1 — Sugar, syrup, honey, jam, jelly, cocoa, 1 level T.

FREE FOODS: negligible calories
Bouillon, broth; Coffee, tea; Herbs, spices — Gelatin, plain, rennet tablets; Lemon juice, lime juice; Pickles, unsweetened; Mustard, soy sauce, vinegar; Diet sodas; Saccharin

BONUS FOODS: See expanded list. Adjust for Fat, Bread, Milk, or Miscellaneous Exchanges as required

Activity Record

Walking	_____ minutes
Golfing	_____ minutes
Cycling	_____ minutes
Swimming	_____ minutes
Jumping Rope	_____ minutes
Tennis, squash, etc.	_____ minutes
Jogging	_____ minutes
Running	_____ minutes

Used by permission from *Taking Charge of Your Weight and Well-Being*, 1978, Palo Alto, Calif., Bull Publishing Co.

228

Figure 12-1b.
The Daily Behavior Record.

DAILY BEHAVIOR RECORD FOR: S   M   T   W   Th   F   Sa   (Circle one)   Date _____

Time of Day	M/S	Food Eaten	Food Quantity		H.R.	No. Min.	Where?	Body Position	Doing what else?	Thoughts, Emotions and Feelings?	Persons, Places Things, Events	Results
			Amt.	Cal.								

Figure 12-2.
The Smoking Diary.

To gather information, you should carry a small (3″ × 5″) notebook with you for at least the next five weeks to record information. You should have a total of at least 13 pages in your smoking diary. Alternatively, you can rule off your own pages on 3″ × 5″ index cards.

The diary page should contain enough room to cover three days. Each day is broken up into hours (A.M. and P.M.) so that you can record the time you smoked each cigarette as well as when you experienced each smoking urge. One helpful way to remember to record your smoking is to attach the record notebook or cards to your cigarette pack—perhaps with a rubber band.

Smoking Urges

Start by paying attention to the experiences that occur prior to having a cigarette. This feeling is defined here as a smoking urge. The system for noting your urges is presented below. You will use an urge rating scale with five levels of intensity.

Urge Rating Scale: "I want a cigarette . . ."
1. a little ("not really at all").
2. somewhat ("perhaps").
3. a moderate amount ("vague desire").
4. much ("need").
5. very much ("craving").

Once you experience an urge to smoke, you should pick a number from the rating scale that best describes how much you want that cigarette. Then write the number into the diary on the appropriate page and in the appropriate time slot. Different people evaluate their smoking urges in somewhat different ways. Your task is to be as consistent with your own personal ratings as possible.

Cigarettes Smoked

The smoking urges that lead to your having a cigarette should be indicated, too. All you need to do is draw a circle around the urge rating you selected according to the rules just mentioned. At the end of the day, add up all of the cigarettes you smoked that day and write this total in the top section of the data page. Draw a circle around it as well.

Sleeping. It is helpful to pick out the patterns of your activities as they relate to your smoking. Cross out those hours during which you sleep.

Situations. By "situations," we mean any activities, events, or feelings that consistently seem to signal your smoking. You should think about which situations stand out and then describe them briefly on the back side of the data page. Do this at least three times each day. Information about the links between situations and your smoking will be important in the strategies that will be presented later.

From B. G. Danaher and E. Lichtenstein, *Become an Ex-Smoker: With This Book You Will*, pp. 16–18. Copyright © 1978. Reprinted by permission of Prentice-Hall, Inc., Englewood Cliffs, New Jersey.

when and how behaviors occurred instead of as indictments of themselves. Records are not tests with right and wrong answers; they can only provide information. It is especially important for the information to be as complete as possible. Students need to make an extra effort to keep complete records when they are having a bad day. Then they can begin to discover the patterns that cause bad days.

ANALYZING THE PROBLEM. The daily records for eating, smoking, stress, or any other specific behaviors provide the basis for determining the patterns of the behaviors. The questions that need to be asked are implicit in the forms:

Does the behavior occur at particular times during the day?
Are you engaged in similar types of activities?
Are you usually alone or with specific people?
Do certain thoughts or feelings trigger the behavior?
Do certain places or events trigger the behavior?

Other kinds of situations are unique to a specific problem area. For example buying and storing food, cooking and entertaining, and both the speed with which a person eats and the size of the portions selected all influence patterns of eating behaviors. The Problem Analysis Form (on pp. 45–51 of *Taking Charge of Your Weight and Well-Being*) was designed to be used with the Daily Behavior Record (fig. 12-1). The Problem Analysis Form first refers students to specific columns in the Daily Behavior Record to help them discover patterns and then refers them to related problems in other sections of the Problem Analysis Form. It is a valuable tool to teach students how to use the data they have so conscientiously collected. Discover-

Figure 12-3.
The Stress Log.

Date and Time	What cued me to my stress? (Physiological and cognitive cues.)	What stressed me: Where was I? What was I doing? Who was I with? What did I say to myself?	What did I do about it?	What can I do to avoid or reduce the stressor the next time?

NAME:

DATE(S):

Reprinted by permission of Virginia A. Price, Stanford University.

ing patterns is also a skill that most of my students have needed to learn. In the Taking Charge program, students are urged to go back to the Problem Analysis Form from time to time to discover how the nature of their problems has changed. As some patterns are eliminated or changed other problems become more obvious. I would recommend developing a similar form to accompany any self-monitoring forms that are developed for a behavioral self-management program.

SETTING REASONABLE GOALS. Learning to set reasonable goals —small steps that focus on specific behaviors—is one of the most important elements of a behavioral self-management program. It is also one of the most difficult things for people to do. Our culture sets a high value on achievement, on striving for the highest goal possible. Even when students realize the value of small steps, it is still hard for many of them to put the principle into practice.

Why are reasonable goals—small steps—so important? The answer is in a process psychologists call "shaping." Consider a sculptor with a mound of clay from which to create a bust. One large stroke will not produce the bust. Instead it takes countless small strokes over a period of time. Behavior change occurs in much the same way. Dramatic life-style changes can be produced with one large stroke, but they seldom, if ever, persist. That is the fate of almost every New Year's resolution and many a crash diet or other crash program. The dramatic changes are usually very much like a house of cards.

Enduring behavior change occurs when one structures one's program to ensure gradual success. The first step is to choose an aspect of the problem that is challenging but definitely not the most difficult aspect. Undoubtedly one has tried before to tackle the most difficult part of the problem without success. One needs to override the feeling, "If I can just lick this part of the problem, I will have it made," and choose instead a part of the problem that is challenging but manageable, an area in which one is likely to succeed. For example if one has trouble with frequent snacking, trying to limit the number of snacks at first may be asking for trouble. Instead, one could set as a goal sitting down at the kitchen or dining room table for each snack, then persist with this particular tactic until one feels comfortable with it, until it no longer requires a major effort to remember and perform.

Success with the first tactic provides the incentive to move on to a slightly more challenging tactic. The process is repeated again and again. Finally the series of small steps amount to major changes in behavior patterns. However, at no time should one have felt deprived or overwhelmed. Those feelings are a sure sign that the immediate goals were too high.

Flexibility is essential for appropriate goal setting. In spite of the best intentions, stringent goal setting is such an ingrained habit that people often underestimate the difficulty of the task they have set for themselves. When a goal that seemed to be appropriate proves to be more difficult than anticipated, one needs to reevaluate. Either redefine the goal or even decide to postpone adopting the tactic for awhile. Mental rehearsal, imagining the situation beforehand, is a useful technique for testing out goals.

ADOPTING TACTICS FOR CHANGE.   People are ready to adopt specific tactics for change after they have determined the patterns of the problem behaviors. The choice of tactics goes hand in hand with appropriate goal setting. Certain tactics are challenging whereas others would prove too difficult. Most tactics can be scaled down or up to create the desirable challenge. For example in weight management, students often decide to begin to manage their snacking. One of the specific tactics suggested is to have a "planned snack." At first the planned snack is often in addition to whatever unplanned or spontaneous snacks occur. The following week the planned snack may continue accompanied by a limit on the number of snacks eaten during a specific period of time. As the weeks progress the unplanned snacks are gradually eliminated and, depending on individual preferences and needs, the number of planned snacks may be increased.

The strategies for change in any behavioral self-management program should cover:

1. Managing the external environment
2. Developing positive alternatives to present coping methods
3. Changing self-perceptions and thoughts
4. Developing social support
5. Using self-reward

Each of these is a major concern. In fact an entire chapter is devoted to each in *Taking Charge of Your Weight and Well-Being*. The chapters provide a springboard for students to explore and discuss strategies and alternatives that are uniquely suited to their own needs and priorities. Group discussion, as opposed to a lecture format, is invaluable in bringing students to the point where they can identify their own problems and patterns and devise their own solutions.

In the Taking Charge program we provide the Weekly Tactics

Record (fig. 12-4). Students are encouraged to adapt this form to meet their own particular needs. They are urged to revise any tactic that is listed or to devise their own tactics. The form is keyed to the Daily Behavior Record (fig. 12-1) and the Problem Analysis Form (*Taking Charge of Your Weight and Well-Being*, pp. 45–51) that is meant to be a starting point.

Managing the external environment. The external environment is the source of innumerable signals that trigger the problem behavior: The sight of a bowl of nuts on the table is a signal to eat; holding a drink is a signal to light up a cigarette; being stopped by the *long* red light near your home is a signal to start drumming your fingers on the steering wheel. Tactics for managing or controlling these signals generally fall into two areas: eliminating the signal and consciously altering the response to the signal.

The sensitivity to specific signals is learned and is a part of a person's history. People with eating problems will continue to be very sensitive to food signals in their environment. The sensitivity may diminish over time. In the meantime, however, it is good planning rather than a sign of weakness to deliberately avoid food signals. In the Taking Charge program participants are advised to store food in opaque containers, avoid leaving food lying about on countertops after meals, and avoid bringing problem foods into the house in the first place. If problem foods are available for whatever reason, participants are encouraged to throw them away. Many of the same tactics could be adapted to a smoking program, and similar tactics could be devised for other programs.

Familiar signals that have triggered problem behaviors in the past can become signals for more appropriate or adaptive behaviors. For example, the person who usually becomes uptight at that long red light can *choose* to make the redlight a signal for a short relaxation exercise, with one stroke eliminating a problem behavior and instituting a helpful behavior.

Another aspect of signal control or managing the external environment is deliberately creating new signals for behaviors people are attempting to learn. For example an important part of weight management is exercising more, in addition to learning ways to eat less. The form of exercise advocated at the beginning of the Taking Charge program is walking. This is chosen specifically because it is a nondemanding form of exercise. Nevertheless it is a new behavior for most participants. Each student is given a pedometer to wear. The first week or two, the pedometers serve merely as an assessment device while people record their activity baselines. Then curiosity leads

Figure 12-4.
The Weekly Tactics Record.

Week of _____

Under each of the following **PROBLEM AREAS** are a number of "tactics" you might use in your behavior change efforts. In the left-hand column, write in a number to indicate how many days during the coming week you will use one of these tactics. (For example, you might write 5 next to the tactic "Use Menu Planner" to indicate that out of the next 7 days your goal is to use the Menu Planner at least 5 of those days.) In the right-hand columns, place a check for each day that you actually implement the tactic. At the end of the week, count up the number of tactics chosen for the week and the total number of tactics used. You should begin by choosing *no more than* one or two tactics. Remember to set small, realistic goals — don't try for 7 out of 7 days yet. With each new week of the program, you may add additional tactics (no more than one at a time) or increase your goal for the number of times during a particular week that you will use a tactic you have already chosen previously. Stop using a tactic if you find it is not helping you. Revise your goal downwards if you find you are not implementing a tactic as many times as you had indicated you would in the left-hand column.

S	M	T	W	Th	F	S

Time of Day Problems
____ Eat three regular, planned meals.
____ Eat breakfast.
____ Eat lunch.
____ Have a planned snack between meals.
____ Eliminate snacks between meals.
____ Use a Menu Planner.
____ Eat meals at scheduled times.
____ Eat only planned snacks.

Problem Food Problems
____ Drink sugarless, diet drinks.
____ Don't eat my problem food,_____.
____ Use a sugar substitute.
____ Eat a low-cal snack instead of usual.
____ Chew sugarless gum while cooking.
____ Don't sample food while fixing it.

Food Intake Problems
____ Serve meals hotel-style.
____ Measure all portions.
____ Take one portion only.
____ Share a single serving with another.
____ Leave some of the serving uneaten.
____ Put left-overs away immediately.
____ Put utensils down between bites.
____ Take 20 minutes to finish main meal.
____ Sit down while eating.
____ Use separate dishes or smaller ones to make quantity look larger.

Environment Problems
____ Be more assertive.
____ Avoid place that gives me trouble.
____ Eat low-calorie things before eating out.
____ Take my own diet drinks to the party.
____ Tell workmates not to offer me food.

Figure 12-4. *(continued)*

	S	M	T	W	Th	F	S

Emotion and Thinking Problems
_____ Use relaxation techniques.
_____ Express my feelings objectively.
_____ Choose an alternative interpretation.
_____ Go for a walk instead of eating.
_____ Avoid person that upsets me.
_____ Avoid something that upsets me.
_____ Mentally change temptation into something
I wouldn't eat.

Location, Position, Activity Problems
_____ Eat only at my designated eating place.
_____ Do nothing else while eating.
_____ Eat only while sitting down.
_____ Let others get their own snacks.
_____ Don't eat in the car.
_____ Remove food from hiding places.

Buying and Storing Problems
_____ Shop after having eaten.
_____ Shop from a list.
_____ Don't buy troublesome food.
_____ Avoid troublesome aisles.
_____ Use opaque instead of clear wrap.
_____ Turn pictures so I can't see them.
_____ Make food hard to get.

Cooking and Entertaining Problems
_____ Broil or bake instead of frying.
_____ Substitute lower calorie ingredients.
_____ Try new, low-calorie recipe.
_____ Fix low-calorie food for company.

Eating Out Problems
_____ Ask for salad dressing "on the side."
_____ Have bread and butter removed.
_____ Order low-calorie item.
_____ Remove top slice of bread from sandwich.
_____ Order skim milk or diet drink.
_____ Avoid reading dessert list.
_____ Call hostess about her menu.
_____ Eat low-calorie snacks before eating out.
_____ Take own diet drinks or food.

Your Individual Tactics (Write in)

_____
_____
_____

_____ = Total Tactics Chosen

_____ - _____ = _____

| Total Tactics Chosen | Total Tactics Used | If answer is "0," you are on target. If answer is more than "0," you are setting goals that are too high—choose fewer tactics or lower goals next week. If answer is less than "0," you may be pushing too hard—take it easier. |

+ + + + + +

_____ = Total Tactics Used

Used by permission from *Taking Charge of Your Weight and Well-Being,* 1978, Palo Alto, Calif., Bull Publishing Co.

people to check their pedometers a few times during the day. Many people report, sometimes to their own surprise, that checking their pedometers at noon or some other time and realizing their mileage is running a little below normal becomes a signal for them to take a walk.

Group discussion is vital in creating a setting in which each person can devise those signals that will be especially appropriate for him or her. It is a very individual matter; what works or seems like it might work for one person sounds ridiculous to another person. Yet one person alone cannot begin to generate the range of possibilities from which to choose. While group members are brainstorming they demonstrate to themselves their own abilities instead of depending solely on the "expert," the group leader, for ideas. They carry this knowledge of their own abilities with them after the formal end of the program.

Developing positive alternatives to present coping methods. Habits quite frequently develop or persist in response to a need created by a life-style. People with weight problems frequently eat in response to boredom, anxiety, loneliness, depression, excitement, and other emotions. The same is also true for people who smoke, have trouble managing their time, or become stressed. Emotional states as well as environmental signals can trigger problem behaviors. The first step is to eliminate the inappropriate coping behavior, whatever it may be. But this is not enough. It is not usually possible to eliminate the situation that is triggering the emotions. Some coping behavior is necessary. Eliminating the inappropriate coping behavior leaves a vacuum.

The next step is to help people learn more appropriate coping behavior. For this reason behavioral self-management programs become involved in teaching people relaxation techniques and also in helping them explore individual coping behaviors that are particularly suited to them. Given a chance people come up with very unusual but effective alternatives: taking a walk, playing the piano, meditating, doing yoga exercises, devising a room in their homes that is private and off-limits at least at times to other family members, gardening, hiking, cleaning out closets, lighting lots of candles, taking a bubble bath. All of these alternatives have been suggested by students. All of them have seemed absurd to some students. The point is that there are alternatives for each person.

Changing self-perceptions and thoughts. The things people say to themselves, how they interpret situations, how they feel about the goals they have set provide some of the internal signals that trigger behaviors. Consider humans as information processors—human computers if you will. The things that happen to us and the events that go on around us provide input for the computers. Information in computers is processed by a program. Our programs for processing input are the interpretations we make, our thoughts and feelings. There does not need to be anything arbitrary about the way we interpret events. Interpretations, thoughts, and feelings are learned behaviors. Each of us can identify present patterns and choose to change them or to adopt new ones. Each person can exert a great deal of control over the nature of her or his own internal signals.

The first step is becoming aware of private monologues, of self-talk. A worthwhile exercise is described in detail in the chapter "Managing Your Thinking" in *Taking Charge of Your Weight and Well-Being*. Briefly, students are asked to place stickers in conspicuous places such as on the face of their watchs, on the rearview mirrors of their cars, on the refrigerator doors, and on the bathroom mirrors. During the first stage students are asked to stop for a moment each time they notice a sticker and recall what comments they have made to themselves about themselves during the past several minutes. If the statements were positive and appropriate they are to record them on 3" × 5" cards. If the statements were negative or inappropriate they are to think of a positive alternative and record it instead. After a few days they go on to the next stage: Each time they notice a stricker they read one of the statements from their cards. During the last stage they dispense with the cards and generate new self-statements each time they see a sticker. Students typically resist this assignment. It seems silly and a bother. However, those students who overcome their resistance and give the exercise a fair trial consider it one of the most valuable techniques they learn.

We all unwittingly subscribe to a number of unwritten rules. Two typical examples are: (1.) Success is an all-or-nothing proposition, and you don't suceed if you improve a little bit. (2.) It is necessary to be perfect in order to be acceptable or lovable. There are many, many others. They can be challenged if we become aware of them. The chapters "Managing Your Thinking" and "Coping with Emotions" in *Taking Charge of Your Weight and Well-Being* and *A New Guide to Rational Living* by Ellis and Harper (1975) provide useful guides for identifying and altering some of these thought patterns.

Developing social support. Most people find it very difficult to sustain the continued effort necessary for gradual behavior change by themselves. Social support from within the group helps a great deal, particularly in those areas where substantial changes in thought patterns are being made. It is a radical approach to emphasize the positive steps that have been taken, rather than the mistakes that have been made or the changes that still need to be made. It is also radical to set small goals, to view mistakes as learning experiences instead of guilt-inducing failures, to deliberately choose to take a time-out from your tactics, and to choose not to be bothered by events that you previously found very distressing. Group support provides the encouragement and gentle reminders at times when individuals can't provide it for themselves.

Support from within the group also provides an area removed from the scrutiny of family and friends where people can experiment without fear of being ridiculed or judged. Within the group setting, each participant learns to deal individually with his or her own behavior patterns. The Taking Charge program relies heavily on individual problem solving whereby individuals develop their own tailor-made programs designed to fit their own priorities and life-styles. At the same time, they share their experiences and proposed goals and strategies with group members in a situation in which they can both give and get feedback, in a situation in which they can practice and develop new skills. These group experiences give members valuable experiences in problem solving for situations other than the ones they are encountering at the moment. As a result they are better prepared to handle new situations when they arise both within the initial problem area, such as weight management, and in new problem areas.

The group approach also provides a social support system during the program and often for extended periods after the formal program ends. Participants in the Taking Charge program are encouraged to develop support systems within the group from the beginning of the program. Recently when this program was being taught to a fairly large group (forty-five members) at a junior college, seven or eight of the members continued to meet weekly without the group leader for two months between the time when one class series ended and another began. This ongoing support for continued change and maintenance is very important.

A group setting also provides an opportunity to help participants attribute their successes to their own skills and efforts. Such an attribution is very important in promoting continued use of the new skills after the formal program ends. When a group leader acts as a catalyst for group discussion, the group members themselves take responsibility for problem solving for themselves and for helping others; and they demonstrate to themselves their new skills, not just their ability to follow directions.

Family members and friends can also provide valuable social support. Some students feel comfortable in taking advantage of this potential support from the beginning of the program; others need to wait awhile. The types of social support can range all the way from asking people to avoid tempting behaviors such as smoking or eating snacks in your presence to asking them to be actively involved in rewarding specific behavioral changes. A contract that specifies very clearly the behaviors involved for both the student and her or his support person is advisable. It is important to remember that being supportive may not be a habit for other people; that behavior may need to be shaped.

Using self-reward. One's most consistent and reliable source of reward and positive feedback is oneself. One can plan positive thoughts to follow specific behaviors, and one can also externally reward oneself in some way such as with some free time, an enjoyable activity, or a material reward. Either type of self-reward is especially important to maintain new behaviors that have not yet become habits.

Rewarding oneself with thoughts is typically the most effective type of self-reward and at the same time the most difficult to practice. Our culture tends to teach critical skills and frown on positive self-evaluations. Many of us still ascribe to the Puritan ethic that says you should leave well-enough alone and only take notice when things are not going as they should. It takes time and effort for people to realize that being honest with themselves means giving credit where credit is due as well as assiduously pointing out every shortcoming. Yet practical experience and a substantial body of experimental research in psychology make it clear that rewards are much more effective than punishments for teaching new behavior.

External self-rewards such as time, activities, and material things are also effective and also meet with resistance. A typical remark from students is, "I'm already being very nice to myself." If that statement is true, they can begin to make some rules about how and when they get some of those "nice things." They can also develop some new rewards themselves. Something as apparently silly as putting silver stars on a calendar for practicing a particular tactic each day has proved to be very effective for many adults in the Taking Charge program. Other alternatives for self-reward include permitting yourself to read in bed when you don't snack between dinner and bedtime, wearing a favorite piece of jewelry after you have handled the irritation from a difficult phone call by going for a walk instead of going to the refrigerator, or buying a magazine you enjoy but don't subscribe to as you finish up your daily walk.

EVALUATING PROGRESS. The seventh element of a behavioral self-management program, following adopting tactics for change, is developing a means of evaluating progress. Continued self-monitoring provides a basis for a behavioral measure of change. The forms provide a record of change in frequency of both the behaviors one is attempting to decrease and the behaviors one is attempting to increase.

Several of my students have taken this one step further and devised a weekly summary sheet of their own that shows for weight management the tactics mastered that week, the tactics that need additional work, the average daily mileage on their pedometers, the average daily caloric intake, successes of the week, problems of the week, and proposed goals for the coming week. The weekly summaries taken as a group clearly illustrate the progress that has been made.

Periodic evaluation helps maintain motivation. It also points out where certain aspects of a problem such as weight management or stress management have been adequately handled and points the way to the areas to address next. This is an ongoing process that sends one back to the steps of analyzing the problem, setting goals, and adopting tactics.

PLANNING FOR MAINTENANCE. The requirements for continuing and maintaining a behavioral self-management program are built into the program itself. As one nears one's long-term goals one needs gradually to phase out the self-monitoring while maintaining the social support established within the group and among family and friends. One also needs to arrange one's environment to support the changes made and to continue to practice the skills acquired.

A final, but essential, requirement for a maintenance plan is the development of an "early warning system" to help detect new problems or the recurrence of old ones. The best alternative for such a system seems to be a commitment to self-monitoring with the original forms for three to seven days at specified internals such as every three months. A periodic return to record keeping will point out as no other method can the subtle changes in patterns of coping, and a periodic return to the thought awareness exercise discussed earlier will point out changes in thought patterns. It is much easier to deal with slight changes in behavior patterns than to wait until you have started smoking again or gained a fair amount of weight; by that time significant changes in behavior have already occurred.

Other Problem Areas

Self-management skills cannot be taught in a theoretical context where the skills are outlined in a general sense. These skills must be taught within the context of a particular problem area. However, as the Taking Charge data suggests, once a person has acquired the skills in a particular problem area, they become useful tools in other problem areas. The skills can be applied to any problem that can be defined in behavioral terms.

I have used the weight management program described in *Taking Charge of Your Weight and Well-Being* as a model of a behavioral self-management program and given examples from two other problem areas: smoking and stress management. Other potential areas for behavioral self-management programs include assertiveness, insomnia, female sexual responsiveness, fears and phobias, and drinking. There is a list of resource materials for all of these problem areas at the end of this chapter. The chapter "Taking Charge of Your Well-Being" in *Taking Charge of Your Weight and Well-Being* contains a more extensive list of problem areas and resource materials.

The weight management program used here as a model for a behavioral self-management program is, in fact, much more than a weight management program. Students of the program report that they use their new skills for managing other areas of their lives, and the manual has been used as a general self-management manual for problem areas where there is not a good program available. It is not that difficult to substitute another problem for a weight management problem and proceed with the program.

Using Your Information about Behavioral Self-management Programs

There are several ways you can use this information about behavioral self-management programs. First of all you can help promote a behavioral self-management program in your area of interest using some of the existing resource material or developing your own program. *Taking Charge of Your Weight and Well-Being: Leader's Guide* is a separate publication with helpful information about establishing a group, group dynamics, and other techniques for leading a group. After a group is established, the program can be continued by using graduated group members as group leaders and assistants. I have found these people to be very motivated and effective.

Second you can carry the principles discussed in this chapter into your contacts with patients. If you have a behavioral self-management program in operation, it is especially important not to undermine or counter the changes that patients are making in that program. Even without such a program the principles discussed in this chapter are valuable tools for working with people. A positive, guilt-free, supportive, gradual approach is always very effective.

Third you can try to implement a behavioral self-management program for yourself to experience firsthand what it is that you are asking of others. The problem area can be as small as letter writing or nail biting or as large as weight or stress management. In any case the experience is invaluable. The fact that I have previously had a weight problem and have had to learn to manage it means much more to my students than the fact that I have a professional degree. They soon discover that I won't judge them but also that they can't con me. It's a very helpful combination.

Fourth and finally you can evaluate programs that come to your attention using the principles and elements of a behavioral self-management program discussed in this chapter. You should pay particular attention to whether the proposed program includes the following features: baseline data, an individualized problem-solving approach in a group setting, positive alternatives to inappropriate coping behaviors, and skills to change patterns for thoughts and emotions.

References

Bandura, A. Efficacy expectancies: Toward a unifying theory of behavior change. *Psychological Review,* 1977, *84,* 191–215. (a)

Bandura, A. *Social learning theory.* Englewood Cliffs, N.J.: Prentice-Hall, 1977. (b)

Coates, T. J., & Thoresen, C. E. Treating obesity in children and adolescents: Is there any hope? In J. M. Ferguson & C. B. Taylor (Eds.), *Advances in behavioral medicine.* Holliswood, N.Y.: Spectrum, in press.

Danaher, B. G., & Lichtenstein, E. *Become an ex-smoker: With this book you will.* Englewood Cliffs, N.J.: Prentice-Hall, 1978.

Ellis, A., & Harper, R. *A new guide to rational living.* North Hollywood, Calif.: Wilshire, 1975.

Mahoney, M. J. *Cognition and behavior modification: An integrative approach.* New York: Plenum, 1974.

Meichenbaum, D. *Cognitive behavior modification: An integrative approach.* New York: Plenum, 1977.

Nash, J. D., & Ormiston, L. H. *Diet and weight control clinic: A status report* (Internal Monograph). Stanford Heart Disease Prevention Program, Stanford University School of Medicine, 1977.

Nash, J. D., & Long, L. Ormiston. *Taking charge of your weight and well-being.* Palo Alto, Calif.: Bull, 1978. (a)

Nash, J. D., & Long, L. Ormiston. *Taking charge of your weight and well-being: Leader's guide.* Palo Alto, Calif.: Bull, 1978. (b)

Nash, J. D. & Long, L. Ormiston. *Quality of change achieved in a clinical weight management program: Six-month follow-up.* Abstract submitted to the Society of Behavior Medicine, 1979.

Squyres, W. D. *A self-management approach to risk reduction.* Paper presented to the Patient Education in the Primary Care Setting III Workshop, Minneapolis, Minnesota, 1979.

Self-management Resources

Joyce D. Nash & Linda Ormiston Long. *Taking charge of your weight and well-being.* Palo Alto, Calif.: Bull, 1978.

David L. Watson & Roland G. Tharp. *Self-directed behavior: Self-modification for personal adjustment.* Monterey, Calif.: Brooks/Cole, 1972.

Dorothy Tennov. *Super self: A woman's guide to self-management.* New York: Funk & Wagnalls, 1977.

Spencer A. Rathus & Jeffrey S. Nevid. *Behavior Therapy: Strategies for solving problems in living.* New York: Doubleday, 1977.

Michael J. Mahoney. *Self-change: Strategies for solving personal problems.* New York: Norton, 1979.

Leading Groups

Joyce D. Nash & Linda Ormiston Long. *Taking charge of your weight and well-being: Leader's guide.* Palo Alto, Calif.: Bull, 1978.

Weight Management

Joyce D. Nash & Linda Ormiston Long. *Taking charge of your weight and well-being.* Palo Alto, Calif.: Bull, 1978.

Joyce D. Nash & Linda Ormiston Long. *Taking charge of your weight and well-being: Leader's guide.* Palo Alto, Calif.: Bull, 1978.

Smoking

Brian G. Danaher & Edward Lichtenstein. *Become an ex-smoker: with this book you will.* Englewood Cliffs, N.J.: Prentice-Hall, 1978.

Stress Management

Meyer Friedman & Ray H. Rosenman. *Type A behavior and your heart.* Greenwich, Conn.: Fawcett, 1974.

Herbert Benson. *The relaxation response.* New York: Avon, 1975.

Changing Thinking Patterns

Albert Ellis & Robert A. Harper. *A new guide to rational living.* North Hollywood, Calif.: Wilshire, 1975.

Mildred Newman & Bernard Berkowitz. *How to be your own best friend.* New York: Random House, Ballantine, 1971.

Alan Lakein. *How to get control of your time and your life.* New York: New American Library, Signet, 1974.

Dorothy Tennov. *Super self: A woman's guide to self-management.* New York: Funk & Wagnalls, 1977.

Assertiveness

A. Bower & G. H. Bower. *Asserting yourself.* Reading, Mass.: Addison-Wesley, 1977.

P. E. Butler. *Self-assertion for women.* San Francisco: Canfield, 1977.

P. G. Zimbardo. *Shyness: What it is and what to do about it.* Reading, Mass.: Addison-Wesley, 1977.

Insomnia

Thomas J. Coates & Carl E. Thoresen. *How to sleep better: A drug-free program for overcoming insomnia.* Englewood Cliffs, N.J.: Prentice-Hall, 1976.

Female Sexual Responsiveness

Julia Heiman, Leslie LoPiccolo & Joseph LoPiccolo. *Becoming orgasmic: A sexual growth program for women.* Englewood Cliffs, N.J.: Prentice-Hall, 1976.

Lonnie Barbach. *For yourself.* New York: Doubleday, 1975.

Fears and Phobias

Gerald Rosen. *Don't be afraid: A program for overcoming fears and phobias.* Englewood Cliffs, N.J.: Prentice-Hall, 1976.

Drinking

William R. Miller & Ricardo F. Munoz. *How to control your drinking.* Englewood Cliffs, N.J.: Prentice-Hall, 1976.

James L. Free. *Just one more: Help for problem drinkers and their loved ones.* Palo Alto, Calif.: Bull, 1977.

13

Women's Self-help Programs

Sheryl Burt Ruzek

Until recently professionals have had little interest in educating women patients regarding sex-related conditions such as pregnancy, menopause, and diseases of the reproductive organs. Indeed many physicians believe that medical information in the hands of patients is hazardous, generalizing from gross examples to support their position. One gynecologist, for example, told a woman she had trichomoniasis (a common vaginal infection); the patient mistakenly read up on trichinosis and called back saying she felt little worms crawling around in her vagina. In this case the doctor generalized that women should not be given information because they get confused and cause unnecessary trouble. An alternate interpretation—one that women themselves offer—is that doctors should give *more*, not less, information; and they should take the time to see that their patients understand their conditions so that these confusions will not arise so often (Ruzek, 1978). The question, of course, is How can patients be more effectively educated so that these unfortunate occurrences are eliminated or minimized?

Professional and Lay Perspectives on Patient Education

"Patient education" is typically something a professional gives to a passive patient—information and advice on preventive measures, diagnosis, prognosis, and treatment regimens to follows. A major goal of such education is to increase patient compliance with professionals' recommendations by providing just enough information to get the patient to do what the professional judges is best, but not so much information as to frighten the patient or to encourage debate.

Much medical communication is ineffective and unsatisfactory to patients and professionals alike. For example in Korsh and Negrete's (1972) study of pediatric consultations, 20 percent of the mothers left without understanding the child's illness and 43 percent failed to follow medical regimens. Reviewing the literature McKinlay (1975) notes that patients are "blamed" for ignorance and failure to comply by both medical professionals and researchers. Most research focuses on the attributes or characteristics of complying compared to noncomplying patients; relatively few studies directly investigate how physician behavior or the structure of medical care affects what patients learn from medical encounters or how their experience motivates them to comply with regimens. It is taken for granted that compliance is always desirable, despite growing evidence that many medical treatments are in fact hazardous and might profitably be avoided (see e.g., Corea, 1977; Haire, 1972/1975; Illich, 1976; Seaman & Seaman, 1977). Thus to measure patient education effectiveness in terms of compliance with professional advice misses an important dimension of educating patients to be competent health consumers—educating them to comprehend, evaluate, and choose or sometimes refuse medical treatment. Whereas professionals primarily focus on education to encourage compliance, patients are educating themselves and each other to be competent consumers in a broader way.

Lay-controlled patient education, generally referred to as self-help health groups, have proliferated in the 1970s. Most are organized by and for people suffering from specific diseases, disabilities, or addictions such as obesity, colostomy, mastectomy, emphysema, or alcoholism (for names and addresses of such groups in the United States, see Gartner and Riessman, 1977, pp. 159–176; for Great Britain see Robinson and Henry, 1977, pp. 143–149, or contact the National Self-Help Clearinghouse). Others serve broader client groups such as women at various stages of the life cycle who need education related to reproductive health (for names and addresses of these groups see Ruzek, 1978, pp. 241–265, or contact the National Women's Health Network).

Self-help health groups emphasize lay, rather than professional, control of organizations, activities, and services. Expertise is based on experience and demonstrated competence rather than on formal credentials, and all participants, including professionals, are expected to accept patients taking an active role in their own health care. Self-help proponents are often critical of traditional medical theories and practices and seek to demystify medical care by encouraging patients to be knowledgeable and be responsible for meeting their own basic health needs. Many self-help groups also function as support systems for individuals attempting to redefine their roles in society, especially groups composed of people whose health condition carries stigma or leads to social or economic discrimination. These groups may additionally serve as a base for political action to improve the quality or availability of services needed by members. In general, participants in self-help groups study their health problems to learn how to care for their basic needs and to improve their ability to negotiate with medical personnel when treatment is needed. Learning to comply with traditional medical advice is not a goal. (See Gartner & Riessman, 1977; Howard, Davis, Pope, & Ruzek, 1977; Hurvitz, 1974; Katz & Bender, 1976; Kleiber & Light, 1978; Levin, Katz, & Holst, 1976; Marieskind, 1975; Robinson & Henry, 1977; Ruzek, 1975, 1978.)

Self-help Gynecology

Women's active involvement in self-help health education grew out of the consciousness-raising groups of the women's movement where women shared their concerns over contraception, abortion, and obstetrical and gynecologic care. Feminists felt that physicians were too often condescending, paternalistic, judgmental, and noninformative; women were offended at being denied the right to participate fully in decisions about abortion, sterilization, contraception, and treatment of routine problems. Women also felt that physicians failed to give them enough information to discuss procedures or make decisions in a reasoned, competent manner. Health education material is rarely available in waiting rooms and hurried, brief visits with physicians make gaining knowledge difficult. Women also feel that the draping of the pevils during obstetric and gynecologic procedures deprives them of the opportunity to learn about their bodies and reinforces negative stereotypes about women's sexual organs (Boston Women's Health Book Collective, 1973, 1976, 1978; Ruzek, 1978).

Feminists want to assume greater responsibility for and control over their health care. To do this they attempt to shift the social distribution of medical knowledge (anatomy, physiology, medical procedures, treatments) from being the exclusive property of certified experts to being the shared property of patients. In feminist health collectives and clinics, a variety of activities that might be termed *patient education* have been developed to do this, although the largely lay organizations refer to these activities as self-help or self-health groups, participatory clinics, study groups, and body classes.

These activities vary from single meetings to six-to-eight week courses on specific topics. Women's health groups cover basic anatomy and physiology of the female reproductive system, routine gynecologic problems and treatments, childbirth and menopause experiences, and gynecological surgery. Individual sessions or series are often devoted to learning to perform pelvic self-examination. Some groups learn to recognize early symptoms of vaginal infections, identify commonly prescribed drugs, and use home remedies. Groups sometimes are organized especially for women in a particular age group, life-cycle stage, or sexual orientation; others are mixed. Some are for well women; others are for women in need of medical services for routine problems.

Advanced health groups research topics and have published highly informative health education material. The Boston Women's Health Book Collective's highly successful *Our Bodies, Ourselves* (1973, 1976, 1978) has gone through several editions, has been translated into twelve languages, and is used now in medical schools as well as in feminist clinics. The San Francisco Women's Health Collective and the National Women's Health Network produce data sheets on topics such as menopause, breast care, and nutrition. The Los Angeles Feminist Women's Health Center is now completing an extensive duty of self-help gynecology with photographs of vaginal and cervical changes throughout the entire menstrual cycle. Feminist health material is so abundant that the National Women's Health Network has established a clearinghouse to collect and disseminate such information, and a new journal, *Women and Health*, was established in 1976 at the State University of New York, College at Old Westbury.

Women argue that these new sources of health information fill a real need, making them more competent health care consumers. Once they learn the names and symptoms of common vaginal infections, they can recognize them early and use home remedies to alleviate discomfort until they can get medical attention (if necessary). If they are familiar with their bodies and standard medical procedures, they can communicate more easily and provide doctors with important information such as which drugs taken previously have been effective and which have had unfortunate side effects. Should a problem such as vaginal infection recur, these women are able to communicate their symptoms in precise terms rather than having to resort to vague descriptions.

This heightened ability to communicate increases self-esteem, breaks down physicians' stereotypes of women as ignorant and dependent, and results in better use of medical resources. Primary diagnosis is always done by patients, and the more knowledgeable they are, the more efficiently they can use available services. For example women who recognize early symptoms can call a physician or clinic during regular hours, instead of in the middle of the night after the problem has gotten worse.

Feminists' belief that women can and should acquire medical knowledge from each other leads to many of the innovative ways in which direct service as well as strictly informational self-help groups are structured. Beginning with the premise that women possess considerable knowledge and expertise, routine care is organized to provide women access to each others' knowledge in groups rather than in one-to-one encounters with professionals. Some self-help groups associated with the Feminist Women's Health Centers offer participatory gynecology clinics where women who need routine care (Pap smears, breast examination, VD testing, contraceptives, lab tests for vaginal and urinary tract infections, sickle cell testing, prenatal care) receive services in groups of six to eight. The women meet with self-help paramedics and a female nurse-practitioner for two hours; professionals are primarily resource people who answer questions, perform legally restricted tasks (e.g., inserting IUDs, prescribing drugs), and assist group participants to carry out pelvic and breast examinations on themselves and each other. Because diaphragms and IUDs are fitted and inserted in the group, women have ample opportunity to learn about the proper use of these devices and how to check on their placement. Women receive detailed information rather than brief answers to routine questions and believe they become better informed consumers of health services by learning with and from each other. In addition, patients can recall symptoms and concerns throughout the two-hour period, during which time valuable information, often skipped in a hurried encounter, is revealed. Professionals are relieved of the tedium and frustration of hurriedly repeating technical information and are freed to offer in-depth informed comment on medical matters. Time spent watching and listening sensitizes professionals to patients' real concerns and aids in diagnosis and planning medical regimens that patients are most likely to follow because they fulfill their subjectively felt needs.

This kind of patient education differs significantly from traditional health education in several ways. As previously noted, encouraging the woman to accept responsibility for her own health and to learn to care for herself is the goal. Whereas traditionally patient education occurs in private encounters between patient and professional, or in a large, impersonal setting where a professional lectures to a group of patients, feminist forms of patient education emphasize the interchange among lay people who come together in a group setting to share their medical experiences and expertise. Professionals are resource people, not authority figures making decisions and passing judgment on others' fears, concerns, and ignorance.

The success and effectiveness of these group educational activities suggest that despite the belief that private is better than public, private sessions with professionals may be less effective than group care for many routine services. In group sessions women have time to think of questions about the advantages and disadvantages of contraceptive methods and childbirth procedures; and treatments for menopausal symptoms or routine gynecologic disorders can be explained better in a group than individually. In addition, the group offers social-psychological peer support simply unavailable in the one-to-one doctor-patient relationship.

Patient receptivity to group care may be greater than might be assumed. In the mental health field, for example, group therapy including peer therapy is accepted today, although initially many doubted patients would reveal emotional problems in groups, especially groups supervised by nonphysicians (Hurvitz, 1974). Resistance to group gynecologic care stems in part from fear that it would be embarrassing. This fear is especially noticeable among professionals, who have been trained to "manage" embarrassment during obstetric and gynecologic examinations by draping the pelvis, minimizing eye contact, and adopting an artificially "jolly" or stoically silent manner. Feminists argue that, rather than decreasing embarrassment, such practices *create* it, conveying to women patients that there is something inherently unacceptable about their bodies. Thus the cycle of managing embarrassment serves to reinforce it and fails to challenge physicians and nurses to confront and examine—and possibly transform or transcend—their cultural conditioning that makes them ambivalent about women's bodies. It also deprives women of the opportunity to learn about their bodies in a positive way.

A striking feature of self-help gynecology clinics is the way they show that exposure of the female body, including one's own, need not be the unpleasant, embarrassing event women routinely experience in traditional health care settings. Several years ago I asked students to attend a self-help clinic as part of a course on women's role as providers and receivers of health care at the University of California in San Francisco. In their written reports nearly all the students, many of them master's degree candidates with years of professional nursing experience, reported feeling uncomfortable, scared, or apprehensive about doing the assignment. Yet without exception, all commented on how the experience was different than they had expected; it was not embarrassing as they feared it would be. The nurses' comments about how different it was to be a participant, rather than either a professional provider or patient, were especially striking. This maternity nurse-practitioner student's report is typical:

> Jane (the self-help leader) was unembarrassed and self-confident, and taught us how to examine our genitals and cervixes with our own speculums, mirrors and flashlights. I was amazed that of all the cervixes I've seen, this one was *mine!* We compared pubic hair, cervixes, looked at each other, exchanged information, ideas and experiences about reproduction, sexuality, menstruation, myths, the experience of growing up female, and menopause. Most central was our underlying common ground of negative experiences with doctors, gynecologists, nurses (even myself) and sometimes parents and teachers, in our struggles to accept and like ourselves and our bodies. I had felt slightly self-conscious at the beginning of the session, but developed a sense of warmth, security, and sisterhood with these other women. . . . We had shared very intimate experiences in our first two hours together and had learned how to examine our own bodies. I was glad to be able to offer additional information from my nursing experience, but found that my "professional" role did not really prepare me for an active and creative role in a lay setting.

Overall, the students found attending self-help groups interesting, informative, and personally as well as professionally valuable. Even the student (a public health nurse) who was somewhat concerned over the antimedical atmosphere and questioned the validity of some of the information, wrote,

> At the end of the session I felt very excited, uplifted and more in control of my body. The experiences of exploring and sharing with other women aspects of our bodies which have been hidden from us was a truly enlightening adventure.

Feminist health groups also address the political and economic context of health care and teach women to question practices and treatments that seem to be more in the interest of health care providers than patients. For example women learn that hysterectomies are sometimes performed for profit, and they learn that they have the right to a second opinion and should not consent to surgery until they are satisfied that a procedure is really necessary.

In short, feminist self-help proponents believe that they—and only they—have the right to decide what care is best for them after assessing available information and obtaining different opinions and suggestions, particularly because medical science (like other branches of science) is always in flux and there are disagreements within the scientific community itself, a fact physicians often ignore or hide from their patients.

Obviously this kind of patient education is most appropriate as a form of preventive education or in situations, such as pregnancy, where the woman is not really "sick." It is very effective for dealing with routine conditions such as vaginitis, cystitis, and menopausal symptoms. Group education and peer counseling also have wide application for helping patients adjust to serious diseases and the aftermath of treatment. Self-help groups such as Reach for Recovery (for mastectomy patients) and DES-Watch (for women exposed to diethylstilbestrol in utero) reveal the deep need of patients for personal contact with others who share a common plight.

Professionals concerned with providing more effective and more meaningful education for their patients might look to lay groups to learn more about how women feel about their medical care. Some of the self-help groups' innovations, such as providing a mirror so that women can watch pelvic examinations and holding group sessions for prenatal or contraceptive care, can be adapted and integrated into conventional medical settings. Nonetheless, while professionals can learn much about educating patients from lay groups, the effectiveness of lay groups lies in their being just that—they neither want nor need professional direction. Thus professionals who recognize the value of self-help health activities can most profitably participate as fellow "learners," adapt whatever they can into their own practices, and refer their own patients who can benefit from the unique learning experience self-help groups offer.

References

Boston Women's Health Book Collective. *Our bodies, ourselves: A book by and for women.* New York: Simon & Schuster, 1973, 1976, 1978.
Corea, G. *The hidden malpractice: How American medicine treats women as patients and professionals.* New York: William Morrow, 1977.

Gartner, A., & Riessman, F. *Self-help in the human services.* San Francisco: Jossey-Bass, 1977.

Haire, D. The cultural warping of childbirth. *ICEA News,* Special Issue (Spring) 1972. Reissued with Postscript, 1975.

Howard, J., Davis, F., Pope, C., & Ruzek, S. Humanizing health care: The implications of technology, centralization and self-care. *Medical Care,* May 1977, *15* (Suppl.), 11–26.

Hurvitz, N. Peer self-help psychotherapy groups: Psychotherapy without psychotherapists. In R. Roman & H. Trice (Eds.), *The sociology of psychotherapy.* New York: Jason Aronson, 1974, pp. 84–138.

Illich, I. *Medical nemesis: The expropriation of health.* New York: Pantheon, 1976.

Katz, A. H., & Bender, E. I. *The strength in us: Self-help groups in the modern world.* New York: New Viewpoints, 1976.

Kleiber, N., & Light, L. *Caring for ourselves: An alternative structure for health care* (National Health Research and Development Project No. 610-1020A of Health and Welfare, Canada). Vancouver: School of Nursing, University of British Columbia, 1978.

Korsch, M. B., & Negrete, V. F. Doctor-patient communication. *Scientific American,* August 1972, *227,* 66–74.

Levin, L. S., Katz, A. H., & Holst, E. *Self-care: Lay initiatives in health.* New York: Prodist, 1976.

Marieskind, H. Restructuring ob-gyn. *Social Policy,* September-October 1975, *6,* 48–49.

McKinlay, J. Who is really ignorant: Physician or patient? *Journal of Health and Social Behavior,* March 1975, *16,* 3–11.

Robinson, D., & Henry, S. *Self-help and health: Mutual aid for modern problems.* London: Martin Robertson, 1977.

Ruzek, S. Emergent modes of utilization: Gynecological self-help. In V. Olesen (Ed.), *Women and their health: Research implications for a new era* [U.S. Department of Health, Education, and Welfare Publication No. (HRA) 77–3138]. Washington, D.C.: National Center for Health Services Research, 1975.

Ruzek, S. *The women's health movement: Feminist alternatives to medical control.* New York: Praeger, 1978.

Seaman, B., & Seaman, G. *Women and the crisis in sex hormones.* New York: Rawson Associates, 1977.

Women's Self-help Resources

Books

Belita Cowan. *Women's health care: Resources, writings, bibliographies.* Ann Arbor, Mich.: Anshen, 1977.

National Women's Health Network. *Clearinghouse on health information.*

NWHN, 2025 I Street, N.W., Parklane Building, Suite 107, Washington, D.C.
Sheryl Ruzek. *Women and health care: A bibliography with selected annotation.* Evanston, Ill.: Program on Women, Northwestern University, 1976.

Films

Taking our bodies back. Cambridge Documentary Films, Box 385, Cambridge, Mass. 02139.
Self-health. Multi Media Resource Center, 540 Powell Street, San Francisco, Calif. 94108.
Healthcaring from our end of the speculum. Women Make Movies, Inc., 257 W. Nineteenth Street, New York, N.Y. 10011.
New image of myself (cervical self-exam), *Women-controlled abortion, Mastectomy self-help clinic, Home movies* (lesbianism), *Self-help clinic.* Feminist Women's Health Center, 1112 Crenshaw Boulevard, Los Angeles, Calif. 90019.

Organizations

Boston Women's Health Book Collective, Box 192, Somerville, Mass. 02144
Coalition for the Medical Rights of Women, 4079A Twenty-fourth Street, San Francisco, Calif. 94114
Feminist Women's Health Center, 1112 Crenshaw Boulevard, Los Angeles, Calif. 90019
National Self-Help Clearinghouse, 184 Fifth Avenue, New York, N.Y. 10010
National Women's Health Network, 2025 I Street, N.W., Parklane Building, Suit 107, Washington, D.C. 20024

Feminist Health Periodicals

Health Right, Women's Health Forum, 175 Fifth Avenue, New York, N.Y. 10010
The Monthly Extract, New Moon Communications, Box 3488 Ridgeway Station, Stamford, Conn. 06905
Network News, National Women's Health Network, 2025 I Street, N.W., Parklane Building, Suite 107, Washington, D.C. 20024
Women and Health, Issues in Women's Health Care, SUNY/College at Old Westbury, Old Westbury, N.Y. 11568

14

Active Patient Participation and Dental Health Education

Dorothy S. Oda and Jared I. Fine

It is generally acknowledged that dental disease is one of the most widespread health problems in our nation's population and that the cost of dental care is currently rising steadily along with all other health care services. Despite the universal prevalence of dental disease, it is virtually preventable with few exceptions. Therefore the need for greater understanding and appreciation of patient behavior as a contributory factor is crucial to effecting optimal oral health. In this context patient education and preventive dental services become increasingly important in concerted efforts toward cost containment and for improved dental health.

Because of the many factors that contribute to dental problems as well as the multiple consequences, preventive dentistry would, ideally, be a collaborative and collective endeavor with active patient participation and interdisciplinary cooperation. Patient behavior is itself determined by socioeconomic and cultural influences, among numerous other factors, and these must interface with health care systems that have a variety of delivery modes including solo practitioners, group practices, prepaid plans, health maintenance organizations, satellite clinics, and large medical centers, to name a few.

The health care team centered on the patient now includes professionals and paraprofessionals as well as those functioning in expanded roles. While acknowledging the important contributions of all of these health care workers, the emphasis in this chapter is on health professionals generally recognized as providing primary health care including dental services. Toward this multifaceted perspective of preventive dentistry involving the patient and the health practitioner, a review of selected literature provides a conceptual background. Patient education in preventive dentistry is defined by a working model. As a collaborative approach to preventive dental health, an interdisciplinary dental health service chart is presented. Finally there are examples to illustrate the application of the patient education process.

Review of Literature

If preventive dentistry is indeed a mutual endeavor between patient and provider, the utilization of dental services becomes a fundamental consideration. Bauer, Pierson, and House (1978) point out that utilization is not synonymous with demand; it simply measures the number of individuals using dental services, not the quantities of services. They further state that, as costs decrease, the quantity of demand normally increases, but this does not necessarily mean that more people are seeking care. Of particular interest in their literature review report were the top five equally ranked factors strongly affecting utilization of dental services: socioeconomic area, voluntary versus automatic coverage (prepaid dental insurance), degree of employer contribution to premium (insurance), preventive orientation of mothers (pertaining to children), and presence or absence of dental symptoms. These significant influences can be seen to range from external factors dealing mainly with economic and financial matters (socioeconomic areas and dental insurance) to the more internal motivational areas (mother's prevention orientation and presence or absence of dental symptoms).

Larger issues such as socioeconomic conditions, environmental influences, and community issues deserve attention and are included later in the chapter, particularly in the systems analysis section. However, the aspect of primary importance in patient education, individually or collectively, is motivation to seek some form of positive change as needed (such as diet modification or improved plaque control) to prevent or retard undesirable change (such as dental caries or gum problems) by preventive measures.

For the patient to be appropriately motivated to learn about changes and their effects, the process must be a reciprocal one. It is unrealistic and unworkable (not to mention stressful) for the dentist to assume the total responsibility for a patient's dental health. Technical and laboratory procedures are within the dentist's area of responsibility, but patients must be educated to understand that dentistry has its limitations and that success or failure cannot be placed entirely on the shoulders of the dentist (Dobyns, 1978).

In order for patients to become dentally informed, patient responsibility can be emphasized at the outset of the contact with the dentist. Patient education means patient involvement and is a team effort for the patient, who is the constant in the team, and all others providing or assisting in the provision of dental care services. Audiovisual aids, pamphlets, posters, and teaching aids ("What's New," 1978) as well as verbal communication are useful in promoting dental health information.

Communication is a key concept in patient education. The dentist's efforts to meet the patient's need for preventive care and the time expended to motivate the patient must necessarily be viewed in terms of economics and efficient utilization of practice time (Lefer, 1972). Yet in this age of dehumanization and litigations brought on by misunderstandings, it can be argued that it may cost more in time, stress, and even economic loss if effective communication does not take place. The difficulties of evaluating the value and effect of health education are acknowledged (Green, 1977).

The goal of patient education in dentistry is to influence the patient to behave in ways conducive to positive oral health and to avoid behaviors that are detrimental. Obviously almost all of this occurs outside of a dental office. Behavioral assessment of a patient need not be a sophisticated process reserved for highly skilled social scientists. It can be applied to an adequate degree by careful questioning by the practicing dentist and auxiliaries (Clark & Morton, 1977). From a practical standpoint, within their competence and time available, the dental practitioner and staff can evaluate the patient and possible influences such as disposition, attitude, social and cultural values, work and economic situation, and expectations of treatment. A caring interaction and a feeling of personal interest can do more to motivate the patient than the best and most accurate information provided in a perfunctory and depersonalized manner.

Effectiveness of practitioner-patient communication is in large measure related to a common frame of reference. In referring to physicians one author states that, when role expectations of both conform, the practitioner will be more helpful and the patient more likely to conform (Mechanic, 1968). In an ideal situation it would be expected that those patients with the greatest need for preventive dental health information would receive the most and that those patients with the least need would receive the least amount. One study revealed that such was not always the case. The characteristics of the dentist and his or her dental practice, such as treatment for that day, length of treatment, dentist's busyness, type of presentation (lecture, responses to questions), and year of graduation were important factors. Patient characteristics were not highly significant in the provision of preventive information (Hellman, 1976).

Basic to patient motivation is the fact that the patient must have a reason meaningful to her or him (Nizel, 1972). "[Health] education provided to learners must be perceived by them as relevant to their values, concerns, goals, past experiences, and present circumstances" (Simmons, 1977, p. 1138). The patient with his or her particular background and personality must be viewed as undergoing a process wherein the precursors to and consequences of dental problems develop. Blum's (1974) analysis of dental caries is an approach to viewing the causes and effects in a systematic manner (table 14-1).

Preventive Dentistry and Patient Education

Based on the fact that dental problems occur in patients as a result of biophysiological, genetic, sociopsychological, ethnic, and cultural, as well as environmental factors, patient education must take these into account to the extent possible. The purpose of patient education in dentistry is to achieve the highest level of oral health possible for a given person. Active and ongoing participation on the part of the patient is essential, and the patient must seek to use the information appropriately to effect his or her own maximum level of dental health. Various strategies are employed depending on the person, family, or aggregate pattern of behavior.

A conceptual model depicting this dynamic process involved in patient education is given in figure 14-1. The operational diagram in figure 14-2 depicts the interrelationship of preventive interventions and patient actions. For any preventive dental care service to be optimally effective, active participation by the patient is crucial. The preventive interventions in figure 14-2 are currently accepted procedures to prevent or reduce oral health problems.

Table 14-1.
Systems Analysis of Dental Caries

Input to problem		Problem	Output from problem	
Secondary precursors	Primary precursors		Primary consequences	Secondary consequences
Ignorance	Poor diet	D	Pain	Distress
Mass media advertising	Inadequate dental care	E	Inflammation	Pain
Inadequate funds	Low priority	N	Infection	Loss of teeth
Cost of food		T		Systemic effects
		A		
		L	Loss of teeth	Loss of function
Geographic location	Lack of fluoride	C		Low self-esteem
	Inaccessibility of dental care	A		Aesthetic effect
		R		
		I		Malnutrition
Lack of information	Poor oral hygiene	E		
	Genetic factors	S		

Adapted from Henrick Blum, *The Planning of Health.* Copyright 1974 by Human Sciences Press. Reprinted by permission. This adaptation was developed in a small group session at the Second Annual National Symposium of Patient Education, San Francisco, California, October 1978.

Figure 14-1.
Patient education in preventive dentistry.

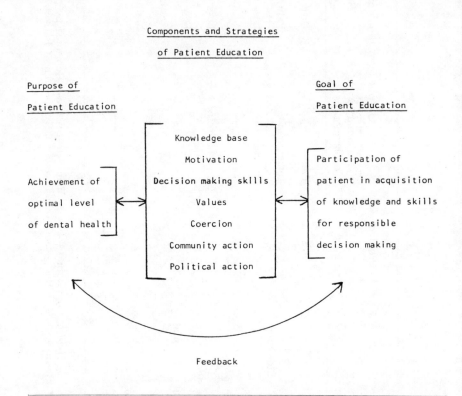

Components and Strategies

of Patient Education

Purpose of   Goal of

Patient Education   Patient Education

Knowledge base

Motivation

Participation of

Achievement of   Decision making skills   patient in acquisition

optimal level   Values   of knowledge and skills

of dental health   Coercion   for responsible

Community action   decision making

Political action

Feedback

Developed in a small group session at the Second Annual National Symposium on Patient Education, San Francisco, California, October 1978.

Comprehensive Perspective and
Interdisciplinary Collaboration

Thus far, emphasis has been placed on individual patient education by the dentist and auxiliary. Dental health is, of course, of primary concern to the dental provider whether general practitioner or specialist. However, health care services are often accused of being fragmented and overly specialized. There is a need for health professionals of various disciplines to function cooperatively and collaboratively for

Figure 14-2.
Relationship between preventive intervention and patient action.

Preventive Intervention		Patient Action
Fluoridation of community water supply	< - - - - ->	Political, educational, financial activism
Occlusal sealants	< - - - - ->	Access to provider, oral hygiene, education, knowledge
Topical fluoride	< - - - - ->	Access to provider, oral hygiene
Fluoride mouth rinse	< - - - - ->	Political activism in school health, motivation
Prophylaxis	< - - - - ->	Motivation, education, knowledge, values, priorities, peer influences
Diet control	< - - - - ->	Same as above
Plaque control	< - - - - ->	Same as above
Treatment (e.g. endodontics)	< - - - - ->	Access to provider, follow-through

the benefit of the patient as consumer. Dental problems can and do occur in virtually all ages from the very young to the elderly. The early identification of dental health conditions by any health practitioner for treatment or referral contributes to the overall health level of a patient. Table 14-2 is a flow chart of age-appropriate dental health services and associated health care settings and providers in the community.

Case Examples of Patient Education

The following three examples demonstrate the application of the dental health education process. The first is a single-patient situation; the second deals with a small group; and the third is an example of community involvement in dental health.

Table 14-2.
Collaborative Dental Health Care Service

Age level/Population	Dental care needs	Service setting	Disciplines	Collaborating/Referral disciplines
Infant	Developmental surveillance	Office, Clinic, OPD	MD, PNP, FNP	DDS–pedodontics, oral surgery; MD–pediatric/plastic surgery
Preschool	Developmental surveillance, prevention, maintenance, restoration	Office, Clinic, OPD preschool, child care center	DDS, MD, RDH, PNP, SN, FNP	DDS–general practice, pedodontics
School-age (including pregnant adolescent, educationally handicapped, developmentally disabled)	Developmental surveillance, prevention, maintenance, restoration, rehabilitation	Office, clinic, OPD, school	DDS, MD, RDH, SN, SNP, PNP, FNP	DDS–general practice, pedodontics, orthodontics
Young adult/college	Prevention, maintenance, restoration, rehabilitation	Office, campus, health service, clinic, OPD	DDS, MD, RN, RDH, FNP, AHP	DDS–general practice, endodontics, periodontics, prosthodontics, oral surgery
Middlescent	Prevention, maintenance, restoration, rehabilitation	Office, clinic, OPD, hospital	DDS, MD, RDH, FNP, AHP	DDS–general practice, endodontics, periodontics, prosthodontics, oral surgery
Senior	Prevention, maintenance, restoration, rehabilitation	Office, clinic, OPD, hospital, extended care facility	DDS, MD, RDH, RN, FNP, AHP	DDS–general practice, endodontics, periodontics, prosthodontics, oral surgery

OPD = outpatient departments; PNP = pediatric nurse practitioner; FNP = family nurse practitioner; RDH = registered dental hygienist; SN = school nurse; SNP = school nurse practitioner; AHP = adult health practitioner.

Nutrition Counseling of an Individual Patient

Nizel (1972) provides an illustration of patient education that emphasizes the need for personalized communication in diet counseling. A positive attitude on the part of the dentist, current scientific knowledge, and realism in diet prescription are also mentioned as necessary attributes to motivate the patient to try to control caries through diet. The motivation bases may be the desire to avoid dental restoration expenses, fear of dental pain, social acceptance, and aesthetic values, among others.

> Robert F. is a 35-year-old single salesman who was concerned about areas of gum line sensitivity and numerous cavities in his teeth. This condition was first noticed six months ago and seemed to be increasing in rate and severity; now 12 surfaces need to be restored.
> Robert lived alone and prepared his own meals. He prided himself on his vigor, which he attributed to the natural foods that he ate. He was willing and could afford to spend significant amounts of money for his wheat germ, blackstrap molasses, kelp, ascerola cherry juice, etc.
> Because he had recently taken on a new line of binoculars which were not selling very well, he had become rather edgy and anxious about business and meeting quotas. To deal with this anxiety and frustration, he was constantly nibbling between meals. The kinds of snacks that he enjoyed and ate were honey on whole wheat crackers, figs, dates, and raisins.
> An analysis of his usual dietary intake indicated an emphasis on yogurt, whole grain cereals, soybean meatlike dishes, alfalfa, wheat germ, tiger's milk, and purified vitamins, especially vitamin E.
> We attempted to explain that he would feel just as good if he ate the less expensive, nutritious foods that could be bought at any supermarket. Further, we suggested that he could substitute noncariogenic snacks like nuts and fruits for his sticky dried fruit. He did not accept our advice. (Nizel, 1972, p. 215)

The author points out that failure in this case was due to a disregard of the patient's emotional dependence on certain foods and that a more gradual educational process may have met with more success.

Dental Health Education of a Small Group

Group dental health education programs such as the Alabama Smile Keeper (ASK) program (Rose, Rogers, Kleinman, Shory, Meehan, & Zumbro, 1979) are often provided in school settings. This one, according to the authors, was a comprehensive school education program designed to improve dental health through teachers teaching preventive dentistry. The program was established at Maxwell Air Force Base Elementary School, where 475 students in grades one through six were examined to determine their oral hygiene status. The Simplified Oral Hygiene Index (OHI-S proposed by Greene and Vermillion (1964) was used prior to the program, immediately after it, and four months later without reinforcement. A written examination (dental aptitude indicator) served to test knowledge of dental health. The same examination was given four months later to check for retention.

The education program for the teachers consisted of a four-hour workshop that included intensive review of courses and prevention of oral disease, discussion of diet and its effect on oral health, plaque removal, and review of related educational material. Teachers were advised to have a humanistic approach, taking into consideration students' self-images, peer group pressure, and well-being, in order to instill the values of good oral health. They were also advised to integrate the dental health material in the regular curriculum during the testing period but not after the second test, when retention without reinforcement was measured.

The results showed that a school dental health education program utilizing teachers to teach preventive dentistry improved the oral hygiene and dental health knowledge of elementary school children. An interesting finding was that the level of dental health knowledge was not directly correlated with application of this information. That is, there was no significant correlation between scores on dental health examinations and the OHI-S scores. The need for continual reinforcement for retention of knowledge was also pointed out.

It should be noted that, whereas the ASK program utilized teachers to teach preventive dental health to students, another method of small group dental health education is direct teaching and supervision of oral care techniques by health practitioners (Meskin, Kenney, Martens, & Meskin, 1977; Silverstein, Gold, Heilbron, Helms, & Wycoff, 1977).

Community Fluoridation

The fluoridation of community water supplies as a preventive measure for dental caries is widely accepted by scientific groups as well as health organizations and agencies. However it also has strong and vocal opponents who are determined and persevering in their efforts to prevent or stop fluoridation in communities. The following is a case history of a successful fluoridation campaign using minimal labor and budget but a conjoint effort of professionals and consumers (Boriskin, 1979).

In a multicounty water district with 1,100,000 customers and about 500,000 registered voters, a fluoridation campaign was begun after two prior election defeats. The district population was extremely diversified, with severe poverty areas as well as affluent sections. There was a wide economic, educational, and cultural spectrum reflected in those who were served by the water district. An analysis of past election failures revealed that: Grass-roots voters were not reached, possibly because most of the campaigning was done by health professionals; the campaign had relatively low visibility; debate forums were rarely beneficial and may have unwittingly aided the opposition; expenditures were not used in the most effective manner; technical language was used in messages; elections were consolidated with statewide primary, rather than general, elections, when voter turnout is usually greater; lead time was too short (six months and one year); and the ballot proposition wording was ambiguous and negative in tone.

With a discouragingly slow start, a core committee had worked for six months when the addition of a key new member renewed the committee, which then became a steering committee. This knowledgeable and dedicated nonhealth professional with significant expertise added critical strength to the group. A singular insight was the recognition that a fluoridation election is a *political campaign* and must be handled as such and not as an educational effort.

The first step was to get the issue on the ballot. Toward this end six goals were established:

1. To obtain 50,000 petition signatures
2. To obtain endorsements from all city councils and county boards of supervisors in the water district
3. To conduct a public opinion poll that would reflect a significant majority of residents favoring a fluoride vote
4. To encourage private citizens to deluge individual water dis-

trict board members with letters encouraging them to call a
vote

5. To obtain endorsements from all state and federal elected
    officials who represent the water district
6. To obtain endorsements from all health groups and commu-
    nity leaders urging the board to call a vote

Fifteen months after the first meeting of the committee, which was
later reorganized and called People for Fluoridation, the deadline for
ballot requirements was met.

The wording of the ballot proposition itself then became of critical importance, for it had to be both informational and educational
about the purposes and benefits of fluoridation. Considerable disagreement occurred between the water district staff and the People for
Fluoridation, but in the end a compromise was reached. The next
two months were occupied with intensive campaigning on both sides
once the water district had publicly announced its intent to place
fluoridation on the upcoming ballot.

Fund raising was a necessity and a major problem. The only organizations to respond to pleas were the local dental society chapters
and one dental insurance corporation with a majority of dentists on
its board of directors. Financial commitment was not forthcoming
from political, religious, health, or community organizations, although
support existed. Many individuals, both lay and professional, donated
smaller sums. A valuable, nonmonetary contribution was 3,000 square
feet of prime-location work space. The money-tree concept of fund
raising was used. A "seed" dentist contacted ten other professional
acquaintances, who in turn contacted ten others. The appeal was for
the fixed sum of $100, and its success depended on the initial selection
of a concerned member of the dental profession who was well known
and commanded respect. The entire campaign budget was $27,000,
of which $26,000 came from dentists and their organizations.

Careful consideration was given to utilizing these limited funds
to the best advantage, and six guidelines were developed:

1. Get maximum visibility during the last two weeks before
    election.
2. Concentrate energies in the low-income areas of the com-
    munity, which would benefit most from the program.
3. Keep campaign messages short and simple.
4. Refuse invitations to participate in any public debate forums
    for television, radio, or before large groups.

5. Keep public image 100 percent positive.
6. Emphasize endorsements of prominent local individuals and organizations with which all segments of the community can identify.

The proposition won by a close margin of only 3,096 votes. The largest city in the water district, one with low-income, high-density areas, accounted for 51 percent of the Yes votes, although in the past it had been decisively negative toward fluoridation. Hence the concentration of campaign efforts on specific areas was clearly justified, according to the author of the report.

As a final note, Boriskin (1979) relates that antifluoridationists immediately began concerted efforts to impede the implementation of the program, and a postelection "public health liaison committee" to the water district functions to keep a watchful eye on the fluoridation program. Opponents continue to try to undo the program. A total of $10,000 was spent *after* the election to preserve the victory, which underscored the need to be diligent in efforts following as well as prior to a community fluoridation vote.

Summary

A multidimensional perspective of patient education emphasizes the importance of the active participation of the ultimate consumer—the patient—in the educational aspect of preventive dentistry. As with all health care services the highest level of health status attainable for each patient is the continuing goal. A collaborative interdisciplinary approach will increase patients' access to care, thereby enhancing the probability of success. The providing of preventive dental health information to patients and their appropriate use of it should be a shared experience between patients and practitioners.

References

Bauer, J. C., Pierson, A. P., & House, D. R. *Factors which affect utilization of dental services* (No. 78–64, Health Resources Administration, U.S. Public Health Service). Washington, D.C.: U.S. Government Printing Office, 1978.

Blum, H. *The planning of health.* New York: Human Sciences, 1974.

Boriskin, J. M. *The winning of a large fluoridation campaign utilizing minimal manpower and budget* (unpublished report). People for Fluoridation Committee, Oakland, California, 1979.

Clark, J. D., & Morton, J. C. Behavioral assessment: An appraisal of beliefs and behaviors relating to treatment. *Dental Clinics of North America,* 1977, *21*(3), 515–530.

Dobyns, R. Patient responsibility. *Dental Clinics of North America,* 1978, *22*(2), 279–284.

Green, L. Evaluation and measurement: Some dilemmas for health education. *American Journal of Public Health,* 1977, *67,* 155–161.

Greene, J. C., & Vermillion, J. R. The simplified oral hygiene index. *Journal of the American Dental Association,* 1964, *68,* 7–13.

Hellman, S. The dentist and preventive dental health information. *Health Education Monographs,* 1976, *4*(2), 132–176.

Lefer, L. Failures in motivation of dental home care. *Dental Clinics of North America,* 1972, *16*(1), 3–11.

Mechanic, D. *Medical sociology: A selective view.* New York: Free Press, 1968.

Meskin, L. H., Kenney, J. B., Martens, L., & Meskin, E. R. A preventive dental program for "high risk" children. *Journal of School Health,* 1977, *47,* 293–295.

Nizel, A. E. Why and how diet counseling might fail in dentistry. *Dental Clinics of North America,* 1972, *16*(1), 209–216.

Rose, C., Rogers, E. W., Kleinman, P. R., Shory, N. L., Meehan, J. T., & Zumbro, P. E. An assessment of the Alabama Smile Keeper school dental health education program. *Journal of the American Dental Association,* 1979, *98,* 51–54.

Silverstein, S., Gold, S., Heilbron, D., Helms, D., & Wycoff, S. Effect of supervised deplaquing on dental caries, gingivitis and plaque (IADR abstract). *Journal of Dental Research,* 1977, *56* (Special Issue A).

Simmons, J. Lessons for health educators. *American Journal of Public Health,* 1977, *67,* 1137–1138.

What's new in preventive dentistry. *Journal of the California Dental Association,* 1978, *6,* 49–52.

15

Patient Compliance and Patient Education: Some Fundamental Issues

Carol N. D'Onofrio

What are the relationships between patient compliance and patient education? Anyone straddling the fields of health and education will be familiar with this question, but the way it is asked depends on where one's primary allegiance lies. Those whose first concern is with the aims of education inquire whether compliance is a proper goal, whereas those who are dedicated to medical care wonder whether education can influence compliance anyway.

The real issue, of course, is power and control—a theme that surfaces in many forms during serious discussion of patient education. As Mattei (1978) has pointed out, thinking in terms of compliance creates a demand situation that may act as a serious impediment to the educational process. Even the word *compliance* is repugnant to many educators because it implies subservience, dependence, and unquestioning obedience to authority.

This clearly is antithetical to the ideals of American education, rooted in participatory democracy, as expressed by such early educational philosophers as Thomas Jefferson, John Dewey, and Alfred North Whitehead. These leaders did not see the purposes of education as preparing people to fit into an existing system, rather as enabling them to govern their own destinies, both as individuals and as members of a free society. Pragmatically, then, the goals of education were not to prepare people to comply with someone else's dictates but to equip them with problem-solving skills whereby they could gain greater control over the directions of their own lives and participate in shaping and changing their communities and institutions to better serve their needs.

I believe that these ideals are deeply embedded in the American character. In recent years, however, their most eloquent advocate has come not from the United States but from the ghettoes of Brazil, where Paulo Freire (1970, 1973) developed his concepts of education for critical consciousness. Perhaps the loss of this philosophical thrust from the mainstream of American education is why many of us left the bureaucracies of the public school system to work, less encumbered we thought, in community health programs. Nevertheless as we strive to increase individual choice and community participation in the health care system, we find we cannot escape the struggle for control between proponents of existing institutions and those of the concept that education should give power to the people. Nowhere do the issues emerge more sharply than in the discussion of patient compliance with medical advice.

As a consequence patient education practitioners become trapped in some difficult dilemmas. Should education be provided only on the basis of physician prescription or should it be freely available to any health consumer? Should our efforts be targeted to achieve behavior change specified by medical agreement on objectives, or should education be guided by what people want to know? Should we risk losing our credibility with the public by dealing only with the medically approved information each patient is to receive about his or her illness and prescribed regimen, carefully avoiding questions about provider competence, conflicting opinions, and vested interests in the system? Or should we risk losing our jobs by making information openly available on these subjects?

Our own beliefs and values about education, medical care, and human nature affect how we grapple with these questions. Because the issues are not simple, the answers are not easy. Indeed, if we deal with them only on a philosophical basis, we can chase ourselves in circles. At best this keeps us from getting on with the job. At worst this looks like a cop-out to our critics, who doubt that education has much impact upon compliance in any event. We therefore need to parcel out the questions and examine the related evidence in an objective manner. In beginning this inquiry, three matters stand out as critical.

Is Patient Compliance Associated with Positive Outcomes of Medical Care?

Certainly in considering whether to commit ourselves as patient educators to a goal of compliance, we need to ask this question. It would seem indisputable that, if people are to benefit from what medical science has to offer, they must be helped to understand the importance of their cooperation in following medical advice. On the other hand noncompliance in certain cases may be a fortunate occurrence.

Statistics on the incidence of unnecessary surgery and over prescribing of drugs suggest that medical advice is not always offered in the patient's interest. Moreover as Sackett and Haynes (1976) observed in their comprehensive consideration of issues in compliance, we cannot assume that faithful adherence to medical advice guarantees achievement of the treatment goal, even when it is set with the best of intentions, for "in addition to biologic variation . . . patients may be the victims of clinical timidity, homeopathy, or diagnostic inaccuracy."

Glogow (1973) raises other considerations in his suggestion that "the 'bad' patient gets better quicker." While noting that compliant behavior may be easier for providers and institutions to deal with, he cities studies indicating compliance may be costly to the patient's well-being. Thus by labeling the compliant patient "good," medical staff in the long run may tend to reward behavior that requires special attention and service, thereby conditioning patients to an even greater degree of compliance, in which they may stifle their aggression, anger, and fear and suppress their feelings in general. Potential consequences are suggested in research by Dunbar (1947), who found that model patients' "are the ones most likely to die or return later in a more serious phase of their illness" (p. 46), and by Daniels and Davidoff (1950), who suggested that the so-called good patient has a long clinical course and recovers slowly.

In some of his own research Glogow also found that patients who followed medical instructions in a glaucoma study were poor, older, foreign born, or on public welfare, and that careful observation of these people revealed a kind of powerlessness, a fear of authority, and an obedience to medical staff. Conversely, the noncompliants seemed to be more independent and less intimidated, and also to have a greater number of options. Accordingly Glogow suggested that we should replace the concept of compliance with that of participation, so that our goal becomes to involve people actively in decisions about medical care. This approach, then, would support the broader purposes of education by serving to bring power to the people. It also is consistent with legal requirements for informed consent, which brings us to a second critical question.

How Does the Educational Process Influence Compliance?

There is a good deal of objective evidence from a variety of sources to indicate that simply providing patients with information on their illness and how to follow medical advice will have very little effect on compliance. Sackett and Haynes (1976) report from their comprehensive review that "an interesting finding at sharp variance with conventional wisdom is that there appears to be no relationship between patients' knowledge of their disease or its therapy and their compliance with the associated treatment regimen."

This conclusion bears closer scrutiny, for it appears to contradict the common proposition that a more knowledgeable patient will be more apt to recognize the value of adhering to the therapeutic plan. Here we should point out that the requirements of research methodology often necessitate violating much of what we know about the dynamics of the educational process. Thus many of the studies Sackett and Haynes reviewed may have employed only univariate analysis to examine the relationship between knowledge and behavior, whereas theory indicates that the real influence of knowledge on compliance is much more likely to rest in its interaction with other variables affecting learning and change. Perhaps when research methods are more adequately matched to theory, the data will reveal that knowledge does indeed play a critical role in compliance.

I suspect, however, that the key to understanding the seeming conflict between general recognition that information is important and the conclusion of Sackett and Haynes rests in what is meant by "knowledge." Educational specialists emphasize the importance of active patient participation in problem identification and prioritization, in the establishment of change objectives, and in the process of making decisions about how change will be accomplished. This implies, then, that patients should help to define the knowledge that they need in order to cope with their illness and treatment regimen. Nevertheless, all too frequently the information made available to patients—and research measures of knowledge levels—are based solely on what providers decide patients ought to know.

The existence of citizen-initiated mutual aid groups—estimated by Levin (1978) to number over 500,000 and to involve more than 5 million people—indicates that many patients consider the information that providers offer insufficient if not irrelevant. Analysis of these groups reveals rather clearly that they are formed by consumers who have identified deeply felt needs or sources of acute frustration, or in some cases health or medical risks and dangers, that existing approaches to health care and the medical management of the problem have not taken into account (Arthur D. Little, 1976; Tracy & Gussow, 1976). The knowledge these groups generate and exchange therefore may be a much more powerful determinant of compliant or noncompliance than the information provided within the formal health care system.

Nor are the "veterans" of health care experiences and health care providers the only sources of information available to patients. Robinson (1974) identified four additional types of communication that patients use in determining whether or not to follow medical advice. According to her research, *internal sources*, including physiological signals, preexisting knowledge and beliefs, and factors in one's life situation, were much more important influences on the behavior of heart patients than were *external sources* of communication, which included not only what was said by the health care team and what was learned from other patients but also information from the media. Whether we plan it or not, patients weigh all of these inputs and make their own decisions about whether compliance is in their best self-interest.

If patient education is to be effective then, it must assist patients to order and analyze all of this information as part of the problem-solving process. This view is consistent with the theoretical position that, if education is to result in behavior change, internalization of learning must occur (Kelman, 1961). Whereas compliance may result from outside pressure or identification with authority, unless patients come to feel for themselves the importance of the behavior, change will either be short-lived or be patterned after a chronic disease model in which continuing educational intervention is necessary.

Herein lie the principle reasons why educational specialists objected to reliance on media packages for patient education. Although such packages may be effective when combined with interpersonal approaches that elicit active patient participation in problem solving, used alone they simply beam more information at patients without helping them to reconcile the multiple, and often conflicting, messages they are already receiving.

Because internalization is such a necessary and central goal of education, the effects of using external incentives also must be carefully studied. External rewards may be effective when they are consistent with a person's internal value system; however, this is very complex and as yet little understood. As the Indian sterilization program demonstrates, the use of external incentives to motivate action can result in resentment, resistance, and distrust, as people come to understand the full consequences of their action and the fact that they have been coerced (Minkler, 1977).

Now this brings us to a third question—the critical one for health providers who wonder whether education really is an essential component of medical care as patient education practitioners so often claim.

Can Education Improve Compliance?

Sackett and Haynes (1976) are doubtful. From their review and analysis of strategies for improving compliance, they concluded that education had a success rate of only 64 percent in effecting improvements that were both clinically and statistically significant. In contrast they estimated that behavioral and combined behavioral-educational approaches had success ratings of 85 percent and 88 percent respectively. Nevertheless in their classification of strategies they used a very limited definition of education, equating it with information giving. At the urging of Stanley Rosenberg some of us at Berkeley therefore undertook a re-analysis of the interventions that Sackett and Haynes considered.

We began by drawing on educational principles to develop criteria of educational adequacy for interventions directed at improving compliance. Then we assigned scores to each study according to whether the educational problem had been diagnosed prior to intervention, whether clear educational objectives had been set, whether patients had actively participated in these processes, and several other dimensions. Although we have only begun to analyze the data, some of the results are already clear.

First we found that most interventions reported in the compliance literature were generally weak in educational quality. Second we found that, despite their labels, the classifications of interventions adopted by Sackett and Haynes failed to establish mutually exclusive categories for educational strategies and also failed to distinguish education from other activities lacking in educational merit. Finally when we reexamined the relationship of educational adequacy to compliance, using Sackett and Haynes's methodology and measures of the dependent variable, we found that the group of studies scoring above the midpoint on our scale showed a 100 percent success rate in improving compliance as well as therapeutic outcome. Thus we conclude that education can be effective when it meets certain minimal standards of quality.

Summary and Conclusions

To summarize, then, let us return to the fundamental issue of whether education and compliance are compatible. Inasmuch as *compliance* denotes obedience to an external authority, this concept is inconsistent with the purposes of education in a democratic society. Although providers may attempt to use education to increase compliance, this effort is likely to be ineffective as long as they maintain control over the educational process. On the other hand education that involves the patient with the provider in defining and resolving problems in medical care can be very effective in obtaining patient cooperation to achieve the treatment goal.

On another level the relationship between education and compliance involves a power struggle. In order to function as smoothly and efficiently as possible, health care systems and the professionals who work them strain to maintain control over patients. As Lorber (1975) has pointed out, limiting the communication of information to patients is the chief method through which this is accomplished. Withholding information thus serves to prevent the interruption of work routines with questions as well as to mask the shortcomings and failures of providers and to protect the professional stance of detachment. At the same time, compliance is rewarded, whereas noncompliance is quelled in a variety of ways. Thus Lorber reports from her own and other research that patients who do not comform to the expectations of doctors and nurses become known as "problems" and are tranquilized, labeled as irrational and irresponsible, and sometimes discharged early or otherwise subjected to medical neglect.

Patients, however, have access to information from multiple sources and thus their power is not so easily limited. Those who evaluate their treatment and are satisfied will comply. Those who are dissatisfied may also comply because they fear authority or the consequences of not following medical advice. Others will exercise their power in a number of ways. As Hayes-Bautista (1976) has observed, patients may modify their regimens either by adding to them or subtracting from them; they may attempt to renegotiate their treatment with the provider; or they may sever the relationship. In addition, dissatisfied patients in increasing numbers are discovering the power of the courts or banding together in mutual aid groups that often attempt to change the system (Tracy & Gussow, 1976).

Such actions represent not merely noncompliance but an effort by patients to gain control over their own destinies. Relating this thrust to a general loss of faith in U.S. institutions, McKnight (1975) observed that "people apparently want to have more caring, community-connected empowering relationships that do not depend on institutional interventions." Accordingly he argued that, if hospitals and the medical system are to be viewed as credible, health professionals must no longer consider themselves as "producers" of health but rather should think in terms of "institutional limits, low technology, and citizen health action." Among his specific recommendations are policies that emphasize making services understandable, involving people called patients in the repair of their health, and opening up the hospital to the care and curative power of friends and neighbors. On the other hand he contends that "if hospitals treat patients as though they have no role in dealing with their own health, they are health 'miseducators.' "

The answer therefore is clear. Given the existing body of scientific knowledge as well as the mysteries we do not yet understand, the variations and fluctuations in the present health care system, the purposes of education in a free society, the nature of the educational process, and an independent citizenry that in one way or another will exert the right of self-determination, the goal of patient education cannot be to achieve unquestioning compliance with medical advice. Rather, education must foster open sharing of information, questions, doubts, and concerns so that providers and consumers of health care can learn from each other. In this way we can all increase our understanding and our options, decide together how best to resolve the problems of medical care, and pool our resources toward these ends. Through participatory education, then, we can find new power to achieve patient treatment goals. At the same time we will be joining forces to reshape our institutions, empowering them to serve more effectively our society's changing needs.

References

Arthur D. Little, Inc. A summary of women's self-care programs. In *Appendix of project descriptions for a survey of consumer health education programs*. Prepared for the Office of the Assistant Secretary for Planning and Evaluation, U.S. Department of Health, Education, and Welfare. Reproduced by National Technical Information Service, U.S. Department of Commerce, January 1976, pp. 196–201.

Daniels, G. E., & Davidoff, E. The mental aspects of tuberculosis. *American Review of Tuberculosis*, 1950, *62*(5), 532–538.

Dunbar, F. *Mind and body: Psychosomatic medicine*. New York: Random House, 1947.

Freire, P. *Pedagogy of the oppressed*. New York: Seabury Press, 1970.

Freire, P. *Education for critical consciousness*. New York: Seabury Press, 1973.

Glogow, E. The "bad patient" gets better quicker. *Social Policy*, November-December 1973, pp. 72–76.

Hayes-Bautista, D. E. Modifying the treatment: Patient compliance, patient control and medical care. *Social Science and Medicine*, 1976, *10*, 233–238.

Kelman, H. C. Processes of opinion change. In W. G. Bennis, K. D. Benne, & R. Chin (Eds.), *The planning of change*. New York: Holt, Rinehart, and Winston, 1961, pp. 509–517.

Levin, L. S. Patient education and self-care. In *National patient education symposium* (Proceedings), University of California at San Francisco, September 24–25, 1977. Atlanta: U.S. Public Health Service, Center for Disease Control, Bureau of Health Education, 1978, pp. 24–31.

Lorber, J. Good patients and problem patients: Conformity and deviance in a general hospital. *Journal of Health and Social Behavior*, 1975, *16*(2), 213–225.

Mattei, T. J. Meeting patient education outcomes: Patient/provider responsiveness. In *National Patient Education Symposium*, (Proceedings), University of California at San Francisco, September 24–25, 1977. Atlanta: U.S. Public Health Service, Center for Disease Control, Bureau of Health Education, 1978, pp. 104–106.

McKnight, J. L. Hospitals must work to change image. *Hospitals*, May 16, 1975, *49*, 72–74.

Minkler, M. "Thinking the unthinkable": The prospect of compulsory sterilization in India. *International Journal of Health Services*, 1977, *7*(2), 237–248.

Robinson, L. A. Patients' information base: A key to care. *Canadian Nurse*, 1974, *70*(12), 34–36.

Sackett, D. L., & Haynes, R. B. (Eds.). *Compliance with therapeutic regimens*. Baltimore: Johns Hopkins University Press, 1976.

Tracy, G. S., & Gussow, Z. Self-help health groups: A grass-roots response to a need for services. *Journal of Applied Behavioral Science*, 1976, *12* (3), 381–396.

16

The (Already) Activated Patient: An Alternative to Medicocentrism

Patricia Dolan Mullen

The explanation of phenomena that are presently not understood . . . requires the search for processes that are presently known and unidentified.
(Lindesmith, Strauss, & Denzin, 1975, p. 46)

Implicit images of human behavior and of what phenomena constitute "problems" have a profound influence on the choice of program objectives and the information that is collected as a base for planning patient education programs (McHugh, 1968; Ryan, 1972). The associated research and evaluation efforts are also subject to similar limitations of perspective despite their more objective stance (Blumer, 1969; Kuhn, 1962; Stimson, 1974). In patient education this sometimes has led to the exacerbation of the schism between professional and patient viewpoints that already exists owing to large differences in perceptions, knowledge bases, and sociocultural characteristics (e.g., Apple, 1960; Baumann, 1961; Hayes-Bautista, 1978; Jenkins, 1966; Kleinman, Eisenberg, & Good, 1978; Strauss, 1972). One view, that of the health care provider, has tended to dominate patient education programs and research.

To the reader of the current and most often cited patient education literature, several themes predominate. The first is that medical care providers are engaged in a rational process of treating diseases (physical abnormalities), primarily via the prescription of various regimens to be carried out by their patients. One of the challenging tasks for the professional is to ensure compliance with the regimen, for it is now widely acknowledged that patients cannot all be counted on to follow through correctly or at all (Sackett & Haynes, 1976). The second theme is that patients, the targets of educational "strategies," behave less rationally than the providers, particularly when they pose compliance problems and depart from the professional's model of the ideal patient.

This chapter suggests ways to break out of what Green and his colleagues (Green, Werlin, & Avery, 1977) have called the medicocentric perspective. These strategies are based on alternative images and approaches to defining problems and to gathering data. A small but significant group of studies from medical sociology are described in terms of their theoretical underpinnings, methodology, and application to patient education programs. A longer presentation of the results of a study of myocardial infarction (heart attack) patients illustrates what can be learned from the approach being suggested. It is followed by guidelines for applying this approach and a more general conceptual framework for understanding specific chronic illnesses.

Medicocentrism in Patient Education Programs and Research

The patient's perspective has received less emphasis in practice than it has lip service among the planners of patient education programs, clinicians, and researchers. This is seen in the objectives selected for programs and evaluation efforts, in the vocabulary of the field, and in the focus of much of the research being reported in journals and at patient education conferences and symposia.

For example behavior change is viewed as a more important indicator of program success than patient satisfaction or other measures of meeting objectives patients set for themselves (e.g., the review by Green *et al.*, chapter 2 in this volume). Witness the underdevelopment of more patient-centered measures such as "informed decision-making" (regardless of outcome) and the underutilization of quality-of-life scales (Barofsky, Sugarbaker, & Mills, 1979; Bergner, Bobbit, Pollard, Martin, & Gilson, 1976), while drug tracers and other physical tests to avoid self-reports are perfected and widely used. The language used to define the issues in patient education, notably compliance and its synonyms, conjures up an inactive, unknowledgeable person in the patient role, one who is not capable of self-determination. Then there is the question of what is researched and with what methods. The terms *compliance, adherence,* and their opposites imply a motivation for the behavior: conformity and non-conformity or deviance. This is further reinforced by the definition of the patient's behavior in relation to a standard (the medical regimen). In fact the research problem as it is frequently conceived is one of deviance, albeit using an up-to-date, liberal model that blames the delinquent or noncomplier in subtle ways (Matza, 1964; Ryan, 1972).

Historically there have been three sorts of research problems posed (Stimson, 1974): First was the description of the extent of the deviance problem in terms of numbers and proportions. The second, having to do with the characteristics of the deviants, met with little success (Sackett & Haynes, 1976), but it implies that noncompliers were thought possibly to be identifiable types whose behavior in this area was consistent over time. "Why do some patients not follow instructions?" was the third and strikingly less well-covered research issue until the past few years. A broader set of variables is now being investigated, including: (1) the factors in patients' social contexts and perceptions, (2) their material resources, (3) the substance and tone of encounters with professionals, and (4) the organization of the medical care delivery system (Sackett & Haynes, 1976, pp. 34–39). However, the dependent variable continues to be compliance; the perspective, medicocentric, if only benignly so.

An Alternative: The (Already) Activated Patient

The theoretical model underlying a more naturalistic approach is one in which human beings are viewed in active, processual terms and are seen as capable of engaging in self-reflexive behavior. The interplay of a person's self-conceptions with the meaning he or she and important others attach to objects in their worlds is highlighted in this approach (Blumer, 1969; Lindesmith et al., 1975; Mead, 1956; Strauss, 1969).

> Human beings characteristically act with self-awareness, exercise self-control, exhibit conscience and guilt, and in the great crises of life make decisions with reference to some imagery of what they are, what they have been, and what they hope to be. (Lindesmith et al., 1975, p. 301)

Thus to say that someone has a self is to say that one defines or has a meaning for oneself and can interact with this self to attribute meaning to concepts, acts, material objects, and so forth and judge them before deciding on a course of action.

> In any of his countless acts—whether minor, like dressing him-. self, or major, like organizing himself for a professional career—the individual is designating different objects to himself, giving them meaning, judging their suitability to his action, and making decisions on the basis of the judgment. (Blumer, 1969, p. 80)

Objects in and of themselves do not call out a definition or action, for the meaning is not inherent in the object. Thus a pain one identifies and interprets is very different from a mere organic feeling, and this lays the basis for doing something about it instead of merely responding organically to it. For example the pain of childbirth is differently defined than pain experienced on a chronic basis or pain that has been inflicted unexpectedly.

Definitions are emergent and may be transformed over time, because they are socially constructed (e.g., Berger & Luckmann, 1967; McHugh, 1968). To return to the pain example the natural childbirth movement helps women interpret pain differently (as "contractions") than many American women have interpreted it in the past decades (as terrible pain from which anesthetics offer welcome relief). In learning what it is to have a disease that was previously unfamiliar, people take into account what others (including medical personnel) tell them is its meaning. The initial definition will change over time as further experience, information from illness peers, and legitimation or disbelief from others occur.

The implications of this view are that in order to understand an area of human behavior it is necessary to learn something about what people make of their situations, not just at one point, but over time. Furthermore this suggests that it is possible to identify *patterns* of meanings because members of groups with similar backgrounds tend to have similar sets of meanings. Data which are gathered in such a way that response is as open and free as possible would be preferred. Individual and group interviews that have minimal structure and offer sufficient time to develop the "story" and probe differences and discrepancies are desirable. Because people's retrospective accounts of their behavior do not qualify as scientific explanations, it is ideal to have contact at several time intervals or to have more than one version (perhaps that of a family member).

Such analyses are being conducted by medical sociologists and anthropologists, and the results are developing into a body of work that complements the medicocentric view with a patient-centered view. In this literature active people who are coping with illnesses (experiences of disvalued changes in states of being and social function) are depicted in their broad contexts where the regimen and medical care-related factors are not necessarily central even though they may be regarded as highly problematic. These studies use interview and participant observation data to answer the broad analytical questions What are people who have this illness engaged in doing? and What are the stages of that process and which conditions make it vary? For example Charmaz (1972) found out the ways families of the chronically ill shoulder the burden placed on them and how they feel about this burden. Benoliel (1975) studied a special group, families of newly diagnosed diabetic children, and traced their adaptation and its influence on the child over time, with emphasis on two chief issues, managing time and using food. Patient-identified problems such as pollution control with ulcerative colitis (Reif, 1975), funding with chronic renal failure (Suczek, 1975), getting around with emphysema (Fagerhaugh, 1975), and managing unstable symptoms with rheumatoid arthritis (Wiener, 1975) have been investigated by other researchers, who began with the questions such as What it is like to have emphysema? and Are there any special problems you have with the diabetes?

Others have cut across diagnostic categories because patients' problems often have other parameters: Among these are Davis's (1964) classic study on the ways people with visible physical handicaps assert their normality when meeting new people; Charmaz's (1973) more theoretical work on the self-conceptions of chronically ill people; and Fagerhaugh and Strauss's (1977) study of the negotiations between staff and patients over the management of pain.

An extended example of the naturalistic approach is presented in the next pages. It was taken from a study conducted as the basis for an in- and outpatient education program for heart attack victims and their families (Mullen, 1973, 1978).

Cutting Back after a Heart Attack

The heart attack or myocardial infarction (MI) changes or brings into question the basic order of a victim's life, creating a situation in which, temporarily at least, many old norms of behavior and self-conception do not apply. Whether this was the first or the latest of several episodes, the survivor of a heart attack faces the difficult task of resuming life in a new and ambiguous state. Aspects of health, energy, career, finances, social and family relationships, personal identity, and relative position vis-à-vis age peers and other comparison groups that have been taken for granted are thrust into self-conscious consideration. Thus in addition to the problem of survival, the patient is faced with the question of how well she or he will live and what can be salvaged from the former way of life. The MI regimen is characterized generally by cutting back, that is, eliminating and reducing (fatty foods, smoking, competitive or very active sports, heavy work, stressful situations, and excess activity) rather than by adding and increasing.

On another dimension, coronary heart disease is easier for the patient to deal with because the patient has a wide latitude of action compared to other chronic illnesses. Unlike the arthritis or stroke patient most MI patients are not physically forced to cut back. This freedom can be complex and confusing, however, because patients are largely on their own in interpreting the vague and ominous warning "Take it easy." The harder dimension is that sudden death may be the consequence of overstepping the unclear boundary line of safety, and one cannot count on having warning signals. The ability to overdo puts heart patients in jeopardy, so that the challenge becomes reaching one's limit minus one.

In summary, there are three analytically distinct (but practically interrelated) types of cutbacks involved: (1) those actually forced by the MI; (2) those indicated by the appearance of symptoms, either literally (lack of energy stops the activity) or definitionally ("I'd better stop now, because I usually get chest pain when I feel this way and keep going"); and (3) those that are part of the regimen. In finding a new set of guidelines for everyday life, the person who has had an MI must balance these cutback demands against the maintenance of those aspects of life that are personally and socially meaningful.

Minimizing Losses

The chief problem for heart attack victims may be described as minimizing losses, which refers to the decision to make certain unfavorable cutbacks to ward off the perceived probability of larger and more devastating losses in the future. This is done under circumstances of relative ambiguity, autonomy, and anxiety.

While the MI is still prominent, patients reassess their life goals with reference to their personal definitions of the quality of life. As one person put it, "I think it changes your mental outlook a lot. I know it does, in fact. You don't take a self-inventory before like you do afterwards." One concept of quality is expressed in blanket statements such as "Now I don't take for granted the things I used to; I appreciate them more now." This tends to fade with distance from the occurrence of the MI, but the overall assessment and appreciation for "the time I have left" is an important element in decision making.

More specific conceptions of quality are highly idiosyncratic and encompass activities, responsibilities, and relationships that are individual parts of the familiar way of life. It may be the special things a woman does to signify that she is a competent worker or a good wife or mother. It may be a beloved hobby or a pastime that is the focus of the person's companionship with good friends.

In balancing between cutting back and maintaining a certain quality of life, the heart patients develop an ongoing, personal "calculus" from the diverse elements they see as relevant in their unfamiliar and emergent situation. In each of the stages of cutting back the constellation of specific factors and problems changes, and these changes in turn affect the cutting back process. The three stages of cutting back are *immobilization, resumption,* and *new normal.*

IMMOBILIZATION: ESTIMATING AND EXPLAINING THE DAMAGE. Like others struck by sudden illness or personal disaster, MI victims need to explain and estimate the crisis and its consequences. They take stock, develop causal explanations to answer the Why me? and Why now? questions, and seek and screen information using direct and indirect strategies, such as interpreting cues of medical personnel and comparing their experience with that of others.

A patient-epidemiologist's retrospective study often emphasizes events having close temporal proximity. Other properties of causal theories are their faulting emphasis, certainty, and heart imagery. The faulting aspect is important, and it includes positive or ameliorating causes ("I'd be dead now if I hadn't jogged regularly"). Victims compare themselves in numerous ways with others they know who have had similar experiences in order to predict their own prognosis and the quality of life they will be able to lead after they recover. They may use these new peers normatively ("my friend returned to his job, and so can I"), or they may stress the differences ("A business associate had to retire early, but she had a more severe attack than I did").

Assigning cause, gathering and processing information, and selecting comparative predictors all help to establish guidelines for cutting back. They are the foundations of a sense of control. Inability to partial out the factors in one's life according to their probable relationship to the MI may leave a generalized fear that may create a "cardiac cripple." Another response is fatalism that can lead to overstepping proscriptive boundaries ("There's nothing you can do to make a difference").

RESUMPTION: FIGURING THE CALCULUS OF CUTTING BACK. The major work in the resumption stage is using the factors identified earlier together with new ones generated with patients' increased activity levels to figure the calculus to determine what must be cut back, what should be cut back, and what one will and will not cut back. People mobilize themselves and their resources to find out their limits, principally by testing them empirically. The results of this experimentation (which are by no means always clear or definitive) can then become conditions that influence subsequent tests and decisions. The construction and growth of the calculus begins tentatively, with uncertainty the hallmark of nearly all of the elements, most being inferences, estimates, and predictions. Gradually the calculus stabilizes, and new outer limits of action are established.

Resumption usually starts very soon. In fact at an early point MI patients may feel much better than their actual physical state warrants. While still on the coronary care unit, remobilization is guided and protected. Return home, however, is usually accompanied by uncertainty and increased reminders, demands, and temptations from the former way of living. Those who are past this period recall the first weeks at home as being difficult. As one women said, "When you get home you're really alone, and you find that you can't do what you used to do."

The most important tasks in discovering how to cut back are learning to interpret bodily signs, dealing with divergent interpretations of what is possible and expected among various consequential people in one's life, developing balancing equations, and finding specific ways of changing behavior.

After an MI, people are self-consciously aware of bodily sensations. information from diverse comparative sources, and experiential data that might be related to the heart condition. The problem is interpreting vague indicators and correcting these interpretations based on perceived consequences. A sense of confidence in one's ability to read cues is needed not only to assess the degree of impairment and gauge progress but also to anticipate and recognize crises in order to summon help and to establish the boundaries for specific activities.

The major patterns of interpreting signs can be dichotomized according to their degree of discrimination. The more conservative, nondiscriminating mode is likely to limit action severely. As the wife of one patient said, "He interprets any symptom as being related to his heart. I don't think he'll ever be the same." The discriminating stance is much more favorable for cutting back wisely but not unduly. Confidence in one's ability to recognize trouble may be derived from sources such as consultation with other patients or medical personnel or from feeling that there were adequate warnings before the MI.

Two problematic aspects of cutting back are the interdependence of activities and their differential valuation by other people who are involved with them. Changing one activity in isolation is almost never possible. Its consequences resonate throughout a person's life and affect other activities and people. This is the major difficulty of minimizing losses, and it is a factor in choices about cutting back. Even if someone does not care about the activity in question, he or she may care very much about that which is associated with it. Or the activity may be highly prized by an important person so that a change may affect that other person and, potentially, the relationship itself. For example fellow workers may resent the extra load they must carry because of a patient's new limits. When the choice of which activities to eliminate or slow down appears discretionary, even more ill feeling and misunderstanding can develop.

The divergence of opinion about etiology, degree of damage, and activity capacity is exacerbated by the difficulty of assessing exact limits, the invisibility of the impairment to others, and for many patients, the absence of clear symptoms. Thus family members, coworkers, medical personnel, and the patient may all have different definitions of the patient's situation. The magnitude of influence of a given opinion over cutting back varies with the degree of instrumental or sentimental control the other has over the patient's life. For example a boss's disbelief in the face of work pressures may render a light-duty order meaningless, or the prejudice of employers may keep an MI patient from working at all.

Internal control—the can't-say-no pattern and other sources of personal resistance to cutting back and living within prudent limits—may also be a problem. Moreover a chronic overdoer is likely to define "taking it easy" in comparative rather than absolute terms

("I've cut back to only eight hours, six days a week, and I won't touch a crate weighing over 100 pounds"). The comparative cutback may still be too much.

Cutting back equations indicate the manner in which a patient is juggling meanings to minimize losses, manage risks, and estimate the interaction effects of types of cutbacks and of cutbacks in different areas. Equations for cutting back that preserve quality may be general ("I guess I'll follow the doctor's advice, since I want to see my son grow up," or "I lost weight and lowered my cholesterol in order to recover enough to be active in my temple activities again"). Risk management equations may rationalize risks ("Smoking constricts my arteries, so I drink liquor, which dilates them"), and they may justify major cutbacks ("Lifting heavy objects is too dangerous for me now"). Other equations relate the effects of one activity on another ("When I finish losing this weight, I'll feel more like exercising, and my wife has been wanting me to drop fifteen pounds anyway").

Cutbacks vary according to their comparative distance from what was formerly considered normal. With respect to any one activity, the degree of reduction can be complete, partial, nil, or negative. Partial cutbacks are generally the most advantageous for minimizing losses, for they tend to maintain rewards, satisfaction, social interactions, and related activities.

Complete reductions of major life activities, such as early retirement, result in the loss of connected activities and important aspects of identity. However, complete cutbacks are preferred when salvaging a part of an activity creates too great a strain, as for instance when the heart condition is not believed by others, when comparisons with the former way of behaving are too uncomfortable, or when a person's internal governor is easily overcome by the attraction of exceeding the limits. Another consequence of a complete cutback, of course, can be a welcome unburdening of a distasteful chore. Too many choices of this sort tend to require justification and high credibility to retain acceptance by others.

Negative or "supernormal" cutbacks are the other extreme. *Supernormalizing* refers to doing something to an even greater extent than before the onset of the illness (Charmaz, 1973). It may be positive, arising out of a health-optimizing activity such as jogging, or it may be negative, as in exceeding limits to maintain an old identity.

Cutting back is operationalized through strategies such as situational positioning, conserving energy, and health optimizing. For example, patients position themselves with regard to medical resources, temptations or internal triggers to exceed limits, strong external demands toward excess, and conditions that facilitate cutting back.

To conserve energy, patients who feel they can recognize danger signals monitor their expenditure of energy to recognize points at which they should slow down, take a rest, or stop an activity ("I guess I'm a veteran of this heart business, and I take it easy myself. Work on myself, slow down or speed up, depending"). Other tactics include substituting another person to fill in or take over part of an activity, which usually means role reallocation within a family but may include paid helpers or friendly volunteers; diluting or literally lowering the concentration of energy for an activity or routine, as in switching to doubles tennis or allowing extra time between appointments; and budgeting oneself and one's energy.

NEW NORMAL: ADJUSTING TO A NEW IDENTITY. The central question in the new normal stage when resumption has reached its plateau is How do people who must live under this special set of chronic conditions come to view themselves? Some people find that they are better off after than before their MI, and others see little change. The new normal stage, however, often involves renormalizing with lower expectations to accommodate the reduction of former activities and the consequent impact on the quality of life. In Clausen's words, "He must come to terms with the fact that he is not something he was, something to which he was committed" (1968, p. 3).

Some ways in which MI patients reconcile themselves to a problematic new identity are through discovering positive modes of dependence, choosing favorable standards of comparison, finding compensations for cutbacks, and avowing illness at appropriate times. The divergent interpretations and valuations of others—real, projected, or anticipated—continue to be significant as mirrors for self-appraisal and, as such, are strongly related to difficuties and choices in this stage.

Some MI patients must come to terms with the need for help from others. Dependence can be financial or related to certain activities and tasks such as carrying groceries or driving a car, and dependence can have pervasive consequences for the personal identity. Their reactions to dependence may push them to exceed limits, or it may prevent them from asking for the assistance needed for partial or nil cutbacks and leave them with complete cutbacks and greater losses. A more positive way of dealing with the repayment issue is to develop other forms of equivalency. Money, talent or ideas, and "credit" from past deeds are all alternate currencies.

Patients also develop preferred helpers whose assistance is especially comfortable because of their cheerful and willing response (which legitimates the request), consistent offers to help, devaluation of the resources they expend ("I have lots of time"), or claims that they are repaid by other aspects of the relationship. Another quality of preferred helpers is the degree to which their perceptions of the patient's disability agree with the patients' view, so that there is belief but not a tendency to be too protective for comfort.

Looking at oneself in relation to someone else is a common method by which people assess their progress, standing, and so forth. MI patients compare themselves with situational (MI) peers, their former selves, their ideal selves, and their age peers. The choice of comparison is not always theirs. Some comparisons, usually unfavorable ones, may be forced on them. Comparisons with others who have had MIs legitimate cutting back decisions and sometimes give rise to new ones.

Three standards for self-comparison commonly used are:

Old normative. The difference between the pre-MI level of activity and the new normal

Improvement. The difference between early resumption and the new normal

Negative. The difference between the new normal and what might have happened.

The improvement standard is usually more favorable than comparison of the old self with the new capacity, but it is used less often than the old normative. This may be because the old activities and their loss stand out too poignantly for long periods of time. The contrast between the two standards is seen in an interview in which a 27-year-old male heart patient spoke of his frustration at not being able to do any of the strenuous sports he used to do. His wife interrupted with, "But you don't get winded anymore carrying a bag of groceries up the stairs." He was using the old normative, whereas she used the improvement standard.

Comparisons with age peers are often a proxy for comparisons with the old self. Heart patients who withdraw from younger or more active peer groups and associate themselves with an older or less active group are literally adjusting their standards of comparison. On the other hand the relative difference between heart patients and their peer groups are not usually as great as, say, the differences experienced by a handicapped child; and MI patients and their groups may accommodate their differences quite easily.

Compensations can be and often are generated from cutting back. This is not a wholly negative process, and in fact it frequently offers opportunities for redesigning a more satisfying life. This is particularly true for Type A people (Friedman & Rosenman, 1974) if they can gain access to new sides of their personalities. Improvement comparison standards and negative comparison standards have compensations. When an important aspect of life appears to be cut out completely, its partial resumption may be appreciated like a gift. Negative standards of comparison set a worse peril against the new normal. People who feel they came close to death are glad to be alive at all; and comfort can be derived from comparing one's own lot with that of another whose fate is even more unfavorable. One way of dealing with unfavorable, forced comparisons is to fashion loss rationales in which compensations outweigh losses. These post hoc equations are like the cutting back equations of resumption except that instead of interrelating cutbacks they involve (1) seeing substitutes as being as good as what they have replaced; (2) emphasizing what they can do over what they cannot; (3) viewing new, valued activities as being facilitated by the cutbacks; and (4) reminding themselves of the distasteful activities they no longer have to do. People who do not find sufficient compensations remain dissatisfied with their new identities and may consequently supernormalize or continue as before (if they can) or live in mourning with the problems of unfavorable comparisons.

MI patients cannot always meet the expectations others form on the basis of their appearance. Whereas visibly disabled people often work at limiting others' judgments about the extent of their "difference" ("Though I may appear to be different, I really am not"), heart patients must sometimes avow illness ("Though I may appear to be the same, I really am not"). How invisibly disabled people respond to others' expectations that they behave in accordance with what they seem to be is a function of their acceptance of their new normal identity, their tolerance for appearing unjustifiably inactive, the possibilities for alternate excuses, their prediction of the likely consequences of revealing their impairment (e.g., being overhelped), and the reaction of others to the initial action.

The decisions made around these factors are fateful when they lead to exceeding limits. Patients may choose to exceed their limits and risk health or life rather than spoil their appearance; they may avoid situations likely to pose such problems; they may develop strategies for making their condition more apparent (advice given one healthy-looking man was "Act sicker than you feel"); they may find ways of explaining their limits on other grounds; they may simply say that they have had a heart attack and cannot do what is expected or can do it only in a limited way; or they may stick to their limits without explanation.

Guidelines for Generating Patient Perspectives

The method for developing the model MI study can be summarized as follows: There were multiple sources of data. These included interviews with patients and with family members, some as individuals and couples and some in groups. First-person written accounts of illness experiences were also used. The medical records were sometimes sources of valuable information about fears, misunderstandings, and problems; and this could be used to formulate specific questions in interviews. Notes from observations made on coronary care and intermediate care units in hospitals and visits to a community coronary club and cardiac exercise program supplemented the interview and record material by giving new views and unique information.

Data were taken from a number of points on the crisis-recovery continuum. Some patients and their spouses were interviewed several times. Questions were open-ended, encouraging responses that could include elaboration of meanings and disclosure of embarrassing or worrisome opinions and behavior, and probing by the interviewer of problematic or contradictory responses.

The analysis emphasized general problems patients identified implicitly as well as explicitly. The range of problems included practical ones involving resources and social arrangements and more profound social and psychological difficulties. The strategies patients and their families used to solve these problems and the consequences of the various approaches were identified.

A main process of core significance was emphasized as an organizing device, which included the stages of the process and the circumstances associated with each. The formulation of hypotheses or statements about the relationships among the variables was the other key feature of the analysis (Glaser, 1978; Mullen & Reynolds, 1978).

A general framework for approaching the ill person's perspective in the case of other chronic conditions is presented below. This was adapted from one developed by Strauss and Glaser (1975), who had studied a number of chronic conditions. The framework contains seven general areas with which a patient (and family) may have to cope, depending on the specific disease and the patient's interpretations of its effects. By asking some of the questions suggested under each area, the patient education program planner will come to understand a good deal more about what it means to be in the patient's role and, it is hoped, about what the goals of the program ought to be.

> *Preventing medical crises and managing them if they should occur.* How likely are they? How serious? Are they apt to have warning signals? Do they require the cooperation of other people or special resources? What do patients think causes them? How do patients feel about them (e.g., embarrassed, very fearful)?
>
> *Controlling symptoms.* How controllable are they? How much do the symptoms interfere with everyday life? How frequent are they? How visible are they to other people? How much does the regimen help? Are there other measures patients could take to control symptoms? How do patients answer these questions?
>
> *Carrying out prescribed regimens.* How much time and money is required? How intrusive are they in daily living? How much cooperation is needed from others? Are there other regimens the patient is also supposed to follow? How effective does the regimen seem to be? Is it additive or is it proscriptive?
>
> *Preventing social isolation or living with it.* Is there a tendency for the ill person to withdraw from contact with others? For others to withdraw? To what extent? Are there symptoms that could be better controlled or regimens that could be made less intrusive to minimize withdrawal?
>
> *Adjusting to the course of the disease.* Is it likely to move downward? At what pace? Does it have remissions? How certain is its course? What can be or has to be done to prepare for the next phases in terms of living arrangements, identity adjustments, and so forth? What do patients believe the course is now and will be in the future?
>
> *Normalizing life-style and interactions with others.* How does the illness affect areas of life such as job, recreation? How great a task is it to normalize? How much tolerance do patients (and families) have for "discrepancies" from normal living? What strategies do patients and families use? What else could they do? Is there a tendency for others to overgeneralize the disability? To underestimate or disbelieve it?

Funding the medical treatments or other economic consequences of the illness. Does the illness affect employment? Is the illness expensive in terms of both direct and indirect costs? Is this cost an undue burden for particular groups of patients? What other resources could be mobilized to help?

References

Apple, D. How laymen define illness. *Journal of Health and Human Behavior,* 1960, *1,* 219–225.

Barofsky, I., Sugarbaker, P., & Mills, M. E. Compliance and quality of life assessment. In S. J. Cohen (Ed.), *New directions in patient compliance.* Lexington, Mass.: Lexington Press, 1979.

Baumann, B. Diversity in conception of health and physical fitness. *Journal of Health and Human Behavior,* 1961, *2,* 39–46.

Benoliel, J. Q. Childhood diabetes: The commonplace in living becomes uncommon. In A. L. Strauss & B. G. Glasser (Eds.), *Chronic illness and the quality of life.* St. Louis: Mosby, 1975.

Berger, P. L., & Luckmann, T. *The social construction of reality: A treatise in the sociology of knowledge.* New York: Doubleday, Anchor, 1967.

Bergner, M., Bobbitt, R. A., Pollard, W. E., Martin, D. P., & Gilson, B. S. The sickness impact profile: Validation of a health status measure. *Medical Care,* 1976, *14,* 57–67.

Blumer, H. *Symbolic interactionism: Perspective and method.* Englewood Cliffs, N. J.: Prentice-Hall, 1969.

Charmaz, K. C. Shouldering a burden. *Omega,* 1972, *3,* 23–33.

Charmaz, K. C. *Time and identity: The shaping of selves of the chronically ill.* Unpublished doctoral dissertation, University of California at San Francisco, 1973.

Clausen, J. A. *Socialization and society.* Boston: Little, Brown, 1968.

Davis, F. Deviance disavowal: The management of strained interaction by visibly handicapped. In H. S. Becker (Ed.), *The other side: Perspectives on deviance.* New York: Free Press of Glencoe, 1964.

Fagerhaugh, S. Getting around with emphysema. In A. L. Strauss & B. G. Glaser (Eds.), *Chronic illness and the quality of life.* St. Louis: Mosby, 1975.

Fagerhaugh, S., & Strauss, A. L. *Politics of pain management: Staff-patient interaction.* Menlo Park, Calif.: Addison-Wesley, 1977.

Friedman, M., & Rosenman, R. H. *Type A behavior and your heart.* New York: Knopf, 1974.

Glaser, B. G. *Theoretical sensitivity: Advances in the methodology of grounded theory.* Mill Valley, Calif.: Sociology Press, 1978.

Green, L. W., Werlin, S., & Avery, C. Measuring the decline of medicocentrism: Research issues in self-care. *Health Education Monographs,* 1977, *5,* 161–189.

Hayes-Bautista, D. E. Chicano patients and medical practitioners: A sociology of knowledges paradigm of lay-professional interaction. *Social Science and Medicine,* 1978, *12,* 83–90.

Jenkins, D. Group differences in perception: A study of community beliefs and feelings about tuberculosis. *American Journal of Sociology,* 1966, *71,* 417–429.

Kleinman, A., Eisenberg, L., & Good, B. Culture, illness and care: Clinical lessons from anthropologic and cross-cultural research. *Annals of Internal Medicine,* 1978, *88,* 251–258.

Kuhn, T. S. *The structure of scientific revolutions.* Chicago: University of Chicago Press, 1962.

Lindesmith, A. R., Strauss, A. L., & Denzin, N. K. *Social psychology* (4th ed.) Hinsdale, Ill.: Dryden, 1975.

Matza, D. *Delinquency and drift.* New York: John Wiley, 1964.

McHugh, P. *Defining the situation: The organization of meaning in social interaction.* Indianapolis: Bobbs-Merrill, 1968.

Mead, G. H. *Mind, self and society: From the standpoint of a social behaviorist* (C. W. Morris, ed.). Chicago: University of Chicago Press, 1956.

Mullen, P. D. Health education for heart patients in crisis. *Health Services Reports,* 1973, *88,* 669–675.

Mullen, P. D. Cutting back after a heart attack: An overview. *Health Education Monographs,* 1978, *6,* 295–311.

Mullen, P. D., & Reynolds, R. The potential of grounded theory for health education research: Linking theory and practice. *Health Education Monographs,* 1978, *6,* 280–294.

Reif, L. Ulcerative colitis: Strategies for managing life. In A. L. Strauss & B. G. Glaser (Eds.), *Chronic illness and the quality of life.* St. Louis: Mosby, 1975.

Ryan, W. *Blaming the victim.* New York: Random House, Vintage, 1972.

Sackett, D. L., & Haynes, R. B. (Eds.). *Compliance with therapeutic regimens.* Baltimore: Johns Hopkins University Press, 1976.

Stimson, G. V. Obeying doctor's orders: A view from the other side. *Social Science and Medicine,* 1974, *8,* 97–104.

Strauss, A. L. *Mirrors and Masks.* Mill Valley, Calif.: Sociology Press, 1969.

Strauss, A. L. Medical ghettos. In E. G. Jaco (Ed.), *Patients, physicians, and illness* (2d ed.). New York: Free Press, 1972.

Strauss, A. L. & Glaser, B. G. (Eds.). *Chronic illness and the quality of life*. St. Louis: Mosby, 1975.

Suczek, B. Chronic renal failure and the problem of funding. In A. L. Strauss & B. G. Glaser (Eds.), *Chronic illness and the quality of life*. St. Louis: Mosby, 1975.

Wiener, C. L. The burden of rheumatoid arthritis. In A. L. Strauss & B. G. Glaser (Eds.), *Chronic illness and the quality of life*. St. Louis: Mosby, 1975.

17

Inquiry into Action:
What Are the Next Steps?

Wendy D. Squyres

On numerous occasions in this book, authors have re-
marked about the rapid increases in health, medical, and educational
technologies; the recent proliferation of patient education media and
materials; and slower, although sustained, changes in consumer and
provider expectations regarding the role of the health care delivery
system in patient education. One senses in all of this that enough is
already known about how patient education can be effective. It's as
if patient education is one enormous jigsaw puzzle with all the pieces
laid out yet many still unassembled. The following is a summary of
the recommendations from the chapters that comprise this book. I
hope they will be steps to action and will lead to further assembling
of the puzzle.

1. Advances in the state of the art of patient education are encouraging. There is a rapidly growing body of empirical literature,
an increased rigor being applied in evaluations, increased sophistication of educational methods being employed and tested, and some
useful findings emerging to strengthen the scientific base of practice
in patient education. The continuing weaknesses are oversimplification of behavior and the causes of behavior that must be influenced
through patient education, a persistent failure to make explicit the
theoretical or assumptive connection between educational interventions and behavioral or health outcomes, and limited analyses leaving many questions untouched that would have been answerable with
further analysis of the data available or a simple modification of the
experimental design (chapter 1). Students and researchers of patient education should create a balanced scientific base from the lit-

erature of medical and nursing care, medical sociology, health education and health psychology and then find innovative forums for the diffusion of these findings for application by practitioners.

2. As quality assurance and risk management interventions are mandated and are accompanied by increased practitioner responsibilities for the development of standards of care and the documentation of care, patient education protocols should be incorporated into standardized care plans. These protocols need to be tested with specific patient populations; the result of such testing should yield a variety of educational variables that can be generalized to most populations. To the extent that such information can be generalized is the extent to which standardized protocols will be appropriate. Protocols should be flexible, capable of some individualization, and regularly updated. Current or former patients may be excellent committee participants in a protocol development process (chapters 2 and 3).

3. Patients cannot be plugged into AV (audiovisual media) like they can to IVs (intravenous solutions). The actual therapeutic value of mediated approaches to patient education depends on the application of sound principles of learning and educational planning. Media programs need to fit into well-organized, systematic programs that include human follow-up and interaction. Local, regional, and national consortia should be formed for reducing unnecessary duplication of media production efforts (chapter 5).

4. Funding issues were barely touched on in this book, but if the current state of the art prevails, there will continue to be situations in which practitioners are forced to set priorities on the allocation of scarce patient education resources. As a precursor to setting these priorities, sound educational diagnoses and planning (chapter 7) need to be conducted. Evaluation of patient education should be undertaken with the consideration of its opportunity to initiate the process of planned social change (chapter 8).

5. The coordination of patient education efforts should be conducted at the administrative level of any organization. This level of coordination will encourage multidisciplinary as well as interdisciplinary planning, evaluation, role clarification, and policy making (chapter 9). In addition such an administrative position would enhance the possibilities for capturing and recording the organization-wide investments and benefits of patient education efforts (chapter 6).

6. Active patient participation should be maintained throughout educational endeavors in health care delivery systems. Actual

problem-solving and problem-delineation strategies are discussed in chapters 10–14.

7. Historically, not only have people involved in patient education been coming up with inappropriate answers to questions regarding the goals of patient education programs, but they have also been asking the wrong questions. An alternative framework for posing the appropriate questions is offered in chapter 16. Practitioners should precede the definition-of-the-problem stage of patient education planning with data-gathering sessions, such as interviews and participant observation. These sessions would yield a more naturalistic view of the patient, and therefore an in-depth look at the patient's experience with coping with the disease. The resulting data would serve to enrich the program planning as well as to highlight the complexity of the specific situation.

In conclusion, D'Onofrio charts the direction for future action as follows: Given

1. The existing body of scientific knowledge as well as the mysteries we do not yet understand
2. The variations and fluctuations within the present health care system
3. The purposes of education in a free society
4. The nature of the educational process
5. An independent citizenry that in one way or another will exert the right to self-determination

the goal of patient education cannot be to achieve unquestioning compliance with medical advice. Rather, education must foster open sharing of information, questions, doubts, and concerns so that providers and consumers of health care can learn from each other. In this way we can all increase our understanding and our options, decide together how best to resolve the problems of medical care, and pool our resources toward these ends. Through participatory education, then, we can find new power to achieve patient treatment goals. At the same time, we will be joining forces to reshape our institutions, empowering them to serve more effectively our society's changing needs (chapter 15).

APPENDIX
A Resource Guide

Wendy D. Squyres with Thomas G. Flora

Position Statements

The following three position statements are "classics" in that they have dominated decision making and policy making in patient education over the last five years. Patient educators in many settings have used the philosophical positions of these papers as a part of their rationale for offering educational services and have quoted them in their proposals to administration. As the state of the art in patient education practice changes, it is imperative that practitioners, individually or collectively, keep the trade organizations and third-party payers informed.

1. American Medical Association. Statement on Patient Education Adopted by the AMA House of Delegates, June 1975*

Resolutions 37 and 41 (C-74) dealing with patient education were referred to the Board of Trustees for study and report at the 1975 Annual Convention.

Both resolutions called for planned programs of patient education developed and supervised by patient education committees whose membership would include health professionals, educators, and consumers. Both would have required that such programs be prescribed by a physician and documented on the patient's charts, as a basis for third-party reimbursement.

*Printed with the permission of the American Medical Association, 535 North Dearborn Street, Chicago, Illinois 60610.

The American Medical Association's Department of Health
Education and Division of Medical Practice have been exploring the
overall subject of planned patient education programs and have
arrived at the following general findings and recommendations in
response to Resolutions 37 and 41 (C-74).

Definition and Role of Planned
Patient Education Programs

It is recognized that increasingly complex patterns of health care,
along with the patient's environment, attitude, lifestyle, and cooperation, all play an important part in effective treatment. Informed,
motivated, and supportive participation in treatment by patients and
their families can aid the recovery of the patient and enhance the
quality of his health. Patient education, as an integral part of high
quality health care, provides an avenue to such improved participation.

Education of the patient has always been part of the ongoing
professional responsibility of physicians, nurses, dietitians, therapists,
and all other members of the health team. Health professionals have
traditionally provided patients with some information about their illness and the prescribed course of treatment. Some health instruction
has also been provided. In some situations, there is a need indicated
for a structured educational effort beyond that which individual members of the team can provide. It is in these situations that planned
patient education programs may be expected to serve.

The provision of patient education services, designed to assist
the patient and his family in the effective management of individual
health, is a shared and continuous responsibility of both the physician and the patient. Patient education directed toward the effective
management of individual illness and maintenance of health com-
mences with the patient's entry into the health services. A positive
personal experience between the physician and the patient at first
contact will greatly contribute to the success of an effective patient
education program.

The following factors define planned patient education:

1. Programs are distinguished from general health education
    of the public in that they focus on individuals who present
    themselves for medical services in institutions and in phy-
    sician's offices.

2. Programs are directed at the patient's understanding of his specific disease entity or physical or mental disability.
3. Programs assist the patient (and/or sometimes family members) to cooperate in the treatment of the disease or disability.
4. Programs involve patients with diseases or disabilities in which there are substantial grounds for belief that the patient will be better able to participate in treatment and that the treatment will be more effective with such a planned program than without it.

It should be clear from these four factors that planned patient education programs are distinct from general health education programs for the public and from programs intended as education for prevention of disease or for health maintenance. The planned program is for patients under treatment.

As the relationship between the physician and the patient is established, the physician determines the patient's level of knowledge concerning his illness or health, and the patient's educational needs. In this relationship, it is incumbent upon the patient to provide the necessary health history and medical information, and to comply with the prescribed medical regimen. Adherence to a prescribed treatment program is dependent upon the patient's understanding and acceptance of his condition, recognition of the importance of his role in the daily management of his prescribed treatment and satisfaction with health services provided. It is in these areas that a planned patient education program can enhance quality care.

Reimbursement

Planned patient education is a legitimate reimbursable item of patient care, when prescribed by a physician, appropriate to the patient's condition and substantiated by entries on the patient record. Planned patient education should be eligible for reimbursement under the various health insurance and other third-party payment programs.

Benefits

Properly planned programs of this type will improve care and can reduce the overall cost of treatment. Enabling patients to play a greater part in their own treatment can reduce unnecessary utilization of trained health professionals and of health care facilities. However, potential benefits such as cost containment, shortened recovery time and improved patient morale may not be immediately achievable. Any new interdisciplinary program takes time to develop and to become effective.

Content and Organization

Planned patient education programs should be based on identified objectives; should make use of sound educational methods; should have approved content that is scientifically accurate; and should be adaptable to the individual needs of patients.

Objectives need to be clarified at the outset along with specific criteria for measuring their achievement. The success or failure of the program should be determined by how well the objectives are realized.

Recommendations

The Board of Trustees believes the general findings and recommendations contained in this report respond to Resolutions 37 and 41, and recommends that the report be adopted and Association activities to improve effective patient education be continued.

2. American Hospital Association. Health Education: Role and Responsibility of Health Care Institutions°

Since the release of the Report *of the President's Committee on Health Education, much attention has been given to defining the scope of health education, how it should be done, and by whom. It has become apparent that various organizations in the community have roles to play in educating the public about its health. It is also apparent that unless these organizations define these roles and responsibilities and begin to work toward meeting them, health education efforts will continue to be unplanned, uncoordinated, and sporadic. This statement was developed by a special committee of the American Hospital Association's Council on Manpower and Education to help hospitals and other health care institutions define their health education roles, recognize the importance of planned health education programs, and set policies concerning health education. It was approved by the AHA Board of Trustees May 15, 1974, and became S83 in the AHA's S series leaflets. S83 is superseded by this reprinting of the statement.*

Introduction

The following paragraphs from the AHA's *Policy Statement on Provision of Health Services* provide a foundation for the statement on health education.

The system [for the delivery of health services] must be oriented to the maintenance of personal good health and to the prevention of illness rather than being primarily oriented to the treatment of illness after it becomes acute.

The system must include financial incentives for keeping people well and, if they are ill, for making them well as soon as possible.

Every individual shares a responsibility to protect his own health, and proper discharge of the responsibility will reduce the incidence of illness, disease, and injury. In order to encourage individuals to take care of themselves to the maximum extent possible, programs of education to teach people how to exercise this responsibility must be developed, conducted, evaluated, and maintained.

Statement

Health education is an integral part of high-quality health care. Hospitals and other health care institutions, as focal points of community health care, have an obligation to promote, organize, implement and evaluate health education programs. As a part of this process, hospitals should plan with other health care institutions and community agencies to define each organization's role and responsibility in meeting the health education needs of the populations they serve.

In order to improve health and health care services, ongoing systems of health education must be planned, implemented, and documented. The maintenance of health and the prevention of disease can be achieved by a cooperative effort between knowledgeable and motivated consumers and health care personnel. Health education is a planned process that entails the joint identification of needs, the exchange of knowledge and concerns, and the clarification of personal responsibilities for health—all designed to encourage positive health practices and to improve the delivery of health care.

Hospitals and other health care institutions should recognize the opportunity to exercise a role of leadership in the health education of three specific audiences: the patient and his family; personnel, including employees, medical staff, volunteers, and trustees; and the community at large.

The major emphasis of health education is health promotion, which includes health maintenance, disease and trauma management, and the improvement of the health care system and its utilization. Through health education programs, hospitals and other health care institutions can contribute to important health care goals, such as improved quality of patient care, better utilization of outpatient services, fewer admissions and readmissions to inpatient facilities, shorter lengths of stay, and reduced health care costs.

A significant corporate commitment, including staff and financial resources, is essential if hospitals and other health care institutions are to fulfill their leadership role in health education. This commitment involves the acceptance and implementation of health education as an integral component of health care, the designation of specific responsibility for organizing and implementing health education programs, and continuing education. Programs to fulfill this commitment can be developed either independently by hospitals or other health care institutions or through collaboration with health professional groups, consumer groups, health associations concerned with specific diseases, and the educational community.

Financial responsibility for health education that is integral to the treatment and care of the patient is a legitimate part of the cost of caring for the patient. Health education that is designed to maintain the good health of the community at large and to prevent illness should be viewed as a service to the community. Such services are legitimate activities for hospitals and other health care institutions; however, efforts should be made to broaden the base of financial support for them by working collaboratively with other agencies and by seeking funding for health education programs.

3. Blue Cross Association. White Paper on Patient Health Education, Approved by the Board of Governors, August 1974*

The following White Paper addresses the issue of patient health education and the operational role which Blue Cross Plans can assume in this area. It finds that a patient education program, integrated into the routine services of the institution, offers the potential for both cost containment and improved quality of patient care. It concludes with the recommendation that Blue Cross Plans should encourage health care institutions to establish and operate programs in patient education and should support them financially through the existing payment mechanism.

The health care system is being challenged to improve its efficiency and effectiveness. Reforms in the system must forcefully address the need to contain rising health care costs and to assure the quality of health care services.

Given the complexity and the diversity of this challenge, no single response is appropriate. As one mechanism among many, patient health education may contribute to containing health care costs and enhancing the individual's understanding of and compliance with his treatment regimen. Patient education reinforces the patient's awareness of his responsibility for his own health, and self-responsibility is crucial for the ultimate effectiveness of health care.

Patient health education, for the present purpose, is a process comprising several elements: Mutual identification of present and future health care needs by patient and professional, planning for the appropriate mix of professional and patient responsibility for meeting those needs, exchange of knowledge regarding the selected treatment regimen, motivation of patient and professional to perform their respective roles, and continuing evaluation of alternative methodologies. Patient education is part of the total process of patient care. As used here, patient education generally refers to hospital-based programs. However, the locus of the intervention is not as important as its nature.

The purpose of this statement is twofold: To examine the evidence on the impact of patient health education on the cost and quality of patient care, and to recommend an operational course of action to Plans.

*Printed with the permission of the Blue Cross Association. 840 North Lake Shore Drive, Chicago, Illinois 60611.

Issues

The concept of patient health education raises several issues. The principal questions which must be resolved, however, are:

1. Should Plans pay for patient education?
2. What kinds of criteria should be employed to determine the allocability of patient education expenses to Plan reimbursement?
3. What is the appropriate role for Plans in patient health education?

The answers to such questions emerge from an evaluation of the impact of patient education on the cost and quality of health care.

Effects on Costs

In examining the costs of patient care, one may adopt several perspectives: Health care costs per capita in a given service area, costs per admission, costs per service unit, and costs per episode of illness. The development of valid and reliable measures is crucial to the proper evaluation of the patient education program.

Theoretically, patient education might contribute to reduced costs by decreasing the unnecessary utilization of health care services and by encouraging use of the most appropriate locus of care for health problems. These potential effects are critical to improving the efficacy of medical services.

Empirical evidence suggests that structured patient education speeds recovery in certain case types. For example, preoperative instruction has resulted in a significantly higher incidence of early discharge among those receiving intensive preoperative instruction and practice as compared to those not receiving such treatment.[1] Other studies have found similar results. Specific educational interventions can lead to reduced use of postoperative narcotics,[2] decreased emergency room utilization[3] decreased readmissions and patient days for

[1] Healy, Kathryn M. Does preoperative instruction really make a difference? *American Journal of Nursing,* January 1968, pp. 62–67.
[2] Egbert, Lawrence D., et al. Reduction of postoperative pain by encouragement and instruction of patients. *New England Journal of Medicine,* April 16, 1964, pp. 825-827.
[3] Miller, Leona, and Goldstein, Jack. More efficient care of diabetic patients in a county hospital setting. *New England Journal of Medicine,* June 29, 1972, pp. 1388–1391.

readmissions[4] and reduced total admissions for a target population.[5]

Total health care cost for the individual may be reduced by substituting less expensive treatment modalities and loci of care for hospitalization and emergency room use. To assess whether such substitutions really do reduce *total* costs, total utilization of health services by specific groups over a given time frame must be calculated.

While not presenting conclusive evidence of reduced *total* costs of care for specific groups, some studies do suggest large cost savings as a result of changes in the pattern of utilization. For example, the Tufts–New England Medical Center research,[6] using a self-selected sample of male hemophiliac outpatients given postperiod instruction and practice in self-infusion, yielded the following pre–post comparisons: total inpatient days declined from 432 to 42, outpatient visits per patient decreased from 23.0 to 5.5, and total costs per patient went down 45% (from $5,780 to $3,209). At the University of Southern California Medical Center, a reorganization of the diabetic care system, incorporating a telephone "hotline" for information, medical advice, and the filling of prescriptions, counseling by physicians and nurses, and pamphlets and posters to promote the service, was associated with more than a 50% reduction in emergency room visits per clinic patient and the avoidance of approximately 2,300 medication visits.[7] These findings suggest that certain types of patient education do promote the substitution of self-care and information-seeking for acute care services.

On balance, organized patient education has demonstrated its effectiveness in reducing the unnecessary utilization of certain health care services and in encouraging the use of the most appropriate, least-cost settings for care.

Effects on Quality of Care

Patient health education has also demonstrated considerable potential for improving the quality of care.

Several studies have demonstrated the beneficial impact of patient education on the *process* of patient care. The use of an inter-

[4]Rosenberg, Stanley G. Patient education leads to better care for heart patients. *HSMHA Health Services Reports,* September 1971, pp. 793–802.
[5]*Ibid.*
[6]Levine, Peter H., and Britten, Anthony F. Supervised patient management of hemophilia. *Annals of Internal Medicine,* No. 78, 1973, pp. 195–201.
[7]See Miller & Goldstein.

disciplinary team to provide educationally oriented support to patients with congestive heart failure has resulted in increased knowledge among study patients in one sample regarding diet, medications, disease process, and, even more importantly, increased adherence to the treatment regimen.[8] Other research suggests that patient education enhances patient understanding of and compliance with the process of care.[9]

With respect to health care *outcomes*, studies have shown the quality-increasing effects of patient education. At the University of Southern California Medical Center, the reorganization of the system of diabetic care and the initiation of a multi-faceted program of patient education was associated with a reduction of approximately two-thirds in the incidence of diabetic coma from 1968 to 1970.[10] Similarly, in another study, a significantly higher percentage of congestive heart failure patients receiving educational support improved in their ability to function, as measured by the American Heart Association classification. Also, recent work[11] at Massachusetts General Hospital has shown that the provision of intensive preoperative and postoperative information and guidance contributed to reduced pain among surgery patients. These studies point to the potential of patient education in enhancing health status.

Conclusion

The available information regarding patient health education indicates that, where conducted by a coordinated mix of educational and clinical specialists and directed to individual needs and capabilities, it both increases the quality of health care and presents potential cost savings to the health care system and to the public it serves. The Blue Cross system has consistently supported delivery and financing innovations which improve the system's efficiency and effectiveness. As such, patient health education efforts should be encouraged and supported, for they are one promising means of achieving these objectives.

Accordingly, Plans should encouraged health care institutions to establish and operate programs in patient education and should sup-

[8]See Rosenberg.

[9]Green, Lawrence W. Toward cost-benefit evaluations of health education: Some concepts, methods, and examples. The Johns Hopkins University School of Public Health, Division of Health Education, 615 North Wolfe St., Baltimore, Md. 21205. Pp. 36–37 (unpublished paper).

[10]See Miller & Goldstein.

[11]See Egbert, et al.

port them financially through the existing payment mechanism. To realize its full potential for cost savings and quality improvement, it is critical that the patient education function be integrated into the total process of patient care. To assure that sound programs are developed and maintained, the following guidelines are suggested as criteria for determining payment for patient education programs. In applying these guidelines, the variation in programs and population needs for patient education should be considered. Accordingly, a flexible approach to their interpretation should be adopted.

Guidelines for Programs in Patient Education

1. The purpose and operational objectives of the program should be clearly stated, and the techniques for meeting the objectives should be specified.
2. Patient education should be provided as an integral element of the total patient care process within a supportive organizational framework.[12] Existing hospital-based programs in patient education shall be reviewed by either the Joint Commission on Accreditation of Hospitals or the Bureau of Hospitals of the American Osteopathic Association.
3. Necessary and appropriate health education should be developed and financed as a routine element of the care of each patient.
4. Educational methodologies should be directed to specific case types and desired behavioral changes and the results of such interventions as to cost and quality of care should be documented. As in other expenses, continuing management evaluation of the cost effectiveness of the service should be conducted. Programs should be revised over time to reflect the results of such evaluation.

It is appropriate that the Blue Cross system encourage the development of cost-effective programs in patient education. Where patient education is properly related to the other components of the total patient care process, there is clear potential for reduction of health care costs and improvement in the quality of health care processes and outcomes. Blue Cross Plans share responsibility with

[12]Examples of this organizational framework are the hospital, home care program, HMO, or community health education program.

those providing patient education to ensure that this potential is realized. Accordingly, the Blue Cross System should play an active part in the development, implementation, and evaluation of sound programs in patient education.

Health Education Materials and the Organizations That Offer Them

Several health-related agencies, foundations, and private companies publish information concerning themselves or their interests. A wealth of printed material, exhibitions, and audiovisual devices are available to facilitate the learning of various aspects of health, science, and safety. The organizations listed in the next section will provide pamphlets, booklets, brochures, wall charts, models, and filmstrips that can be used in the classroom. Most material is free or inexpensive, and catalogs and sample material will be sent on request. For national organizations,* check for a local office before writing to a national headquarters. Following the alphabetical list is a topical list to aid the patient educator in the task of finding suitable teaching aids to accompany their planned educational interventions. Inevitably, the addresses and companies will change with time. In addition, it is impossible to assume that this list is complete. Hopefully, this list will be the beginning of the educator's search for well-prepared, reasonably priced, and responsible health messages for their patients.

Where to Find Everything (Almost)*

Abbott Film Service
Scientificom Distribution Center
709 N. Dearborn
Chicago, Ill. 60610

Abbott Laboratories
Public Relations Department
North Chicago, Ill. 60604

Adult Education Association
810 Eighteenth Street, N.W.
Washington, D.C. 20006

Aetna Life and Casualty Company
Information and Education
  Department
151 Farmington Avenue
Hartford, Conn. 06115

*"Where to Find Everything (Almost)" was compiled by Kae Hentges, M.S.P.H., Coordinator of Patient Education, Family and Community Medicine, University of Missouri School of Medicine. Reprinted by permission.

Al-Anon Family Group
Headquarters
P.O. Box 182
Madison Square. Station
New York, N.Y. 10010

Alcoholics Anonymous
World Services, Inc.
P.O. Box 459
Grand Central Station
New York, N.Y. 10010

Alexander Graham Bell Association
for the Deaf, Inc.
3417 Volta Place, N.W.
Washington, D.C. 20007

Allergy Foundation of America
801 Second Avenue
New York, N.Y. 10017

American Academy of Dermatology
2250 N.W. Flanders Street
Portland, Ore. 97210

American Academy of Family
Physicians
1740 W. Ninety-second Street
Kansas City, Mo. 64114

American Academy of Neurology
4005 N. Michigan Avenue
Chicago, Ill. 60611

American Academy of Ophthalmology and Otolaryngology
Rochester, Minn. 55901

American Academy of Pediatrics
1801 Hinman Avenue
P.O. Box 1034
Evanston, Ill. 60204

American Academy of Physical
Medicine and Rehabilitation
30 N. Michigan
Suite 922
Chicago, Ill. 60602

American Association for Health,
Physical Education and
Recreation
1201 Sixteenth Street, N.W.
Washington, D.C. 20036

American Association for
Inhalation Therapy
332 S. Michigan Avenue
Chicago, Ill. 60604

American Association for Maternal
and Child Health
P.O. Box 965
Los Altos, Calif. 94022

American Association of Dental
Schools
211 E. Chicago Avenue
Chicago, Ill. 60611

American Association of Nurse
Anesthetists
3010 Prudential Plaza
Chicago, Ill. 60601

American Association of
Ophthalmology
1100 Seventeenth Street, N.W.
Room 304
Washington, D.C. 20036

American Association of Poison
Control Centers
c/o Academy of Medicine of
Cleveland
Poison Information Center
10525 Carnegie Avenue
Cleveland, Ohio 44106

American Association of Retired
Persons
1909 K Street, N.W.
Washington, D.C. 20049

American Association of Workers
for the Blind, Inc.
1511 K Street, N.W.
Washington, D.C. 20005

American Association on Mental
Deficiency
5201 Connecticut Avenue, N.W.
Washington, D.C. 20015

American Baker's Association
Public Relations Department
1700 Pennsylvania Ave, N.W.
Washington, D.C. 20006

American Cancer Society
777 Third Avenue
New York, N.Y. 10017

American Chemical Society
1155 Sixteenth Street, N.W.
Washington, D.C. 20006

American Chiropractic Association
2200 Grand Avenue
Des Moines, Iowa 50312

American College Health
Association
2807 Central Street
Evanston, Ill. 60201

American College of Allergists
2141 Fifteenth Street
Boulder, Colo. 80302

American College of Cardiology
9650 Rockville Pike
Bethesda, Md. 20014

American College of Nurse
Midwives
1000 Vermont Avenue, N.W.
Washington, D.C. 20005

American College of Obstetrics and
Gynecology
One E. Wacker Drive
Chicago, Ill. 60601

American College of Physicians
4200 Pine Street
Philadelphia, Pa. 19104

American College of Preventive
Medicine
801 Old Lancaster Road
Bryn Mawr, Pa. 19010

American College of Sports
Medicine
1440 Monroe Street
Madison, Wis. 53706

American College of Surgeons
Surgical Film Library
Davis & Geck, Distributor
One Casper Street
Darien, Conn. 06810

American Corrective Therapy
Association, Inc.
7631 Willis Avenue
Van Nuys, Calif. 91405

American Dental Assistants
Association
211 E. Chicago Avenue
Chicago, Ill. 60611

American Dental Association
Bureau of Dental Health Education
211 E. Chicago Avenue
Chicago, Ill. 60611

American Dental Hygienists
Association
211 E. Chicago Avenue
Chicago, Ill. 60611

American Diabetes Association, Inc.
600 Fifth Avenue
New York, N.Y. 10020

American Dietetic Association
620 N. Michigan Avenue
Chicago, Ill. 60611

American Dry Milk Institute
130 N. Franklin Street
Chicago, Ill. 60606

American Egg Board
205 Touhy Avenue
Park Ridge, Ill. 60068

American Foundation for the
Blind, Inc.
15 W. Sixteenth Street
New York, N.Y. 10011

American Freedom from Hunger
Foundation
1100 Seventeenth Street, N.W.
Suite 701
Washington, D.C. 20036

American Group Practice
Association
P.O. Box 949
20 S. Quaker Lane
Alexandria, Va. 22313
American Health Foundation
1370 Avenue of the Americas
New York, N.Y. 10019

American Heart Association
Inquiry Section
44 E. Twenty-third Street
New York, N.Y. 10010
or 7320 Greenville Avenue
Dallas, Tex. 75231

American Home Economics
Association
2010 Massachusetts Avenue, N.W.
Washington, D.C. 20036

American Hospital Association
840 N. Lake Shore Drive
Chicago, Ill. 60611
(Elizabeth Lee, Staff Specialist for
Health Education)

American Human Association
Children's Division
P.O. Box 1266
Denver, Colo. 80201

American Industrial Hygiene
Association
66 South Miller Road
Akron, Ohio 44313

American Institute of Baking
Consumer's Service Department
400 E. Ontario Street
Chicago, Ill. 60611

American Institute of Biological
Sciences
1401 Wilson Boulevard
Arlington, Va. 22209

American Institute of Family
Relations
5287 Sunset Boulevard
Los Angeles, Calif. 90027
American Insurance Association
Engineering and Safety
Department
85 John Street
New York, N.Y. 10038

American Lung Association
G.P.O. 596
New York, N.Y. 10001

American Meat Institute
59 E. Van Buren Street
Chicago, Ill. 60605

American Medical Association
Order Department
535 N. Dearborn Street
Chicago, Ill. 60610

American Medical Students
Association
1400 Hicks Road
Rolling Meadows, Ill. 60008

American Medical Women's
Association, Inc.
1740 Broadway
New York, N.Y. 10019

American Museum of Natural
History
Film Library
Fifty-eighth and Central Park West
New York, N.Y. 10027

American National Red Cross
Office of Public Information
Seventeenth and D Street, N.W.
Washington, D.C. 20006

American Nurses' Association
2420 Pershing Road
Kansas City, Mo. 64108

American Occupational Therapy
   Association
6000 Executive Boulevard
Suite 200
Rockville, Md. 20852

American Optometric Association
Department of Public Affairs
7000 Chippewa Street
St. Louis, Mo. 63119

American Orthopsychiatric
   Association, Inc.
1790 Broadway
New York, N.Y. 10019

American Orthotic and Prosthetics
   Association
919 Eighteenth Street, N.W.
Washington, D.C. 20006

American Osteopathic Association
212 E. Ohio Street
Chicago, Ill. 60611

American Pharmaceutical
   Association
2215 Constitution Avenue, N.W.
Washington, D.C. 20037

American Physical Therapy
   Association
1156 Fifteenth Street, N.W.
Washington, D.C. 20005

American Physiological Association
9650 Rockville Pike
Bethesda, Md. 20014

American Podiatry Association
20 Chevy Chase Circle, N.W.
Washington, D.C. 20010

American Psychological
   Association
1200 Seventeenth Street, N.W.
Washington, D.C. 20036

American Public Health
   Association
1015 Fifteenth Street, N.W.
Washington, D.C. 20005

American Rehabilitation
   Foundation
1800 Chicago Avenue
Minneapolis, Minn. 55404

American School Health
   Association
515 E. Main Street
Kent, Ohio 44240

American Social Health
   Association
1740 Broadway
New York, N.Y. 10019

American Society for Pharmacology
   and Experimental Therapeutics,
   Inc.
9650 Rockville Pike
Bethesda, Md. 20014

American Society for
   Psychoprophylaxis in Obstetrics
1423 L Street, N.W.
Suite 410
Washington, D.C. 20005

American Society of Biological
   Chemists
9650 Wisconsin Avenue
Washington, D.C. 20014

American Society of Clinical
   Pathology
2100 W. Harrison Street
Chicago, Ill. 60612

American Society of Hospital
Pharmacists
4630 Montgomery Avenue
Washington, D.C. 20014

American Society of Plastic and
Reconstructive Surgeons, Inc.
29 E. Madison
Suite 812
Chicago, Ill. 60611

American Society of Radiological
Technologists
645 N. Michigan Avenue
Room 620
Chicago, Ill. 60611

American Speech and Hearing
Association
9030 Old Georgetown Road
Washington, D.C. 20014

American Toy Institute, Inc.
200 Fifth Avenue
New York, N.Y. 10010

American Veterinary Medical
Association
600 S. Michigan Avenue
Chicago, Ill. 60605

American Video Network
660 S. Bonnie Brae Street
Los Angeles, Calif. 90057

Ames Company
Division of Miles Laboratories
1127 Myrtle Street
Elkhart, Ind. 46514

Armour and Company
Consumer's Services Department
Greyhound Towers
Phoenix, Ariz. 85077

Arthritis Foundation
3400 Peachtree Road
Atlanta, Ga. 30326

Association for the Aid of Crippled
Children
Division of Publications
345 E. Forty-sixth Street
New York, N.Y. 10017

Association for Voluntary
Sterilization, Inc.
14 W. Fortieth Street
New York, N.Y. 10018

Association of American Medical
Colleges
2530 Ridge Avenue
Evanston, Ill. 60201

Association of Rehabilitation
Centers, Inc.
7979 Old Georgetown Road
Washington, D.C. 20014

Association of Teachers of
Preventive Medicine
William Marine, M.D.
University of Colorado Medical
Center
Room C245
4200 E. Ninth Avenue
Denver, Colo. 80262

Athletic Institute
805 Merchandise Mart
Chicago, Ill. 60654

Audience Planners
208 S. LaSalle Street
Chicago, Ill. 60604

Ayerst Laboratories
685 Third Avenue
New York, N.Y. 10017
Attention: Carmen Vellon,
Professional Services
West Hall

Becton Dickinson and Company
Rutherford, N.J. 07070

Beecham-Massengill
Division of Beecham, Inc.
Bristol, Tenn. 37620

Best Foods
Consumer Service Department
Englewood Cliffs, N.J. 07632

Better Vision Institute, Inc.
230 Park Avenue
Suite 3157
New York, N.Y. 10017

Bicycle Institute of America, Inc.
122 E. Forty-second Street
New York, N.Y. 10017

Blue Cross-Blue Shield
Director of Public Relations
425 N. Michigan Avenue
Chicago, Ill. 60690

Bluestone Video Makers
4018 Twenty-second Street
San Francisco, Calif. 94114

B.N.A. Communications, Inc.
8371 Bernice Drive
Strongville, Ohio 44136

Borden Company
Marketing Services
50 W. Broad Street
Columbus, Ohio 43215

Boy Scouts of America
New Brunswick, N.J. 08903

Brady Company, Robert J.
Route 197
Bowie, Md. 20715

Brand Names Foundation
Department C5
P.O. Box 678
Maple Plain, Minn. 55359

Brookhaven Memorial Hospital
101 Brookhaven Hospital Road
Patchogue, N.Y. 11772

Bureau of Health Education
Center for Disease Control
Atlanta, Ga. 30333

Burroughs Welcome Company
Research Triangle Park, N.C.
27709

Campbell Soup Company
Food Service Products Division
375 Memorial Avenue
Camden, N.J. 08101

Candlelighters
123 C Street, S.E.
Washington, D.C. 20003

Carnation, Inc.
Medical Marketing Division
5045 Wilshire Boulevard
Los Angeles, Calif. 90036

Carolina Population Center
Educational Materials Program
University Square
University of North Carolina
Chapel Hill, N.C. 27514

Center for Disease Control
Teaching Resources
Instructional Systems Division
Bureau of Training
Atlanta, Ga. 30333

Center for Health Administration
  Studies
5720 S. Woodlawn Avenue
University of Chicago
Chicago, Ill. 60637

Center for Mass Communication
  of Columbia University Press
440 W. 110th Street
New York, N.Y. 10025

Center for Science in the Public
  Interest
1779 Church Street, N.W.
Washington, D.C. 20036

Cereal Institute, Inc.
135 S. LaSalle Street
Chicago, Ill. 60603

Channing L. Bete Company, Inc.
45 Federal Street
Greenfield, Mass. 01301

Child Study Association of
America
9 E. Eighty-ninth Street
New York, N.Y. 10028

Child Welfare League of America,
Inc.
1145 Nineteenth St., N.W.
Suite 618
Washington, D.C. 20036
(Consortium on Early Childbearing
and Childrearing)

Children's Asthma Research
Institute and Hospital
3401 W. Nineteeth Street
Denver, Colo. 80204

Children's Foundation
1028 Connecticut Avenue, N.W.
Washington, D.C. 20036

Children's Hospital Medical Center
Health Education Department
300 Longwood Avenue
Boston, Mass. 02115

Churchill Films
662 N. Robertson Boulevard
Los Angeles, Calif. 90069

Ciba Pharmaceutical Products, Inc.
556 Morris Avenue
Summit, N.J. 07901

Cleveland Health Museum and
Education Center
8911 Euclid Avenue
Cleveland, Ohio 44106

Commonweal Productions
71 Ellery Street
Cambridge, Mass. 02138

Community Nutrition Institute
1910 D Street, N.W.
Washington, D.C. 20006

Connecticut General Life Insurance
Company
Advertising and Public Relations
Room 319
Hartford, Conn. 06115

Consumer Advocate
Ralph Nader
53 Hillside Avenue
Winston, N.C. 06098

Consumer Directory of Federal
Offices
Request from: Public Documents
Center
Department 016F
Pueblo, Colo. 81009

Consumer Federation of America
1012 Fourteenth Street, N.W.
Suite 901
Washington, D.C. 20005

Consumer Product Safety
Commission
Washington, D.C. 20207

Consumer's Union of U.S., Inc.
256 Washington Street
Mount Vernon, N.Y. 10550

Council for Exceptional Children
Educational Research Information
Center
1201 Sixteenth Street, N.W.
Washington, D.C. 20006

Cutter Laboratories
Fourth and Parker Streets
Berkeley, Calif. 94001

Del Monte Kitchens
Del Monte Corporation
215 Premont Street
San Francisco, Calif. 94119

Distilled Spirits Council of the
United States, Inc.
Suite 1300
Pennsylvania Building
425 Thirteenth Street, N.W.
Washington, D.C. 20004

Do It Now Foundation
Institute for Chemical Survival
P.O. Box 5115
Phoenix, Ariz. 85010

Drug Abuse Council
1828 L Street, N.W.
Washington, D.C. 20036

Eastman Kodak Company
Health Education Service
Teaching Films Division
343 State Street
Rochester, N.Y. 14608

Eaton Labs Division
Morton-Norwich Products, Inc.
Medical Film Library
Norwich, N.Y. 13815

Educational Materials Program
Carolina Population Center
University of North Carolina
Chapel Hill, N.C. 27514

Educator's Progress Service
Randolph, Wis. 53956

Eli Lilly and Company
Educational Resources Program
P.O. Box 100B
Indianapolis, Ind. 46206

Emko Company
5912 Manchester Avenue
St. Louis, Mo. 63143

Employer's Insurance of Wausau
Safety and Health Services
Wausau, Wis. 54401

Encyclopedia Britannica Films,
Inc.
Public Relations
425 N. Michigan Avenue
Chicago, Ill. 60611

Epilepsy Foundation of America
1828 L Street, N.W.
Suite 406
Washington, D.C. 20036

Equitable Life Assurance Society
of America
1285 Avenue of the Americas
New York, N.Y. 10019

Evaporated Milk Association
228 N. LaSalle Street
Chicago, Ill. 60601

Fairview General Hospital
c/o The Greater Cleveland
Hospital Association
1021 Euclid Avenue
Cleveland, Ohio 44115

Family Communications, Inc.
4802 Fifth Avenue
Pittsburgh, Pa. 15213

Family Planning and Population
Information Center
960 Ostrom Avenue
Syracuse, N.Y. 13210

Fleishman's Margarine
P.O. Box 1407
Elm City, N.C. 27822

Florida Citrus Commission
P.O. Box 1720
Lakeland, Fla. 33802

Food Council of America
1750 Pennsylvania Avenue, N.W.
Washington, D.C. 20005

Ford Foundation
320 E. Forty-Third Street
New York, N.Y. 10017

Foundation Center
888 Seventh Avenue
New York, N.Y. 10019

Geigy Pharmaceuticals
Ardsley, N.Y. 10502

General Foods Corporation
Consumer Service Division
250 North Street
White Plains, N.Y. 10602

General Mills
Nutrition Department
P.O. Box 113
Minneapolis, Minn. 55440

Gerber Products
Professional Service Department
445 State Street
Freemont, Mich. 49412

Gerontological Society
One Dupont Circle
Suite 520
Washington, D.C. 20036

Good Housekeeping Institute
Good Housekeeping Bulletin
  Service
959 Eighth Avenue
New York, N.Y. 10019

Green Giant Company
Home Services Department
5601 Green Valley Drive
Minneapolis, Minn. 55437

Griggs Film Library
The Clarement Foundation, Inc.
P.O. Box 187
Claremont, Calif. 91711

Group for Advancement of
  Psychiatry
419 Park Avenue South
New York, N.Y. 10016

Guiding Eyes for the Blind
11 West Forty-second Street
New York, N.Y. 10036

Hazelden
P.O. Box 176
Center City, Minn. 55012

Health Films Library
P.O. Box 309
One Wilson Street
Madison, Wis. 53701

Health Insurance Institute
Department H
277 Park Avenue
New York, N.Y. 10017

Health Research Group
2000 P Street, N.W.
Suite 708
Washington, D.C. 20036

Heinz, H. J.
Consumer Relations
P.O. Box 57
Pittsburgh, Pa. 15230

Hogg Foundation for Mental
  Health
University of Texas
Austin, Tex. 78712

Holister, Inc.
211 E. Chicago
Chicago, Ill. 60611

Holland-Rantos Company, Inc.
P.O. Box 5
Piscataway, N.J. 08854

Hospital Audio-Visual Education
606 Holstead Avenue
Mamaroneck, N.Y. 10543

Human Relations Media
175 Thompkins Avenue
Pleasantville, N.Y. 10570

Imagination, Inc.
2651 University Avenue
Minneapolis, Minn. 55114

Indiana University School of
  Medicine
Medical Education Resources
  Program
1100 W. Michigan Street
Indianapolis, Ind. 46202

Industrial Hygiene Foundation of
  America, Inc.
5231 Centre Avenue
Pittsburgh, Pa. 15232

Institute for the Crippled and
  Disabled
400 First Avenue
New York, N.Y. 10010

Institute of Food Technologists
221 N. LaSalle Street
Chicago, Ill. 60601

Institute of Makers of Explosives
420 Lexington Avenue
New York, N.Y. 10016

Institute for Sex Education
22 E. Madison Street
Suite 805
Chicago, Ill. 60602

International Apple Institute
2430 Pennsylvania Avenue, N.W.
Washington, D.C. 20037

International Association for
  Medical Assistance for Travelers
350 Fifth Avenue
Suite 5620
New York, N.Y. 10001

International Association for
  Suicide Prevention
2521 W. Pico Boulevard
Los Angeles, Calif. 90006

International Society for the
  Rehabilitation of the Disabled
219 E. Forty-fourth Street
. New York, N.Y. 10017

Johnson and Johnson, Inc.
Educational Services
Patient Care Division
501 George Street
New Brunswick, N.J. 08901

Kellogg Company
Department of Health Economics
  Services
Battle Creek, Mich. 49016

Kemper Insurance Company
4750 N. Sherisan Road
Chicago, Ill. 60640

Kenny Rehabilitation Institute
1800 Chicago Avenue
Minneapolis, Minn. 55404

Kimberly-Clark Corporation
Life Cycle Center
P.O. Box 551
Neenah, Wis. 54956

Knox Gelatin, Inc.
Johnston, N.H. 12095

Kraft Foods Corporation
500 Penstigo Court
Chicago, Ill. 60690

La Leche League International, Inc.
9616 Minneapolis Ave.
Franklin Park, Ill. 60131

Lederle Laboratories
Film Library
One Casper Street
Danbury, Conn. 06810
or Pearl River, N.Y. 10965

Lee Creative Communications
P.O. Box 1367
5 S. St. Regis Street
Rochester, N.Y. 14618

Libby, McKeil and Libby
200 S. Michigan Avenue
Chicago, Ill. 60604

Licensed Beverage Industries, Inc.
Division of Educational Study
485 Lexington Avenue
New York, N.Y. 10017

Martland Hospital
College of Medicine and Dentistry
65 Bergen Street
Newark, N.J. 07107

Maternity Center Association
48 E. Ninety-second Street
New York, N.Y. 10028

McDonald's, Inc.
McDonald's Plaza
Oak Brook, Ill. 60521

McNeil Laboratories, Inc.
Camp Hill Road
Fort Washington, Pa. 19034

Mead Johnson Laboratories
2404 W. Pennsylvania Street
Evansville, Ind. 47721

Medcom, Inc.
1633 Broadway
New York, N.Y. 10019

Medfact Films
420 Lake Avenue, N.E.
Massillon, Ohio 44646

Medic Alert Foundation
1000 N. Palm
Turlock, Calif. 95380

Medical Library Association
919 N. Michigan Avenue
Chicago, Ill. 60611

Medidisc Corporation
P.O. Box 14306
North Palm Beach, Fla. 33408

Mental Health Materials Center
419 Park Avenue South
New York, N.Y. 10016

Merck, Sharp and Dohme
Audio-Visual Services
West Point, Pa. 19486

Merrill-National Laboratories
Division of Richardson-Merrill,
Inc.
Cincinnati, Ohio 45215

Metropolitan Life Insurance
Company
Health and Welfare Division
One Madison Avenue
New York, N.Y. 10010

Milex Central
(Doctor Discusses Series)
1873 Grove Street
Glenview, Ill. 60025

Milner-Fenwick
3800 Liberty Heights Avenue
Baltimore, Md. 21215

Muscular Dystrophy Associations
of America, Inc.
Patient Service and Research
Department
1790 Broadway
New York, N.Y. 10019

Myasthenia Gravis Foundation
National Headquarters
2 E. 103rd Street
New York, N.Y. 10029

Nabisco, Inc.
425 Park Avenue
New York, N.Y. 10022

Narcotics Education, Inc.
6830 Laurel Street, N.W.
Washington, D.C. 20012

National Academy of Science
Food and Nutrition Board
2101 Constitution Avenue, N.W.
Washington, D.C. 20418

National Association for Gifted
Children
8080 Spring Valley Drive
Cincinnati, Ohio 45236

National Association for Mental
Health
10 Columbus Circle
New York, N.Y. 10019

National Association for Music
Therapy, Inc.
P.O. Box 610
Lawrence, Kans. 66044

National Association for Practical
Nurse Education and Service,
Inc.
535 Fifth Avenue
New York, N.Y. 10017

National Association for Retarded
Children, Inc.
420 Lexington Avenue
New York, N.Y. 10017

National Association for Retarded
Citizens
Publications Department
P.O. Box 6109
Arlington, Tex. 76011

National Association of Hearing
and Speech Agencies
919 Eighteenth Street, N.W.
Washington, D.C. 20006

National Association of Manufacturers Distribution Services
277 Park Avenue
New York, N.Y. 10017

National Association of Margarine
Manufacturers
545 Munsey Building
Washington, D.C. 20004

National Association of Social
Workers
2 Park Avenue
New York, N.Y. 10016

National Association of the
Physically Handicapped
76 Elm Street
London, Ohio 43140

National Biscuit Company
Consumer Services
425 Park Avenue
New York, N.Y. 10022

National Canners Association
Home Economics Services
1133 Twentieth Street, N.W.
Washington, D.C. 20036

National Center for Health
Education
211 Sutter Street
San Francisco, Calif. 91404

National Commission for Social
Work Careers
2 Park Avenue
New York, N.Y. 10016

National Committee for Prevention
of Child Abuse
111 E. Wacker Drive
Suite 510
Chicago, Ill. 60601

National Congress of Parents and
Teachers
700 N. Rush Street
Chicago, Ill. 60611

National Coordinating Council on
Drug Education
1211 Connecticut Avenue, N.W.
Suite 212
Washington, D.C. 20036

National Council on the Aging
1828 L Street, N.W.
Washington, D.C. 20036

National Council on Alcoholism,
Inc.
730 Fifth Avenue
New York, N.Y. 10019

National Council on Crime and
Delinquency
44 E. Twenty-third Street
New York, N.Y. 10010

National Council on Drug Abuse
Eight S. Michigan Avenue
Suite 310
Chicago, Ill. 60603

National Council on Family
Relations
1219 University Avenue, S.E.
Minneapolis, Minn. 55414

National Cystic Fibrosis Research
Foundation
3379 Peachtree Road, N.E.
Atlanta, Ga. 30326

National Dairy Council
111 North Canal Street
Chicago, Ill. 60606

National Easter Seal Society for
Crippled Children and Adults,
Inc.
2023 W. Ogden Avenue
Chicago, Ill. 60612

National Education Association
1201 Sixteenth Street, N.W.
Washington, D.C. 20036

National Environmental Health
Association
1600 Pennsylvania Avenue
Denver, Colo. 80203

National Epilepsy League, Inc.
203 N. Wabash Avenue
Chicago, Ill. 60601

National Federation of Licensed
Practical Nurses, Inc.
250 W. Fifty-seventh Street
New York, N.Y. 10019

National Fire Protection
Association
60 Batterymarch Street
Boston, Mass. 02110

National Foundation for Sudden
Infant Death, Inc.
1501 Broadway
New York, N.Y. 10036

National Foundation for the Blind
218 Randolf Hotel Building
Des Moines, Iowa 50309

National Foundation-March of
Dimes
P.O. Box 2000
White Plains, N.Y. 10602

National Health and Welfare
Department
Office of Information Service
Ottawa 3
Canada

National Health Council
1740 Broadway
New York, N.Y. 10019

National Hemophilia Foundation
25 W. Thirty-ninth Street
New York, N.Y. 10018

National Inter-agency Council on
Smoking and Health
P.O. Box 3650
Central Station
Arlington, Va. 22203

National Kidney Foundation
116 E. Twenty-seventh Street
New York, N.Y. 10016

National League for Nursing, Inc.
Director of Public Relations
10 Columbus Circle
New York, N.Y. 10019

National Livestock and Meat Board
36 S. Wabash
Chicago, Ill. 60603

National Medical Association
1625 I Street, N.W.
Washington, D.C. 20006

National Multiple Sclerosis Society
205 E. Forty-second Street
New York, N.Y. 10017

National Paraplegia Foundation
333 N. Michigan Avenue
Chicago, Ill. 60601

National Parkinson Institute
1501 N.W. Ninth Avenue
Miami, Fla. 33136

National Psoriasis Foundation
P.O. Box 1365
Portland, Ore. 97207

National Retired Teachers
  Association/American
  Association of Retired Persons
1909 K Street, N.W.
Washington, D.C. 20049

National Save-a-Life League
20 W. Forty-third Street
New York, N.Y. 10036

National Society for Autistic
  Children
1234 Massachusetts Avenue, N.E.
Washington, D.C. 20005
and its Information & Referral
  Service
306 Thirty-first Street
Huntington, W.Va. 25702

National Society for Prevention of
  Blindness, Inc.
Director of Information Services
79 Madison Avenue
New York, N.Y. 10016

New York Life Insurance Company
Public Relations Department
51 Madison Avenue
New York, N.Y. 10010

Nutra-Mate Textured Vegetable
  Protein
A. E. Stanley Company
Food Service Division
2011 Swift Drive
Oak Brook, Ill. 60521

Nutrition Foundation, Inc.
99 Park Avenue
New York, N.Y. 10016

Omni Education
190 W. Main Street
P.O. Box 220
Sommerville, N.J. 08876

Optimists International
4494 Lindell Boulevard
St. Louis, Mo. 63108

Oral Hygiene Publications
911 Pennsylvania Avenue,
Pittsburgh, Pa. 15222

Ormont Drugs and Chemicals
  Company
520 S. Dean Street
Englewood, N.J. 07631

Ortho Pharmaceutical Corporation
Director of Educational Services
Raritan, N.J. 08869

Overeaters Anonymous
3730 Moter Avenue
Los Angeles, Calif. 90034

Parents Anonymous
2930 W. Imperial Highway
Suite 322
Inglewood, Calif. 90303

Parents Magazine Films
52 Vanderbilt Avenue
New York, N.Y. 10017

Parke Davis and Company
Joseph Campau at the River
G.P.O. Box 118
Detroit, Mich. 48232

Parkinson's Disease Foundation
640 W. 168th Street
New York, N.Y. 10016

Patient Education Center
North Carolina Memorial Hospital
Chapel Hill, N.C. 27514

Penwalt Pharmaceutical
    Corporation
P.O. Box 1212
Rochester, N.Y. 14603

Perennial Education, Inc.
1825 Willow Road
Northfield, Ill. 60093

Pet, Inc.
Office of Consumer Affairs
Pet Plaza
400 S. Fourth Street
St. Louis, Mo. 63101

Pfizer Laboratories, Inc.
235 E. Forty-second Street
New York, N.Y. 10017

Pharmaceutical Manufacturers
    Association
Public Information Office
1155 Fifteenth Avenue, N.W.
Washington, D.C. 20005

Planned Parenthood Federation
    of America
810 Seventh Avenue
New York, N.Y. 10019

Playschools Association
120 W. Fifty-seventh Street
New York, N.Y. 10019

Population Reference Bureau
1755 Massachusetts Avenue, N.W.
Washington, D.C. 20036

Pritchett and Hull Associates
2996 Grandview Avenue, N.E.
Atlanta, Ga. 30305

Proctor and Gamble Distributing
    Company
Public Relations Division
P.O. Box 599
Cincinnati, Ohio 45201

Professional Research
660 S. Bonnie Brae Street
Los Angeles, Calif. 90057

Prudential Life Insurance Company
    of America
Prudential Plaza
Newark, N.J. 07010

Public Affairs Committee, Inc.
381 Park Avenue South
New York, N.Y. 10016

Pyramid Films
Box 1048
2801 Colorado Boulevard
Santa Monica, Calif. 90406

Quaker Oats
Consumer Service
Merchandise Mart Plaza
Chicago, Ill. 60654

Ralston Purina Company
Nutrition Services
Checkerboard Square
St. Louis, Mo. 63188

Reader's Digest
Pleasantville, N.Y. 10570

Registry of Medical Technologists
445 N. Lake Shore Drive
Chicago, Ill. 60601

Research Media, Inc.
96 Mt. Auburn Street
Cambridge, Mass. 02138

A. H. Robins Company
1407 Cummings Drive
Richmond, Va. 23220

Roche Laboratories
Division of Hoffman-LaRoche, Inc.
Nutley, N.J. 07110

Ross Laboratories, Educational
   Services
Department 441
625 Cleveland Avenue
Columbus, Ohio 43216

Sandoz Pharmaceuticals
East Hanover, N.J. 07936

Saunders Company, W. C.
W. Washington Square
Philadelphia, Pa. 19105

Schering Corporation
Union, N.J. 07083

Science Research Associates, Inc.
57 W. Grand Avenue
Chicago, Ill. 60610

Scientists Institutes for Public
   Information
30 E. Sixty-eighth Street
New York, N.Y. 10017

Scott Paper Company
Home Service Center
Philadelphia, Pa. 19113

Sealtest Foods
Consumers Service
605 Third Avenue
New York, N.Y. 10016

Searle Company
P.O. Box 5110
Chicago, Ill. 60680

Sex Information and Education
   Council of the United States
1855 Broadway
New York, N.Y. 10023
and its Publications Office
1825 Willow Road
Northfield, Ill. 60093

Sister Kenny Institute
1800 Chicago Avenue
Minneapolis, Minn. 55404

Smith, Kline and French
   Laboratories
Services Department
Room E10
1500 Spring Garden Street
Philadelphia, Pa. 19101

Society for Nutrition Education
2140 Shattuck Avenue
Suite 1110
Berkeley, Ca. 94704

Society for Public Health
   Education, Inc. (SOPHE)
655 Sutter Street
San Francisco, Ca. 94102

Society for Visual Education, Inc.
1345 Diversy Parkway
Chicago, Ill. 60614

Society of Teachers of Family
   Medicine
1740 W. Ninety-second Street
Kansas City, Mo. 64114

Society of the Plastics Industry,
   Inc.
250 Park Avenue
New York, N.Y. 10017

Source, Inc.
P.O. Box 21066
Washintgon, D.C. 20009

Squibb and Sons, Inc.
General Offices
P.O. Box 4000
Princeton, N.J. 08540

Standard Brands
D.M.S., Inc.
22 East Twenty-second Street
New York, N.Y. 10010

Stuart Pharmaceuticals
Division of I.C.I. United States
Wilmington, Del. 19897

Sugar Information, Inc.
52 Wall Street
New York, N.Y. 10005

Sunkist Growers Consumer Services
P.O. Box 7888 Valley Annex
Van Nuys, Calif. 91409

Swift and Company
Public Relations Department
115 W. Jackson
Chicago, Ill. 60604

Syntex Laboratories
3401 Hillview Avenue
Palo Alto, Calif. 94304

Tampax, Inc.
5 Dakota Drive
Lake Success, N.Y. 11040

Teach 'Em, Inc.
625 N. Michigan
Chicago, Ill. 60611

Train-Aide
1015 Grandview Avenue
Glendale, Calif. 91201

Trainex Corporation
P.O. Box 116
12601 Industry Street
Garden Grove, Calif. 92641

Trainex Patient Video Corporation
10 Perimeter Place, N.W.
Atlanta, Ga. 30339

Union Central Life Insurance
Company
Medical Department
Southwest Corner, Fourth and Vine
P.O. Box 179
Cincinnati, Ohio 45201

United Cerebral Palsy Association
Public Relations Director
66 E. Thirty-fourth Street
New York, N.Y. 10016

United Fresh Fruit and Vegetable
Association
777 Fourteenth Street, N.W.
Washington, D.C. 20005

United Fruit Company
Educational Department
Pier 3
Prudential Center
Boston, Mass. 02199

United Nations
Office of Public Information
New York, N.Y. 10017

United Ostomy Association, Inc.
1111 Wilshire Boulevard
Los Angeles, Calif. 90017

University of Illinois Medical
Center
Public Information Office
P.O. Box 6998
1737 W. Polk Street
Chicago, Ill. 60608

University of Minnesota
Center of Death Education and
Research
1167 Social Science Building
Minneapolis, Minn. 55455

University of Toronto
Division of Instructional Media
Services
8 Taddlecreek Road
Toronto,
Ontario, Can. M5S 1A8

Upjohn Company
7000 Portage Road
Kalamazoo, Mich. 49001

Vidcom
10 Perimeter Place
Suite 150
Atlanta, Ga. 30339

Vitamin Information Bureau, Inc.
383 Madison Avenue
New York, N.Y. 10017

Walmat Company
3430-32 Illinois Street
Indianapolis, Ind. 46208

Warner/Chilcott
Division of Warner-Lambert
    Company
Creative Services Department
Morris Plains, N.J. 07950

Wells National Services
    Corporation
200 Park Avenue
New York, N.Y. 10017

Westwood Pharmaceuticals
468 Dewitt Street
Buffalo, N.Y. 14213

Wheat Flour Institute
14 E. Jackson Boulevard
Chicago, Ill. 60604

World Health Organization
    Publications
c/o Columbia University Press
International Documents Service
2960 Broadway
New York, N.Y. 10027

Wyeth Laboratories
Philadelphia, Pa. 19101

Zero Population Growth
1346 Connecticut Avenue, N.W.
Washington, D.C. 20036

United States Government Agencies*

Center for Disease Control
Training Resources
Instructional Systems Division
Bureau of Training
Consumer Information Center
Pueblo, Colo. 81009

Consumer Product Safety
    Commission
Washington, D.C. 20207

Department of Housing and Urban
    Development
451 Seventh Street, S.W.
Washington, D.C. 20410

Department of Agriculture
Office of Information
Washington, D.C. 20250

Department of Health, Education,
    and Welfare
Public Health Service
Washington, D.C. 20204

Division of Facilities Development
Health Resource Administration,
    PHS
Department of Health, Education,
    and Welfare
Public Health Service'
5600 Fishers Lane
Rockville, Md. 20852

*National headquarters have an asterisk beside them.

National Agriculture Library
Food and Nutrition Information
and Educational Materials
10301 Baltimore Boulevard
Room 304
Beltsville, Md. 20705

National Audio-Visual Center
(GSA)
Sales Branch
Washington, D.C. 20409
or N.A.V.C. Annex Station K
Atlanta, Ga. 30324

National Cancer Institute
Office of Cancer Communication
Bethesda, Md. 20014

National Caries Program
National Institutes of Health
National Institute of Dental
Research
Westwood Building
Room 549
Bethesda, Md. 20014

National Center for Health
Statistics
Room 8-20
5600 Fishers Lane
Rockville, Md. 20852

National Clearinghouse for Alcohol
Information
P.O. Box 2345
Rockville, Md. 20805

National Clearinghouse for Drug
Abuse Information
P.O. Box 1635
Rockville, Md. 20805

National Heart, Lung and Blood
Institute
Heart Information Center
Superintendent of Documents
U.S. Government Printing Office
Washington, D.C. 20402

National High Blood Pressure
Information Center
120/80 National Institutes of
Health
Bethesda, Md. 20014

National Institutes of Health
Office of Information
Bethesda, Md. 20014

National Technical Information
Service
Operations Division
Department of Commerce
Springfield, Va. 22151

Occupational Safety and Health
Administration
1726 M Street, N.W.
Room 1020
Washington, D.C. 20210

Office of Consumer Affairs
H.E.W. Building
Room 330
330 Independence Avenue, S.W.
Washington, D.C. 20201

Superintendent of Documents
U.S. Government Printing Office
Washington, D.C. 20402

Veterans' Administration
810 Vermont Avenue, N.W.
Washington, D.C. 20420

Vital and Health Statistics
Department of Health, Education,
and Welfare
Public Health Service
Health Resources Administration
National Center for Health
Statistics
Rockville, Md. 20852

And, if you can't find it here, try: *National Directory of Addresses and
Telephone Numbers*   Published by
Bantam Books, Inc. 666 Fifth Avenue, New York, N.Y. 10019

Accident Prevention

*Aetna Life and Casualty
Public Relations and Advertising
   Department
151 Farmington Avenue
Hartford, Conn. 06115

American Association of State
   Highway Officials
National Press Building
Washington, D.C. 20004

American Automobile Association
1712 G Street, N.W.
Washington, D.C. 20006

American Driver and Traffic Safety
   Education Association
1201 Sixteenth Street, N.W.
Washington, D.C. 20036

American Insurance Association
Engineering and Safety
   Department
85 John Street
New York, N.Y. 10038

American Motorcycle Association
5655 N. High Street
Worthington, Ohio 43086

*American National Red Cross
Seventeenth and D Street, N.W.
Washington, D.C. 20006

American Society for Safety
   Engineers
850 Busee Highway
Park Ridge, Ill. 60068

American Transit Association
299 Madison Avenue
New York, N.Y. 10017

Auto Dealers Traffic Safety Council
1776 Massachusetts Avenue, N.W.
Washington, D.C. 20036

Automotive Industries Division
Highway Users Federation for
   Safety and Mobility
1776 Massachusetts Avenue, N.W.
Washington, D.C. 20036

Bicycle Institute of America, Inc.
122 E. Forty-second Street
New York, N.Y. 10017

*Center for Disease
   Control/CEMA
1600 Clifton Road, N.E.
Atlanta, Ga. 30333

Center for Safety
New York University
329 Shimkin Hall
Washington Square
New York, N.Y. 10003

Channing L. Bete Company, Inc.
45 Federal Street
Greenfield, Mass. 01301

*CNA Financial Corporation
Communications Department
310 S. Michigan Avenue
Chicago, Ill. 60604

*Connecticut General Life
   Insurance Company
Advertising and Public Relations
Room 319
Hartford, Conn. 06115

Employer's Insurance of Wausau
Safety and Health Services
Wausau, Wisc. 54402

Eno Foundation for Highway
   Traffic Control
Saugatuck, Conn. 06880

Ford Motor Company
Educational Affairs Department
Dearborn, Mich. 48120

Highway Research Board
2101 Constitution Avenue
Washington, D.C. 20418

Highway Traffic Safety Center
Michigan State University
East Lansing, Mich. 48823

Highway Users Federation for
Safety and Mobility
1776 Massachusetts Avenue, N.W.
Washington, D.C. 20036

*The Institute for Safer Living
American Mutual Liability
Insurance Company
Wakefield, Mass. 01880

Institute of Traffic Engineers
2029 K Street, N.W.
Washington, D.C. 20006

*Insurance Institute for Highway
Safety
711 Watergate Office Building
2600 Virginia Avenue, N.W.
Washington, D.C. 20037

*Kemper Insurance Company
Advertising and Public Relations
Department
110 Tenth Avenue
Fulton, Ill. 61252

*Liberty Mutual Insurance
Company
Public Relations Department
175 Berkeley Street
Boston, Mass. 02117

Motorcycle, Scooter and Allied
Trades Association
5665 N. High Street
Worthington, Ohio 43085

Motor Vehicle Manufacturers
Association of the United States
320 New Center Building
Detroit, Mich. 48202

*National Easter Seal Society for
Crippled Children and Adults,
Inc.
2023 W. Ogden Avenue
Chicago, Ill. 60612

National Fire Protection
Association
60 Batterymarch Street
Boston, Mass. 02110

National Highway Traffic Safety
Administration
U.S. Department of Transportation
Washington, D.C. 20509

*National Safety Council
Director of Public Information
425 N. Michigan Avenue
Chicago, Ill. 60611

New York Life Insurance Company
Public Relations Department
51 Madison Avenue
New York, N.Y. 10010

Safe Winter Driving League
520 N. Michigan Avenue
Chicago, ill. 60611

Society of the Plastics Industry,
Inc.
250 Park Avenue
New York, N.Y. 10017

*The Travelers Insurance
Companies
Marketing Services
One Tower Square
Hartford, Conn. 06115

*Union Central Life Insurance
Company
Medical Department
P.O. Box 179
Cincinnati, Ohio 45201

*U.S. Department of Agriculture
Independence Avenue
Washington, D.C. 20250

U.S. Department of Defense
Office of Civil Defense
Washington, D.C. 20301

U.S. Department of Labor
Occupational Safety and Health
   Administration
1726 M Street, N.W.
Room 1020
Washington, D.C. 20210

Aging

*Administration on Aging
Office of Human Development
U.S. Department of Health,
   Education, and Welfare
Washington, D.C. 20201

*National Council on the Aging
1828 L Street, N.W.
Washington, D.C. 20036

Child Care

See also Family Life.

American Academy of Pediatrics
1801 Hinman Avenue
P.O. Box 1034
Evanston, Ill. 60204

The American Legion
National Headquarters
700 N. Pennsylvania Street
Indianapolis, Ind. 46206

Association for the Aid of Crippled
   Children
Division of Publications
345 E. Forty-sixth Street
New York, N.Y. 10017
Books, pamphlets, reprints

Canadian Department of National
   Health and Welfare
Child and Maternal Health
   Division
Ottawa, Ontario, Can.
*Catalog and materials on child
care, pregnancy, home safety for
children*

Child Study Association of
   America, Wel-Met, Inc.
50 Madison Avenue
New York, N.Y. 10010
Pamphlets, book lists

Child Welfare League of America,
   Inc.
67 Irving Place
New York, N.Y. 10003
*Pamphlets and periodicals dealing
with medical facilities for children
receiving welfare, research goals of
the league, adoption services*

*Community Services
Administration
Social and Rehabilitation Service
U.S. Department of Health,
Education, and Welfare
Washington, D.C. 20201
Pamphlets, leaflets

Consumer Information
Public Documents Center
Department O16F
Pueblo, Colo. 81009
*Index of publications on energy
conservation diet, food labeling,
child care, consumer safety*

*John Hancock Mutual Life
Insurance Company
Manager, Community Relations
200 Berkeley Street
Boston, Mass. 02117

*Johnson and Johnson, Inc.
Educational Services, Patient Care
Division
501 George Street
New Brunswick, N.J. 08901

Maternity Center Association
48 E. Ninety-second Street
New York, N.Y. 10028
*Brochures, pamphlets, teaching aids
describing reproduction and birth*

National Congress of Parents and
Teachers
700 N. Rush Street
Chicago, Ill. 60611
*Pamphlets on children, school
problems*

*National Easter Seal Society for
Crippled Children and Adults,
Inc.
2023 W. Ogden Avenue
Chicago, Ill. 60612
*Reprints, leaflets, pamphlets,
bibliographies*

TAMA Division of Profesional
Productions
Northstar Medical Offices
7615 Metro Boulevard
Edina, Minn. 55435
*Catalog on self-contained classroom
screens with films, and kits on
teaching human screenability (five
levels)*

Dental Health

See also Nutrition.

American Dental Association
Bureau of Dental Health
  & Education
211 E. Chicago Avenue
Chicago, Ill. 60611
*Catalog listing pamphlets, charts,
posters, audiovisual materials*

*National Dairy Council
Nutrition Education Division
111 N. Canal Street
Chicago, Ill. 60606
*Contact nearest dairy council or
national headquarters. Material by
grade level.*

Environmental Pollution

*Aetna Life and Casualty
Public Relations and Advertising
   Department
151 Farmington Avenue
Hartford, Conn. 06115
Pamphlet, film

*American Lung Association
1740 Broadway
New York, N.Y. 10019
*Contact local Lung Association
chapter*

Bethlehem Steel Corporation
Bethlehem, Pa. 18016

*CNA Financial Corporation
Communications Department
310 S. Michigan Avenue
Chicago, Ill. 60604

*Public Health Service
Environmental Health Service
U.S. Department of Health,
   Education, and Welfare
Rockville, Md. 20852
Reprints, pamphlets

Eyesight

American Association of
   Ophthalmology
1100 Seventeenth Street, N.W.
Room 304
Washington, D.C. 20036
*Pamphlets and films on contact
lenses, common eye diseases such
as glaucoma, identification of sight
problems in children*

*American Foundation for the
   Blind, Inc.
15 W. Sixteenth Street
New York, N.Y. 10011
*Books, pamphlets, journals,
newsletters, films*

American Optometric Association
Division of Public Information
7000 Chippawa Street
St. Louis, Mo. 63119
*Catalog and pamphlets, posters,
films, transcriptions, scripts for
broadcast use*

*Better Vision Institute, Inc.
230 Park Avenue
Suite 3157
New York, N.Y. 10017
Packet of materials

*National Society for the
   Prevention of Blindness, Inc.
Director of Information Services
79 Madison Avenue
New York, N.Y. 10016
*Films, pamphlets, exhibits, radio
and television spots*

Family Life Education

See also Child Care; Mental Health.

American College of Obstetricians and Gynecologists
One East Wacker Drive
Chicago, Ill. 60601
Catalog of booklets, reprints, pamphlets dealing with pregnancy, labor, childbirth

American Institute of Family Relations
5287 Sunset Boulevard
Los Angeles, Calif. 90027
Pamphlets on marriage, family life, personality problems

American Medical Association
Department of Health Education
535 N. Dearborn Street
Chicago, Ill. 60610
Pamphlet series

American Social Health Association
1740 Broadway
New York, N.Y. 10019
Pamphlets, posters

Birth Control Handbook
P.O. Box 1000
Station G
Montreal 130, Quebec, H2W2N1
Canada
Excellent handbook on birth control

Canadian Department of National Health and Welfare
Child and Maternal Health Division
Ottawa, Ontario, Canada
Catalog and materials on child care, pregnancy, home safety for children

Child Welfare League of America, Inc.
67 Irving Place
New York, N.Y. 10003
Pamphlets and periodicals dealing with medical facilities for children receiving welfare, research goals of the league, adoption services

*Kimberly-Clark Corporation
Life Cycle Center
P.O. Box 551
Neenah, Wis. 54956
Materials to supplement health and family life education courses

Margaret Sanger Center
380 Second Avenue
New York, N.Y. 10010
Pamphlets from Planned Parenthood relating to the center

Maternity Center Association
48 E. Ninety-second Street
New York, N.Y. 10028
Brochures, pamphlets, teaching aids describing reproduction and birth

Mental Health Materials Center
419 Park Avenue South
New York, N.Y. 10016
Selective reference guides, plays, and other publications for mental health and family life education programs

National Council on Family Relations
1219 University Avenue, S.E.
Minneapolis, Minn. 55414

*Planned Parenthood Federation
    of America
Publication Section
810 Seventh Avenue
New York, N.Y. 10019
*Pamphlets, reprints, posters, films.
Some Spanish-language material
available*

Public Affairs Committee, Inc.
381 Park Avenue South
New York, N.Y. 10016
*Pamphlets on child guidance,
family well-being, marriage, special
family concerns*

SIECUS
1855 Broadway
New York, N.Y. 10023
*Booklets, leaflets, pamphlets,
catalog on films available*

Smart Family Foundation
65 E. South Water Street
Chicago, Ill. 60601

First Aid

See also Accident Prevention.

*American National Red Cross
Office of Public Information
Seventeenth and D Street, N.W.
Washington, D.C. 20006
*Contact Local Red Cross chapter.
Films, pamphlets, textbooks,
exhibits, radio scripts*

*Johnson and Johnson, Inc.
Attention: Miss Anne Williams
Health Care Division
501 George Street
New Brunswick, N.J. 08901
Folder, chart

Foot Health

*American Podiatry Association
20 Chevy Chase Circle, N.W.
Washington, D.C. 20010
Leaflets, pamphlets, films, exhibits

General Motors
Department of Public Relations
3044 W. Grand Boulevard
Detroit, Mich. 48202
*Materials on foot care, mental
health, allergies*

Health

*Aetna Life and Casualty
Public Relations and Advertising
    Department
151 Farmington Avenue
Hartford, Conn. 06115
Leaflets, posters, films

American Medical Association
Department of Health Education
535 N. Dearborn Street
Chicago, Ill. 60610
Films, pamphlets, posters

*American National Red Cross
Seventeenth and D. Street, N.W.
Washington, D.C. 20006
*Contact local Red Cross chapter.
Films, pamphlets, textbooks*

American Osteopathic Association
Editorial Department
212 E. Ohio Street
Chicago, Ill. 60611
Pamphlets, reprints, publications

American Public Health
    Association
1015 Eighteenth Street, N.W.
Washington, D.C. 20036
*Educational qualifications of health
workers, reprints, health guides,
control handbooks, housing
manuals, standard laboratory
procedures*

Bethlehem Steel Corporation
Bethlehem, Pa. 18016
Ecology pamphlet

Cleveland Health Museum and
    Education Center
8911 Euclid Avenue
Cleveland, Ohio 44106
*Catalog of nontechnical pamphlets,
books, models dealing with
reproduction, drug use, nutrition,
mental health*

*CNA Financial Corporation
Communications Department
310 S. Michigan Avenue
Chicago, Ill. 60604
Booklet

Commercial Union Assurance
    Company
Public Relations Department
One Beacon Street
Boston, Mass. 02108
Books, pamphlets, posters

Consumer Information
Public Documents Center
Department O16F
Pueblo, Colo. 81009

Consumers Union of U.S., Inc.
256 Washington Street
Mount Vernon, N.Y. 10550
*Reprints, books, booklets, consumer
education materials for classroom
use*

Eli Lilly and Company
Educational Resources Program
P.O. Box 100 B
Indianapolis, Ind. 46206
*Pamphlets about molecular
medicine, protein synthesis, viral,
bacterial infection*

Good Housekeeping Institute
959 Eighth Avenue
New York, N.Y. 10019
Catalog

Institute of Life Insurance
277 Park Avenue
New York, N.Y. 10017
Catalog

*Kimberly-Clark Corporation
Life Cycle Center
P.O. Box 551
Neenah, Wis. 54956
*Material to supplement health and
family life courses*

*Liberty Mutual Insurance
    Company
Public Relations Department
175 Berkeley Street
Boston, Mass. 02117
Pamphlets

*Medical Services Administration
Social and Rehabilitation Service
U.S. Department of Health,
    Education, and Welfare
Washington, D.C. 20201

Mental Health Materials Center
419 Park Avenue South
New York, N.Y. 10016
*Selected reference guides, plays,
other publications for education
programs; leaflets*

*Metropolitan Life Insurance
   Company
Health and Welfare Division
One Madison Avenue
New York, N.Y. 10010
*Catalogs and pamphlets, films,
filmstrips related to personal,
family, school, and community
health*

National Center for Solving Special
   Social and Health Problems
169 Eleventh Street
San Francisco, Calif. 94103

New York Times
Book and Educational Division
229 W. 43rd Street
New York, N.Y. 10036
*Films, filmstrip, cassettes, resource
material*

Pan American Health Organization
World Health Organization
525 Twenty-third Street, N.W.
Washington, D.C. 20037
*Booklets, world health magazine,
pamphlets*

*Pharmaceutical Manufacturers
   Association
Public Information Office
1155 Fifteenth Street, N.W.
Washington, D.C. 20005
*Variety of publications on
prescription drug industry, drug
abuse, other health-related subjects*

*Prudential Insurance Company
   of America
Public Relations Department
Prudential Plaza
Newark, N.J. 07010
Leaflets

Public Affairs Committee, Inc.
381 Park Avenue South
New York, N.Y. 10016
Pamphlets, films (list available)

Scott Education Division
Holyoke, Mass. 01040
*Catalogs on materials and prices
and a series on health adventures
with films*

*Social and Rehabilitation Service
U.S. Department of Health,
   Education, and Welfare
Washington, D.C. 20201
*General information, films, exhibits,
radio-TV spots*

Tampax Inc.
Department HI
Educational Director
5 Dakota Drive
Lake Success, N.Y. 11040
*Educational material on
menstruation and the menstrual
cycle*

U.S. Department of Health,
   Education, and Welfare
Public Health Service
Health Services and Mental
   Health Administration
Office of Information
5600 Fishers Lane
Rockville, Md. 20852
*Catalog of government publications
covering all aspects of health*

*U.S. Government Printing Office
Public Documents Department
Washington, D.C. 20402
*Large selection of pamphlets on
most aspects of health; lists of
government publications on health,
smoking and health, baby and child
care, etc.*

Health Careers

*American Association for
  Rehabilitation Therapy
Box 93
North Little Rock, Ark. 72115
Pamphlets

*American Dental Association
Division of Career Guidance
211 E. Chicago Avenue
Chicago, Ill. 60611
Career information

*American Dietetic Association
620 N. Michigan Avenue
Chicago, Ill. 60611
Careers in dietetics

*American Hospital Association
Division of Health Careers
840 N. Lake Shore Drive
Chicago, Ill. 60611
Pamphlets, posters

American Medical Association
Department of Health Education
535 N. Dearborn Street
Chicago, Ill. 60610
Health career information

*American Medical Women's
  Association, Inc.
1740 Broadway
New York, N.Y. 10019
Pamphlets, films

American Osteopathic Association
Office of Education
212 E. Ohio Street
Chicago, Ill. 60611
Pamphlets, reprints

*American Physical Therapy
  Association
1156 Fifteenth Street, N.W.
Washington, D.C. 20005
Career information

*American Podiatry Association
Council on Education
20 Chevy Chase Circle, N.W.
Washington, D.C. 20010
Leaflets, pamphlets, films, exhibits

*American Public Health
  Association
1015 Eighteenth Street, N.W.
Washington, D.C. 20036
*Educational qualifications on
health workers, reprints*

*Association for the Advancement
  of Health Education
1201 Sixteenth Street, N.W.
Washington, D.C. 20036
*Careers in health education and
school nursing*

*CNA Financial Corporation
Communications Department
310 S. Michigan Avenue
Chicago, Ill. 60604
Reprints

*National Association for Retarded
  Citizens
P.O. Box 6109
2709 Avenue E, East
Arlington, Tex. 76011
Pamphlet on mental retardation

*National Easter Seal Society for
  Crippled Children and Adults,
  Inc.
2023 W. Ogden Avenue
Chicago, Ill. 60612
Pamphlets

*National Health Council
1740 Broadway
New York, N.Y. 10019
*Guidance to many sources of
information on health careers*

*National League for Nursing
10 Columbus Circle
New York, N.Y. 10019
*Lists of accredited nursing
programs and scholarship sources*

Registry of Medical Technologists
P.O. Box 4872
Chicago, Ill. 60680

Rockefeller Foundation
111 W. 50th Street
New York, N.Y. 10020
*Resource films, books on doctor's
assistants*

*Social and Rehabilitation Service
U.S. Department of Health,
  Education, and Welfare
Washington, D.C. 20201

Hearing

American Speech and Hearing
  Association
9030 Old Georgetown Road
Washington, D.C. 20014

*National Association of Hearing
  and Speech Agencies
919 Eighteenth Street, N.W.
Washington, D.C. 20006
*Information on speech and hearing
problems. Pamphlets, posters,
television spots, films. Postcard
requests preferred*

*National Easter Seal Society for
  Crippled Children and Adults,
  Inc.
2023 W. Ogden Avenue
Chicago, Ill. 60612
*Pamphlet on "do's" and "don'ts"
for deaf children*

Sonotone Corporation
Saw Mill River Road
Elmsford, N.Y. 10523
*Pamphlets and charts dealing with
the structure and mechanics of the
human ear*

Hospital Services

*American Hospital Association
Director of Public Relations
840 N. Lake Shore Drive
Chicago, Ill. 60611
Pamphlets, posters

American Osteopathic Association
Office of Hospital Affairs
212 E. Ohio Street
Chicago, Ill. 60611
Pamphlets

Mental Health

See also Child Care; Family Life; Health.

CANHC
P.O. Box 111
Escondido, Calif. 92025
Catalog and materials on dyslexia and mental disabilities

Connecticut Mutual Life Insurance Company
Human Relations Program
140 Garden Street
Hartford, Conn. 06115
Cartoon booklets available to teachers. Hartford lectures by professional staff of Institute of Living

Hogg Foundation for Mental Health
University of Texas
Austin, Tex. 78712

Mental Health Materials Center
419 Park Avenue South
New York, N.Y. 10016
Selective reference guides, plays, other publications for mental health and family life education programs

*Metropolitan Life Insurance Company
Health and Welfare Division
One Madison Avenue
New York, N.Y. 10010
Booklets, films

*National Association for Mental Health and its affiliated state and local associations
43 W. Sixty-first Street
New York, N.Y. 10019

National Association for Retarded Children, Inc.
420 Lexington Avenue
New York, N.Y. 10017
Periodicals, pamphlets, fact sheets dealing with research, education, and general information about mental retardation and the lives of retarded people

National Association for Retarded Citizens
P.O. Box 6109
2709 Avenue E, East
Arlington, Tex. 76011

*National Institute of Mental Health
5600 Fisher Lane
Rockville, Md. 20852
Pamphlets, bibliographies, bulletins

U.S. Department of Health, Education, and Welfare
Office of the Secretary
Secretary's Committee on Mental Retardation
Washington, D.C. 20201
Annotated bibliography of books and periodicals dealing with mental retardation

Nutrition

American Dietetic Association
620 N. Michigan Avenue
Chicago, Ill. 60611
Booklets and material for teachers

American Home Economics Association
2010 Massachusetts Avenue, N.W.
Washington, D.C. 20036
Pamphlets, reprints

American Institute of Baking
400 E. Ontario Street
Chicago, Ill. 60611
Catalog, pamphlets

American School Food Service
Association
4101 E. Gliff Avenue
Denver, Colo. 80222
*Materials on nutrition, school
lunch programs*

*Cereal Institute, Inc.
135 S. LaSalle Street
Chicago, Ill. 60603
*Leaflets, source books, charts,
filmstrips on breakfast and cereals*

Florida Citrus Commission
P.O. Box 148
Lakeland, Fla. 33802

Food and Agriculture Organization
of the United Nations
1335 C Street, S.W.
Washington, D.C. 20437
Catalog

General Mills
9200 Wayzata Boulevard
Minneapolis, Minn. 55440
Pamphlets

H. J. Heinz Company
P.O. Box 57
Pittsburgh, Pa. 15230

National Biscuit Company
Consumer Services
425 Park Avenue
New York, N.Y. 10022
Booklets, charts, leaflets

National Canners Association
1133 Twentieth Street, N.W.
Home Economics Services
Washington, D.C. 20036

*National Dairy Council
Nutrition Education Division
111 N. Canal Street
Chicago, Ill. 60606
*Contact nearest dairy council or
national headquarters. Material,
films, filmstrips, displays, by grade
level*

National Livestock and Meat
Board
36 S. Wabash Avenue
Room 700
Chicago, Ill. 60603

Nutrition Foundation, Inc.
489 Fifth Avenue
New York, N.Y. 10016
Booklets, films, resource materials

Ralston Purina Company
Nutrition Services
Checkerboard Square
St. Louis, Mo. 63199

Sugar Information, Inc.
254 W. Thirty-first Street
New York, N.Y. 10001

Sunkist Growers Consumer
Services
P.O. Box 7888, Valley Annex
Van Nuys, Calif. 91409

United Fresh Fruit and Vegetable
Association
777 Fourteenth Street, N.W.
Washington, D.C. 20005

U.S. Department of Agriculture
Agricultural Research Service
Washington, D.C. 20250
Publication list, pamphlets

Wheat Flour Institute
Supervisor of Distribution
14 E. Jackson Boulevard
Chicago, Ill. 60604
Pamphlets, posters, filmstrip

Occupational Therapy

*American Occupational Therapy
  Association
6000 Executive Boulevard
Rockville, Md. 20852

Physical Fitness

See also Nutrition; Child Care;
  Health.

American Medical Association
Committee on Exercise and
  Physical Fitness
535 N. Dearborn Street
Chicago, Ill. 60610

Association for the Advancement
  of Health Education
1201 Sixteenth Street, S.W.
Washington, D.C. 20036
Films, pamphlets, award system

Commercial Union Assurance
  Company
Public Relations Department
One Beacon Street
Boston, Mass. 02108
Booklets, posters

*Liberty Mutual Insurance
  Company
Public Relations Department
175 Berkeley Street
Boston, Mass. 02117

Rehabilitation

See also Mental Health;
  Alcoholism; Drug dependence
  and abuse.

*American Association for
  Rehabilitation Therapy
Box 93
North Little Rock, Ark. 72115
Pamphlets

*CNA Financial Corporation
Communications Department
310 S. Michigan Avenue
Chicago, Ill. 60604
Reprints

Kenny Rehabilitation Institute
A/V Publications Office
1800 Chicago Avenue
Minneapolis, Minn. 55404

*Rehabilitation Services
  Administration
Social and Rehabilitation Service
U.S. Department of Health,
  Education, and Welfare
Washington, D.C. 20201
*Leaftlets, pamphlets, reports,
films*

School Health

See also Health.

American Medical Association
Department of Health Education
535 N. Dearborn Street
Chicago, Ill. 60610

Association for the Advancement
  of Health Education
1201 Sixteenth Street, N.W.
Washington, D.C. 20036
*Books, pamphlets, charts, audio-
visuals, catalog of additional
teaching materials*

*National headquarters

Annotated Selected Bibliography

This bibliography was prepared by the chapter authors in order to introduce readers to the patient education literature. It is not meant to be complete or representative of the themes advanced in this book. Refer to chapter references for an up-to-date perspective on the various topics.

Arnold, M. F. Criteria for documentation and education of cancer public education programs. *Health Education Monographs*, 1973, A discussion of the appropriateness and feasibility of evaluating programs is presented along with the factors that influence the impact of the evaluation effort. The author also examines the types and levels of evaluation.

Becker, M. H. (Ed.). The health belief model and personal health behavior. *Health Education Monographs*, Winter 1974, *2*, Twenty years of research on this model is reviewed and synthesized. The several authors examine the studies related to the model and offer their critique on its current applicability and the need for future field studies. It is recommended as "a textbook and as a basic reference for students, practitioners, and investigators."

Becker, M. H., Drachman, R. H., & Kirscht, J. P. A new approach to explaining sick-role behavior in low-income populations. *American Journal of Public Health*, March 1974, *64;* 205–216. The authors are critical of the shotgun method of selecting variables for compliance studies and stress the need to "diagnose the situation." Although directed toward improving research, the suggestions of what to include in a systematic approach that provides for sequential learning experiences are relevant for program planning.

Bernstein, L., & Dana, R. H. *Interviewing and the health professions* (2nd ed.). New York: Appleton Century Crofts, 1973. A good reference in a basic technique needed for effective educational planning on the basis of what exists.

Brown, E. (Ed.). *Oral health, dentistry, and the American Public: The need for an improved oral care delivery system*. Oklahoma: University of Oklahoma Press, 1974; especially chap. 2: S. S. Kegeles, Adequate oral health, blocks, and means by which they may be overcome, pp. 73–128.

Davis, F. *Illness interaction and the Self.* Belmont, Calif.: Wadsworth, 1972 (Paperback). Davis presents medical sociological views on how student nurses come to view themselves as professionals. He also discusses how patients and their families cope with illness.

Dodge, J. S. What patients should be told: Patients' and nurses' beliefs. *American Journal of Nursing,* October 1972, *72,* 1852–1856. The differences between what the patient wants to know and what the nurse thinks a patient wants to know have been identified. The lack of professional awareness of this difference may be a major factor in noncompliant behavior.

Fostering the Growing Need to Learn (Monograph and annotated bibliography on continuing education and health manpower). Regional Medical Programs, U.S. Public Health Service, 1974. A series of papers written by adult educators presents ideas on the management and process of planning in continuing education. Sections are also included on the health care practitioner as instructor and effective caring. The bibliography is very extensive.

Friedson, E. *Profession of medicine: A study of the sociology of applied knowledge.* New York: Dodd, Mead, 1970. A study of the social organization of the medical profession, in which the author examines the formal organization of the profession, the nature of illness, and the limits of professional knowledge and autonomy.

Gatzke, H. K. & Yenney, S. L. Hospital-wide education and training. *Hospitals,* March 1973, *47,* 93–97. The ideas presented on the development of an education and training program in a hospital form a good basis for similar consideration for the creation of a patient education program. Planning, organization, strategy, and commitment are discussed.

Glickman, I. (Ed.). Chairside preventive dentistry. *Dental Clinics of North America,* 1972, *16* (4 whole issues). Glickmen deals with many issues that confront dentists in daily practice, e.g., plaque control, topical fluoride, nutritional guidance, oral cancer, chemoprophylaxis, radiation, orthodontics, and tissue injury.

Green, L. W. Should health education abandon attitude-change strategies? Perspectives from recent research. *Health Education Monographs,* 1970. The internal and external factors influencing the behavior of an individual are discussed and a scheme is presented as a "Classification of Change Process and Social-Psychological Outcomes of Behavior under Different Conditions of Psychological Readiness and Social Support."

Green, L. W. Evaluation of patient education programs: Criteria and measurement techniques. In *Proceedings of a conference on education for the patient.* Southern Illinois University, Carbondale, Ill., June 1974. A didactic summary of definitions, criteria, measurement techniques and designs of material previously published by the author. The balance of the article provides four principles of health education as propositions, along with their implications for evaluative research in patient education.

Green, L. W. Toward cost-benefit evaluation of health education: Some concepts, methods, and examples. *Health Education Monographs,* 1974, *2* (Suppl. 1). The author redefines evaluation, develops a scheme for looking at the relationships among the relevant factors of health education, and specifies the opportunities for evaluation. He proposes a cost-benefit index to identify the specific parameters and statistics required to conduct standardized estimates for comparisons among the factors.

Green, L. W., & Talamanca, I. F. Suggested designs for evaluating patient education programs. *Health Education Monographs,* Spring 1974, *2.* The authors classify patient education studies reported in the literature on the basis of their quasi-experimental designs (as described by Campbell and Stanley). Suggested research designs are proposed and the strengths and weaknesses of each are discussed.

Hamilton, W. P. & Lavin, M. A. *Decision-making in the coronary care unit: A manual and workbook for nurses.* St. Louis, Mo.: Moody, 1975. The original publication in 1972 was developed as a teaching method to use in conferences with coronary care unit nurses. The format is a brief didactic outline of a specific point, followed by cases in which important nursing decisions had to be made. The revised edition has added a chapter on patient education.

Heydebrand, W. *Hospital bureaucracy.* New York: Dunellen, 1973. In this sociological study of the organizational structure of hospitals, the author discusses task structure, complexity, coordination, and bureaucratic theory. It is a good orientation to the "hospital culture."

Jenny, J. A strategy for patient teaching. *Journal of Advanced Nursing* 1978, *3,* 341–348. An interactional model for patient teaching is proposed that relates patient values to patient behavior change through engagement of patient and facilitation by the nurse.

Kelman, H. C. Compliance, identification and internalization. Three processes of attitude change. *Journal of Conflict Resolution,* 1958, *2,* 51–60. This provides an important differentiation of the way social influence occurs and the outcomes of each process. The difficulty of achieving internalization, the most realistic goal in health education, is well presented.

Knutson, A. L. *The individual, society and health behavior.* New York: Russell Sage Foundation, 1965. In this excellent presentation of the theoretical underpinning for perception, motivation, values, attitudes, and beliefs, the author discusses these as they apply to learning, the communication process, and obtaining health action.

Lee, E. A. Annual administrative reviews: Health education. *Hospitals,* April 1974, *48,* 133–139. The variety of educational efforts and other forces which have developed are reviewed. The article contains a long list of references on what a variety of health professionals are saying and doing in patient education.

Redman, B. *The process of patient teaching in nursing.* Saint Louis: Mosby, 1972. This is a classic text for the learner and the practitioner. The teaching-learning process and the role of the nurse in health education are discussed. Some evaluation methodologies are included.

Richards, R., & Kalmer, H. Patient education. *Health Education Monographs,* Spring 1974, *2.* This collection of eleven papers describes a variety of patient education programs in as many different institutions.

Roberts, B. J. Research in educational aspects of health programmes. *International Journal of Health Education,* January-March 1970, *3* (Suppl.). This very comprehensive presentation of the nature of health education and those problems requiring research contains a section devoted to the educational problems requiring research, with illustrations from medical care. A conceptual model to guide health education research is included.

Rosenberg, S. G. Patient education leads to better care for heart patients. *HSMHA Health Reports,* September 1971, *86,* 793–802. This demonstration of an educational program for patients with congestive heart failure shows how the methods employed increased patient knowledge of the disease, the medication, and the diet; increased adherence to the prescribed regimen; and reduced hospital readmissions.

Rosenberg, S. G. A case for patient education. *Hospital Formulary Management,* June 1971, *6.* The rationale for patient education is presented. The article then differentiates between information and education; lists educational methods; and makes the point that planned, organized educational programs can cut readmission days, provide cooperative patients, remove some of the burden of patient information from physicians, and allow for more professional use of staff time.

Ruzek, S. B. *The women's health movement: Feminist alternatives to medical control.* New York: Praeger, Special Studies, 1978. Here is a comprehensive study of the women's health movement as it emerged out of the feminist movement and related consumer health movements during the 1960s. Conventional obstetrical and gynecological services are compared to alternative feminist services, and the feminist critique of health care is discussed. Feminist strategies for change and the response of professionals are included.

Shapiro, I. S. The teaching role of health professionals in a formal organization. *Health Education Monographs,* 1973. The author analyzes an extensive experience in a group health organization in terms of how the structure and function of the various professionals affect the educational efforts.

Shipper, J. K., Jr., & Leonard, R. C. (Eds.). *Social interaction and patient care.* Philadelphia: Lippincott, 1965. This is a good paperback reprinting of articles on the sociology and social psychology of patient care in the hospital.

Steuart, G. Planning and evaluation in health education. *International Journal of Health Education,* 1969, *12,* 65–76. Two models for health education "diagnosis" are delineated. Health educator–client interactions are stressed.

Ulrich, M., & Kelley, K. Patient care includes teaching. *Hospitals,* April 1972, *46,* 59–65. In this detailed description of the health education program at the Charles T. Miller Hospital in Minnesota, where a multidisciplinary team approach is used to coordinate the program, specific operational procedures are described. Benefits to the hospital and the patient are identified.

Winslow, E. The role of the nurse in patient education. *Nursing Clinics of North America,* 1976, *11,* 213–222. The necessity for patient education is emphasized. Several factors that facilitate patient education, as well as those that interfere with it, are discussed.

Wise, H., Beckhard, R., Rubin, I., & Kyte, A. *Making health teams work.* Cambridge, Mass.: Ballinger, 1974. The authors set forth the values implicit in health team operation and offer suggestions of how to cope with the problems health workers face in delivering comprehensive health care. The authors look at the overall administrative structure necessary for the team method, the roles, decision making, power distribution, and staff education. The analysis builds on the Lewian life space model.

Young, M. A. C. Review of research and studies related to health education practice (1961–1966): Program planning and evaluation. *Health Education Monographs,* 1968. The literature is reviewed with regard to the concepts, models, and methods of evaluation. Conceptual studies specifically related to health education are presented along with some early program evaluation efforts.

Index